NEUROSES

A
Comprehensive
and
Critical View

NEUROSES

A Comprehensive and Critical View

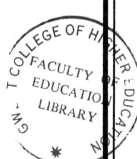

Melvin Gray, M.D.

 VAN NOSTRAND REINHOLD COMPANY
NEW YORK   CINCINNATI   ATLANTA   DALLAS   SAN FRANCISCO
LONDON   TORONTO   MELBOURNE

6 17 12

Van Nostrand Reinhold Company Regional Offices:
New York   Cincinnati   Atlanta   Dallas   San Francisco

Van Nostrand Reinhold Company International Offices:
London   Toronto   Melbourne

Library of Congress Catalog Card Number: 77-25002
ISBN: 0-442-22814-7

Manufactured in the United States of America

Published by Van Nostrand Reinhold Company
135 West 50th Street, New York, N.Y. 10020

Published simultaneously in Canada by Van Nostrand Reinhold Ltd.

15 14 13 12 11 10 9 8 7 6 5 4 3 2 1

Library of Congress Cataloging in Publication Data

Gray, Melvin.
  Neuroses: a comprehensive and critical view.

  Includes index.
  1. Neuroses.   I. Title.   [DNLM: 1. Neuroses.
WM170 G781n]
RC530.G685   616.8'5   77-25002
ISBN 0-442-22814-7

To my wife Leona, our children Janine and Michael;
and in memory of my mother, Esther Grablowsky
and my great nephew, Jay Brendt Scheer.

FOREWORD

It is customary to separate mental disorders into three compartments with considerable overlap. However, these compartments are sufficiently distinct to warrant their description as categories, each with its own characteristics and each with its own subtypes. Yet over many decades there has been a recurrent tendency to lump them all together as one mental disease accepted by only a few psychiatrists. It represents a regression to a pre-Kraepelinian era.

Indeed, the large categories seem to have become more separable as modern research observations, descriptions, and data analyses have extended the ranges of probability. Attention has naturally focused on the most serious and devastating of all, the psychoses. These include the schizophrenias, the unipolar and bipolar depressions, and the organic psychoses. Investigators have been exhorted to study the schizophrenias and funds have been supplied, but their definition (what), their etiology (how), and their teleology (why) have not yet been concluded.

The second category includes the so-called character or personality disorders, which are the object of fresh scrutiny as the histrionic psychoses have declined in intensity and in dramatic behaviors. From this large group, we have now isolated and defined some subtypes such as the borderline, the narcissistic, the delinquent, and some psychopathic personalities.

The third group, which is the largest, the least painful, and the most amenable by psychotherapies, contains the neuroses about which Dr. Gray writes in great detail. The major progress in their therapy has been accomplished during this century by utilizing psychoanalytic theory, which postulates that each type is a way of defending against anxiety. In fact, the subtypes of the neuroses are named according to the methods used in combating or defending against or repressing anxiety.

Accordingly, the author begins his discussion of the neuroses with a chapter on anxiety. The successive chapters describe hysterical, phobic, and obsessive compulsive neuroses. Then follows an extended discussion of depressive illness, which slips into an account of depressive psychoses. Chapters on neurasthenia, depersonalization, and hypochondriasis are considered as neuroses, which they may well be, although these phenomena are observable in almost all psychotics. Certainly, our most recent classification DSM II, and DSM III in the process of reorganizing our concepts, are unclear on these matters.

The author introduces the book with a marvelous and useful historical background to insure the reader's awareness of the mind-body problem as viewed by primitive man, by the ancient Greek philosophers, in the Middle Ages and the Renaissance, and by modern psychiatrists. This introduction stirs the reader's interest with its well-written erudite attention to details. The depth and extent of the author's research is demonstrated by the literature quoted in the bibliography. It is an exciting and stimulating chapter.

This treatise on the phenomenology of the neuroses has long been necessary since very few comprehensive discussions of this category have been published. Its values are multiple: it constitutes a competent overview of the field, it is a powerful stimulation for research into the neuroses not restricted by psychoanalysis, it is a valuable text for students' education, and, in the final chapter, it is an overall eclectic summary of treatment procedures.

This book has obviously required years to research, write, revise, and check. It is doubtful whether such a book could soon be duplicated or extended. It will serve as a monument to excellence and, as well, as a trustworthy reference book.

ROY R. GRINKER, SR.

PREFACE

Psychiatric training is extremely valuable to physicians. Reliable statistics are hard to obtain but indications are that between one third to half of all patients attended by general practitioners are in treatment because of neurotic symptoms. Psychiatry as a clinical subject is initially attractive and intriguing to medical students. As their studies proceed however, many are nonplussed by the conflicting practical and theoretical opinions within the psychiatric community. Thus, early in their medical careers many practitioners and students turn against psychiatry.

Recently, while preparing a series of lectures on neuroses, I experienced some of the same frustration. Research revealed a vast, fascinating literature but also disconcerting and disturbing inconsistencies. In such basic matters as definition, description, theory, and practice a suitable, complete, coherent account of even a single neurotic illness did not exist. A distressing state! Of all the fields of medicine, psychiatry offers some of the best opportunities to teach and illustrate principles of etiology, classification of illness, and principles for examination and treatment of patients.

I hope, therefore, to fill this void by the presentation of an integrated overview of the neuroses. To this end, I have organized the material so as to: (1) clarify terminology; (2) offer a method of organizing data; (3) present a comprehensive picture of each neurosis, encompassing definition, history, classification, etiology, diagnosis, differential diagnosis, course, prognosis, and treatment; (4) summarize major methods of treatment; and (5) trace the historical roots of psychiatric thinking. This approach will help students, psychiatrists, and others in the field of mental health to improve their knowledge and understanding of the neuroses; and will suggest a paradigm for the study of other types of mental illness, such as psychoses, mental deficiency, organic brain disease, and so on.

It is impossible for me to exclude philosophy. In the attempt to answer the traditional questions that philosophy raises—who and what am I?—psychiatrists learn the enormity of the problems involved in the understanding of man. Hence, psychiatry and philosophy are intertwined and cannot be separated.

Psychiatrists and philosophers, at different levels, are searching for the answer to the same conundrum.

The psychiatrist's methods and goals are similar to those of any other physician. He makes a diagnosis and treats, strives to reduce pain, lower discomfort, and improve function. Basically, he deals with individuals: patients in treatment and patients in need of legal testimony.

Since all individuals differ, every case is unique. Paradoxically, all individuals have certain fundamental similarities. All have problems—some seemingly insoluble and others more routine and mundane in nature; and although the psychiatrist is called upon daily to deal with the entire spectrum of man's problems, those conditions that are specifically categorized as "mental" are his major concern. To deal with mental problems effectively the psychiatrist must rely upon certain conceptual guidelines—even theoretical systems—while his efforts center on the individual's experiences in relationship to the self and society. The psychiatrist must correlate the relationship among the individual personality, his experiential response, and the existent conditions in both present and past— a difficult, if not impossible, task to perform.

Abnormal experience and abnormal behavior are the subject matter of psychopathology. Any inquiry regarding cause and effect in abnormal behavior forces examination of the relationship between somatic events and mental phenomena. Because mind and body are an inseparable unity, there are mental states that influence body functions. One can decide to walk, talk, or raise the arms; the thought of food can cause the mouth to water and produce hunger sensations; feelings and thoughts can cause decreased digestive processes, changes in menstrual flow, and alterations in food intake. Anxiety can cause changes in the quality and quantity of milk in a lactating mother. Tension headaches, hyperventilation syndrome, functional tremors, and breath holding in children are psychologically induced. Conversely, no doubt the mind can influence the body and have implications for the body's state of health or disease. There are somatic conditions that can simulate certain mental states. Particular stimuli are associated with certain states of consciousness, e.g., a pinprick causes pain, an alarm clock leads to awakening, hyperthyroidism or pheochromocytom resemble acute anxiety, brain tumors or tranquilizers may precipitate a depression, chronic alcoholism or carbon monoxide intoxication can be manifested by confabulation and so forth. These relationships illustrate the close bond between psychopathology and medicine—the functional-organic interface. Insight into the etiology of abnormal psychic states requires knowledge of the physiology of the nervous system, genetics, neurology, pharmacology, endocrinology, and internal medicine. Thus, medical training is indispensable for proper diagnosis and treatment of the mentally ill and psychiatric training is indispensable for proper diagnosis and treatment of the physically ill. Mind and body are inseparable.

Nothing is more gratifying and reassuring to the physician than to be able to show a one-to-one relationship between cause and effect. However, even in neurology, where a more direct and clean-cut relationship exists between anatomy, physiology, and the clinical picture than in most of medicine, the effect (i.e., clinical manifestation) is nonetheless the result of multiple etiological factors. So, although the neurologist has some advantage over the psychiatrist in validating his diagnoses, it is not as great as might appear. Both subscribe to the comprehensive viewpoint with regard to etiology, diagnosis, and treatment.

The first three chapters of this book—history, etiology, and classification—present a particular theoretical orientation to the study of neuroses.

Just as a thorough examination of each patient is essential to diagnosis and treatment, so too is a knowledge of the history of psychiatry essential to proper practice. Unfortunately, the history of psychiatry is often underrated and overlooked. Yet, its study can aid both students and practitioners in recognizing, and hopefully avoiding, pitfalls and errors of the past. The progression of changing concepts of mental illness that history teaches aids in clarifying some of the confusion surrounding classification, diagnosis, etiology, and treatment of the mentally ill. To trace various aspects of the history of mental illness from their origins is not only a mental exercise but also a path to greater comprehension.

In discussing classification systems, I defend the need for classification as well as the methods involved in constructing such a system. Definitions of prediction, explanation, reliability, homogeneous, heterogeneous, normality, abnormality, and neuroses are presented in order to delineate the limitations and principles of our present classification system. Various diagnostic models are described and evaluated; and in the final analysis the comprehensive model as presented in my article "Principles of the Comprehensive Examination" (*Archives of General Psychiatry,* April 1964) is favored here. Although years have passed since I wrote this article, it remains helpful and relevant. It illustrates a method of organizing data for diagnostic purposes and places the psychiatric examination in its proper perspective as a part of medicine.

The study of etiology includes definitions of explanation, causation, consciousness, and disease. Emphasis is placed on comprehensive multifactorial (multiaxial) analysis which considers constitutional, physical, and psychological factors as well as current life situation and environmental stressors.

The main body of this text is an exposition of individual neurotic conditions as seen from a comprehensive viewpoint. Each neurosis is defined and discussed with regard to history, etiology, diagnosis and differential diagnosis, treatment, course, and prognosis. Hopefully, this type of structural approach will organize, extend, and expand our knowledge of these conditions.

The last chapter describes and evaluates multiple treatment modalities including psychotherapy (individual, group, family, etc.); drugs, physical, surgical, and electrical methods, modes of personal training and practice (e.g., meditation methods, exercise), hypnosis, use of machines and so forth. General principles and goals of treatment as well as the necessity for a treatment plan are discussed. It behooves the student, as well as the general practitioner, to develop a broad knowledge of the many treatment modalities since there is obviously no single, specific treatment applicable to all patients.

Above all, one must recognize that in dealing with neurotic patients we require comprehensive diagnoses and deal with multiple etiologies and therapies. It has been impossible to present a system as broad as this and to be all-inclusive Selection of data necessarily reflects personal bias and limitations. To those whose positions have been neglected, oversimplified, or deleted, I extend my apologies. I have, however, tried to present a fair, balanced overview of neuroses in support of my belief in the validity and necessity of the comprehensive approach.

The author is indebted to many. The manuscript of this book was read in whole or in part by Leona Gray, David Wald, Irving Grablowsky, Phyllis Laszlo, Sidney Gray, Ricky Green, Dr. Lester King, Dr. Venketray Prabhu, and Dr. Philip B. Wahrsinger. I am grateful to each for suggestions, corrections, and criticisms. The ideas came from my students and patients who, by their insights and questions, challenged my every thought and feeling, and my teachers who shared with me their knowledge and friendship. Teachers to whom I owe a special debt are the late Dr. Percival Bailey, the late Dr. Maxwell Gitelson, and Dr. Henry Brosin. Without the encouragement and help of Dr. John Lee this book would not have been written. As an educator, and Chairman of the Department, he provided me with an atmosphere of academic freedom that afforded an opportunity to say and to teach whatever I desired without fear of recrimination. Sheila Denise Hammons had the thankless task of deciphering my handwriting and typing and retyping—to her I am grateful. Natalie Zimmerman and Sharon Wells, librarians at Chicago College of Osteopathic Medicine, saved me endless hours by helping in the collection of research material. Finally—and no words can express this—I appreciate the willingness and understanding of my wife and children to be almost without husband and father for the infinite amount of time that went into preparing this book. To them, I apologize.

MELVIN GRAY, M.D.
Professor of Psychiatry
Chicago College of
Osteopathic Medicine

CONTENTS

Foreword, by *Roy R. Grinker, Sr.* / vii
Preface / ix

1. **Historical Background** / 1

   Early Man / 3
   Dawn of Civilization: Mesopotamian, Egyptian, Hebrew / 4
   Classical Civilization: Greece and Rome / 5
   The Middle Ages and the Renaissance / 12
   The Modern Age / 15
   References / 32

2. **Classification** / 37

   Purposes and Methods / 39
   Pros and Cons / 41
   Definitions / 43
   History / 44
   Normality and Health / 48
   Neuroses / 49
   Diagnostic Models / 51
   References / 56

3. **Etiology** / 59

   Disease Concepts / 62
   Psychiatric Disease Concepts / 65
   Constitutional Factors / 68
   Physical Factors / 71
   Psychological Factors / 74
   Current Life Situations and Stresses / 75
   References / 76

4. Anxiety Neurosis / 79

   Anxiety and Fear, Emotions / 81
   Anxiety, a Neurosis / 82
   History / 83
   Biological Basis for Emotion / 85
   Etiology / 90
   Diagnosis / 96
   Differential Diagnosis / 98
   Course and Prognosis / 100
   Treatment / 101
   References / 103

5. Hysterical Neurosis / 107

   Consciousness and Self / 109
   History / 112
   Etiology / 114
   Diagnosis / 117
   Differential Diagnosis / 121
   Course and Prognosis / 125
   Treatment / 125
   References / 127

6. Phobic Neurosis / 131

   History / 133
   Classification / 135
   Etiology / 137
   Diagnosis / 139
   Differential Diagnosis / 143
   Course and Prognosis / 144
   Treatment / 145
   References / 146

7. Obsessive Compulsive Neurosis / 149

   History / 152
   Classification / 154
   Etiology / 156
   Diagnosis / 162
   Differential Diagnosis / 164
   Course and Prognosis / 166
   Treatment / 166
   References / 168

8. **Depressive Neurosis / 171**

   History / 173
   Classification / 179
   Etiology / 182
   Diagnosis / 190
   Differential Diagnosis / 192
   Course and Prognosis / 194
   Treatment / 195
   References / 199

9. **Neurasthenia / 204**

   History / 205
   Classification / 210
   Etiology / 211
   Diagnosis / 215
   Differential Diagnosis / 215
   Course and Prognosis / 216
   Treatment / 217
   References / 218

10. **Depersonalization Neurosis / 220**

    History / 222
    Classification / 223
    Etiology / 223
    Diagnosis / 228
    Differential Diagnosis / 230
    Course and Prognosis / 231
    Treatment / 232
    References / 232

11. **Hypochondriacal Neurosis / 235**

    History / 239
    Classification / 243
    Etiology / 246
    Diagnosis / 251
    Differential Diagnosis / 255
    Course and Prognosis / 258
    Treatment / 258
    References / 261

12. Treatment / 265

Goals and Principles of Therapy / 266
History / 269
Treatment Plan / 275
PHYSICAL METHODS OF TREATMENT / 277
　　Drug Treatment / 277
　　Specialized Drug Treatment / 287
　　Electrical Treatment / 290
　　Psychosurgery / 294
PSYCHOTHERAPY / 297
　　Individual Psychotherapy / 298
　　Psychoanalysis / 301
　　Behavior Therapy / 302
　　Group Therapy / 304
　　Hypnosis / 306
REFERENCES / 307

Name Index / 315
Subject Index / 319

NEUROSES

A
Comprehensive
and
Critical View

1
HISTORICAL BACKGROUND

Interest in human behavior, what differentiates us from all other forms of life, has been a source of unrelenting curiosity, fascination, supposition, study, and research for millennia. In each generation theologians, philosophers, scientists, poets, writers, and laymen have devoted hours, days, even lifetimes in their search for insight into the workings of the human mind-behavior, thought, volition, feeling—and its connections with the actual physical entity—the body. As a result many "isms" and "ologies" have arisen in an attempt to explain this seemingly unfathomable conundrum.

It is also plain that the history of psychiatry cannot be dissociated from the speculations of leading thinkers, medical and nonmedical, on the nature of man. Accordingly, the object of this chapter is to trace major concepts of the mind in conjunction with psychiatric trends in successive ages. The main emphasis, however, will be relevant to classification, diagnosis, etiology, and the therapeutics of mental disease. From today's vantage point ideas of the past may be considered to be right or wrong. In either instance such studies can provide guidance for comparison with and clarification of current problems.

The term *neuroses** was coined in 1769 by William Cullen (1710-1790), who classified according to botanical principles and followed the methods of François Boissier de Sauvages (1706-1767), Carl von Linné (Linnaeus) (1707-1778), and Hermann Boerhaave (1668-1738). Cullen distinguished four classes of disease: pyrexias, neuroses, cachexias, and local diseases.[1] To him, neuroses were synonymous with nervous system diseases. Subsumed under neuroses were orders—comata, adynamia, spasm, and vesania (insanity)—these orders were further subdivided into genera and species.[2] This resulted in a detailed collection of patients with every possible variation of symptoms and signs and every patient fit a very specific niche within the schema. Slight differences necessitated forming new categories. For instance gout, a neuroses, had 34 varieties of chronic rheumatism subsumed under various genera and species.[3] Some other neuroses such as mania, melancholia, hysteria, epilepsy, and so forth also had many genera and species. It added up to a psychiatric arboretum.

* Cullen used the word *neuroses*, not *neurosis*.

Cullen considered neuroses diseases of sensation and motion (nerve impulse). It was a general, not a local disease of the nervous system, and was without fever.[4]   Underlying his definition and classification of neuroses was Cullen's belief that life is a function of nervous system energy and disease, mainly a disorder of the nerves. He postulated that the brain produced a fluid. The amount of fluid correlated with the amount of available energy which reflected health or disease of the entire body. Neuroses were caused either by an increase or decrease in the tonus of the nervous system. Cullen further thought that a direct relationship existed between the brain and the other bodily organs. Stimulation of the peripheral nervous system or strong emotions could, for example, increase the total nervous energy and lead to mania. This was a mechanistic physiological theory that typified the thinking of his day.[5]

Cullen's definition, classification, and treatment were rooted in the belief that neuroses were disturbances in animal life and that the organ of animal life was the nervous system. The idea that sensation and motion are the basic properties of life dates back to the ancient Greeks and continued to enjoy popularity until relatively recent times. The definition, classification, and treatment as well as the underlying meaning of neuroses has changed since the term was introduced in the eighteenth century.[6] To trace the history of what today are called neuroses, therefore, requires an overview of psychiatric history. Otherwise, it is impossible to understand neuroses or other mental illnesses in their proper perspective. Although the names or labels for the various entities in psychiatry have changed, the phenomena as manifested in the individual have remained more or less consistent—cultural and social conditions do change the form and content of the phenomena. A knowledge of psychiatric history could be extremely valuable in clarifying and interpreting the meaning of the terms in the context in which they are used today and also may have further relevance since a new psychiatric classification system will be introduced in 1979.

Traits or characteristics have always been given names and some were valued more than others. Those traits approved by society were encouraged and considered normal; those traits disapproved were discouraged and considered abnormal. Thus labeling to some extent does reflect the society or culture and cannot be viewed in absolute terms but rather as a relationship between the biological organism and his environment. Psychiatric labeling has today become popular. Ackerknecht writes:

> This trait has become so very common that we are hardly any more aware of it. Persons and crowds, historic personalities and periods, cultures and societies, magic procedures and religions are 'neurotic,' 'sadistic,' 'schizophrenic,' etc., or in the plain and less dignified vocabulary of the common man 'mad,' 'lunatic', and 'crazy.' Even the child in the cradle has not been spared and is supposed by some to undergo a 'normal neurosis.'[7]

Workers in the field of mental health will be in a position to properly evaluate the current status of their discipline only when they are aware of the past as well as the present definitions of terms and their underlying meanings.

EARLY MAN

Primitive man, at the mercy of nature, was confounded by forces he could neither understand nor control. Fear haunted his waking hours and nightmares plagued him while he slept. He stood in superstitious awe of nature and worshiped the elements, animals, totems, fetishes, etc. Even so, he keenly observed and cunningly coped with his surroundings. To ward off and placate the forces of nature he responded by creating illusions of deities, spirits, and magic. On the other hand he empirically devised implements—languages, tools, weapons, societies—for survival.[8]

The primitive relieved his physical pains and mental distresses by turning to rituals of magic, mysticism, and prayer. This was logical since his fate was governed by external forces—wind, rain, storms, sun, moon, volcanoes, earthquakes—as well as diseases that led to pain and death. Thus psychotherapy, the oldest form of medical treatment, began.[9] But he also found beneficial effects in certain plants (drug therapy) and in ritualized deeds of circumcision and trepanation—surgery. Early man believed that plants, herbs, and surgery had curative power. In these treatments the mind was possibly the true healer.

Gods and priest-physicians were also needed to counter or appease the forces of nature; therefore, a priestly caste was created to administer therapeutics. Priests, by divination, were the agents of the gods. Medicine men (shamans) were also agents of the gods but with special potions or magic. Thus the priest-physicians had the power and directed primitive man in his worship of natural forces, animals, and their forms (fetishes). What is currently called "mythology" was primitive man's reality. Man needed gods and priest-physicians to protect him and to insure his survival.

At first, the primitive attributed good and evil to the spirits and then later to the gods. A cause and effect relationship developed between man and the spirits—please the spirits and no evil would fall upon thee but displease the spirits and evil would strike. The spirits helped fertilize the soil, make rain, prevent droughts, increase fertility, and ward off illness or restore health. Sorcerers, seers, magicians, priests, and medicine men practiced black and white magic: black magic brought disease and death whereas white magic averted them. Rigid customs appeared—totems and taboos. The penalties for avoiding custom were disease and death. The supernatural became stratified into gods, devils, and demons.[10] Thus the priest-physician, with his control over life and death, was all powerful. His power was psychological, a most potent tool of man's early discoveries.

DAWN OF CIVILIZATION: MESOPOTAMIAN, EGYPTIAN, HEBREW

The Mesopotamians (Sumerians, Babylonians, Assyrians) developed an advanced culture. They all more or less practiced the same religion and worshiped thousands of different gods. The priests were considered to be of divine origin and nurtured a body of knowledge in which mysticism and magic occupied a prominent role. They placed particular emphasis on demons: a demon for body wasting, one for liver disease, another for woman's disease as well as separate demons for every disease which disturbed them. They believed the ear to be the seat of intelligence. In all matter, animate or inanimate—man, animal, vegetable, and mineral—a will and a personality existed. Therefore, there was no distinction between the various forms of existence.[11]

For the Babylonians, demonology predominated and the priests designed treatments to drive the demons out of the body. Elaborate exorcism and incantation rituals were administered including the use of water, poultices, bandages, and certain plants and minerals. Their priests were also prophets. Disease was believed to be of divine origin and by certain god-given signs the priest could predict its future (divination). They got those signs from the stars, sun, water, moon, planets, organs of animals, and the size and shape of the ears of newborns. The priests also interpreted dreams. The Mesopotamians were the first to elaborate a "system" of medicine and to attempt to diagnose, treat, and prognosticate. They did this mainly on the basis of their religious or astronomical knowledge.[12]

Egyptian theological beliefs have two aspects that are pertinent. First, the immortality of the soul and the resurrection of the body were emphasized. The shape of the pyramids developed from the idea of a rising hill which promised the Egyptian buried within that he would reemerge as a new being. Second, the heart was viewed as the organ that conceived thought and the tongue as the organ that related the conceived thought. The Egyptians mechanistically explained the relationship of the other senses to the heart and tongue. The purpose of the eyes seeing, the ears hearing, and the nose smelling was to report to the heart. The heart, then, released its concepts to the tongue. The tongue announced the heart's thoughts. This explanation associated creation with the functions of the senses, processes of thought, and speech and connected this with god and not to physical being.[13]

The Egyptians improved medicine through observations of embalmed bodies, anatomical studies of animals, and development of medical specialists. Each physician specialized in only one disease. Treatment included recitals (similar to, but not quite, incantations), drugs, surgery, and worship. The Egyptians deified Imhotep, the earliest known physician, into a demigod. Apparently a rational form of medicine was practiced.[14]

About 1200 B.C. the ancient Hebrews, greatly influenced by their powerful neighbors, made their greatest contribution with the concept of Yahweh or

Jehovah—the one and only God. They formulated the soul as that which makes the body alive. The Hebrew word for "breath" is used to refer to soul because it is one of the vital signs of life.[15]

The Hebrew contribution to medicine came primarily through their hygienic laws, descriptions of many diseases, and ethical practices. They had laws and regulations regarding clean and unclean animals, diet, ritual circumcision, menstrual hygiene, sexual behavior, and so on. The Hebrews did not regard physicians highly since the power to make one ill and to cure was solely in God's hands.[16] Dreams were prophetic and of divine origin. God warned Abimelech in a dream not to take Sarah, wife of Abraham. Examples were given of mental illness brought forth when man displeased God; Nebuchadnezzar lived with the beasts and ate grass like the oxen; Saul had periods of excitement and depression; Ezekiel was coprophagic. Therapy, essentially consisted of sacrifice, prayer, magic, incantation, and exorcism.[17,18]

CLASSICAL CIVILIZATION: GREECE AND ROME

The Greeks, originally a collection of barbaric tribes, came from the north and invaded the eastern part of the Mediterranean. There they mixed with and learned from the advanced civilizations of Egypt and the other empires of the ancient East. About 1000 B.C. those empires fell into ruin and from their ashes emerged a distinct Greek civilization.

In the Homeric age the usage of the term *psuche*, defined as the breath of life, was similar to the Hebrew word for breath. Yet for Homer (c. 900 B.C.) the term *nous* (mind) "subsumes a mental structure, an organ, and the end result of the functioning of the organ. . .By the time of Plato (429-347 B.C.) *nous* is a sub-division of *psuche*, a structure that is part of a larger structure."[19]

The idea of the soul continued with such Greeks as Heraclitus (540-475 B.C.) and Pythagoras (570-489 B.C.), early philosophers who made the change from myth to intellect. Their concern was with the ultimate reality of the universe and of man. Heraclitus taught that nothing has permanence or stability; everything was in constant movement and change.[20] He wrote, "One cannot step twice in the same river, for fresh waters are forever flowing in upon you."[21] Since all was in constant change, there was neither beginning nor end—only existence. Being was appearance (becoming), and warm exhalation was the essence (soul) that formed all else. Exhalation is incorporeal, in ceaseless flux, and in movement. Since movement existed there had to be a knower of the movement that was also in movement: hence, all that existed had its being essentially in movement.[22] Pythagoras, a contemporary of Heraclitus, disagreed with him. Pythagoras, and his followers while accepting the reality of opposites conversely believed in the static and unified aspects of being as it appeared to the intellect, not the senses, and proposed the theory of the transmigration of the soul (metapsychosis).[23]   Opposing viewpoints, materialism and idealism, were present with Heraclitus and Pythagoras.

Democritus (c. 460-370 B.C.) proposed an atomistic explanation of man and nature. He speculated that all things were made of indivisible bits of matter called atoms and that these atoms were the only existence. Atoms could neither be created nor destroyed, could only change their form, and were constantly in motion. The interaction between atoms was responsible for all phenomena. Democritus imagined that the soul was a sort of fire and the atoms of the soul were constantly emitted from the body and other atoms replaced them through inhalation. Therefore, the soul was perpetually renewed with fresh atoms and when respiration ceased, life and soul departed from the body: thus "life, mind, and soul" were the same. Besides his materialistic ideas of the soul, he believed in spiritual beings and revelations; and in what appears to be a contradiction, he denied that divine beings exist. The indestructibility of the atom accounts for his belief in immortality.[24, 25]   After Democritus the atomic theory came to an end for a time but reemerged with Epicurus (341-271 B.C.) and the Roman Lucretius (98-55 B.C.).

Plato, who inherited the speculations of Pythagoras, reintroduced idealism and duality. In his theory of ideas or forms (prototypes, paradigms, archetypes) Plato held the view that the universe consisted of two worlds, a world of being or essence (reality) and a world of becoming or existence (appearance). The world of being was occupied by static, changeless, perfect, eternal ideas or forms that existed in isolation, apart from the minds of men; the world of becoming contained perceived or sensible things that were in constant motion and change, and were mere copies of the prototypes. For illustration, all horses or trees were mere copies of the one ideal horse or tree. Man differed from all other material things, however, in having a faculty of reason that by means of thought reflects true knowledge of the essences. But his lower faculties (passion and appetite) were susceptible to sense-impressions that could only give the appearance of things.[26]

Plato divided the soul into mortal and immortal aspects. The immortal (rational) soul was located in the head and there found true or perfect reality. The mortal (irrational) soul he located in the two parts of the body separated by the diaphragm. The neck separated the mortal from the immortal soul and protected the immortal soul from pollution. The noble part of the mortal soul, feelings, he located in the chest and the baser parts, appetites and desires, in the abdomen. Thus Plato proposed a tripartite division of soul and a soul-body dualism.[27]

Aristotle (384-322 B.C.) was dissatisfied with the Platonistic views that ideas exist apart from sensible things and that the soul is separated from the body. He also disagreed with the mechanical atomistic explanation of Democritus. Aristotle viewed the body and soul as an inseparable whole, a conception of matter or functioning living form. He did not localize the soul in any one part of the body but extended it to each and every part of the living organism with the center of all sensations, the seat of the soul, in the heart. Further, for Aristotle the form that matter took was important because as form evolved and became less encumbered with matter, it approached the perfect form, or God. He considered God as pure form (i.e., without any of the potentiality of matter to limit the form) toward which all being was directed. The Aristotelian concept of matter and form thus encompassed a teleological explanation of being. In addition it implied that the soul was the source or cause of the living body and was located in each and every part. In Aristotle's words:

> . . .what has souls in it differs from what has not in that the former displays life. Now this word has more than one sense, and provided any one alone of these is found in a thing we say that thing is living. Living, that is, may mean thinking or perception of local movement and rest, or movement in the sense of nutrition, decay and growth.[28]

Unlike Plato, Aristotle did not consider the soul of man to be separable; he rather postulated a unifying action of the vegetative, sensitive, rational, and motor functions of the soul.[29]

Medicine, art, and science in ancient Greece did not develop suddenly; indeed, they evolved slowly. Greek mythology contains not only an overview of their gods, beliefs, and religion but also an insight into their medicine. To the Greeks some insane people and those who suffered from fits or seizures were blessed by visits from the gods; hence, those persons became demigods. Epilepsy was called the sacred disease. Coronis, the nymph, and Apollo, the chief god of healing, had a son Asklepios. While visiting Hades, Asklepios was so skillful in curing the sick that Pluto, the god of the underworld, complained that his realm would be depopulated. Zeus, king of the gods, then let loose a thunderbolt and killed Asklepios. Afterwards Asklepios was worshiped as a god. Temples of health called Asklepieia were built in his honor and the sick came to these temples to be cured through prayer, sacrifice, and purification. These sanctuaries were probably the first hospitals and were administered by the physician-priests. Arriving at an Asklepian a new patient would see a votive tablet of a previously healed person. The priest then greeted him, consulted with him on his illness, and offered medication and advice. After religious services and further purifications, the patient under the influence of a priest went to sleep. While asleep the patient was supposed to dream; afterwards the priest interpreted the dream and prescribed the proper treatment—baths, massages, purgatives, emetics, concoctions, drugs, etc.[30]

Greek medical schools were first established at Cnidus and Cos (c. 600 B.C.). Previously all medical writings were anonymous.[31] There were also medical schools in Croton, Sicily, Cyrene, Asia Minor, and Rhodes. At these institutions doctors were trained and their writings were identified with various schools of thought.

Hippocrates, the father of medicine, was born in Cos in 460 B.C. He separated medicine as an independent study from philosophy and theology. He was famous as a medical practitioner and teacher and studied medicine at the Asklepian temple. He died around 370 B.C.

The Hippocratic writings are a collection of monographs, textbooks, manuals, speeches, extracts, and notes. Scholars are not certain if one man or many authored these writings. Nonetheless most agree that the "Hippocratic writings" represent the works of many men: thus it would be more appropriate to refer to the school of Hippocratic writings rather than to the man himself.[32] The great advance they made was to explain that all diseases have natural causes and that the starting point of all theory is observation. Even epilepsy, then known as the sacred disease, was considered to be no more divine than any other disease. Garrison said:

> The Law, the Oath, and the opening chapters of the discourse *On the Sacred Disease* are the loftiest utterances of Greek medicine and, whether due to Hippocrates or not, they are informed with the spirit of his ethical teaching.... The argument of the 'Sacred Disease,' which ridicules the supposedly divine origin of epilepsy, was the highest reach of free thought for centuries, and had it been heeded, would have done away forever with the foolish idea that human ills are caused by gods or demons.[33]

The most significant contribution of the Hippocratic writings was the humoural theory that explained constitution, causation, and treatment of disease. In pre-Hippocratic writings it was supposed that all matter was made up of four elements: earth, water, air, and fire. These elements were either in opposition or in alliance with each other—water was opposed to fire but allied with earth. To each of these four elements was appended a pair of primary qualities—heat and cold, moisture and dryness. Building on these ancient beliefs, the Hippocratic writers supposed that all living bodies were made up of four humours: blood (sanguine), yellow bile (cholera), black bile (melancholia), and phlegm (pituita). Health depended on a proper mixture of the humours. The terms used in ancient times, and synonymous with the modern term "mixture," were "tempered" or "complexioned." Diseases were classified according to the superabundance of one or another humour (viz., sanguine, choleric, melancholic, phlegmatic). Moreover, the classification of the humoural theory was physiological inasmuch as each humour was associated with an organ: blood with liver, black bile with spleen, phlegm with lungs, and yellow bile with the gall bladder (Fig. 1-1). Although contemporary psychological terminology includes the four terms—

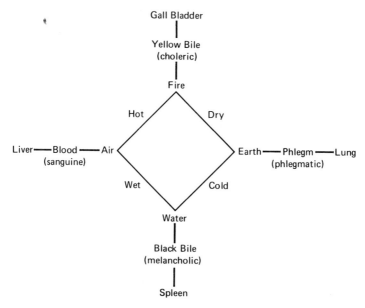

Fig. 1-1. Relationship of elements, qualities, humours, and organ source.[35]

choleric, melancholic, phlegmatic, and sanguine—they do not have the same meaning or connotations in the Hippocratic writings.[34]

Hippocrates classified mental illness as follows: mania, melancholia, dementia, phrenitis, epilepsy, hysteria, and Scythian disease.[36] Veith maintains that Hippocrates did not consider hysteria a mental illness but a disease in which the uterus wandered through the body and exerted pressure on other organs giving rise to symptoms such as palpitations (pressure on the heart) and dyspnea (pressure on the lung).[37] Hippocrates contributed four factors to the understanding of psychiatric illness: (1) a description based on observation;(2) a cause explained by natural phenomena; (3) a position that mental illness could be cured like all other illness; (4) a relationship between heredity and mental disease.

Civilizations, like great ideas, evolve, rise to high peaks, fall into ruin, only to be revived again. By the end of the fifth century B.C. Greek genius reached the height of originality and creativity providing future mankind with models in philosophy, medicine, literature, arts and sciences. It remained, however, for Alexander the Great (355-322 B.C.) to conquer the known world before Greek achievements could spread to the rest of humanity. Soon after Alexander's death his empire fell apart but became the framework for the later Roman empire. In the Hellenistic Age that followed, the Greek heritage was assimilated everywhere.

In 146 B.C. the Romans conquered Greece and gradually absorbed its intellectual and artistic knowledge. Not only did the Romans make the Hellenistic culture their own and give it some new twists but they also accepted the Greek gods and religion thereby assuring the continuity of the Grecian heritage in what is called the Greco-Roman culture.

Philosophy flourished. Besides the Epicurean, Stoic, and Cynic philosophical molds, there was Neoplatonism which affected thought for the next thousand years. Even Galen (129-c. 199 A.D.), the famous Greek physician living in Rome, emulated Plato. He divided the soul into three types of pneuma or spirits: the lowest—natural or physical—dominated the liver and veins (principal organs of nutrition, growth, and reproduction); the middle—vital—dominated the heart, lungs, and arteries (organs concerned with vital functions and locomotion); the highest—psychical—dominated the brain and nervous system (organs concerned with motor function, sensation, feeling, memory, and intellectual life). In essence Galen subscribed to three different seats of the soul. However, he viewed the living organism as a dynamic interplay of naturalistic causes and effects. In Galen's view, a faculty (of the soul) was the cause of motion or activity. He felt structure did not explain the faculty but rather that the faculty gave its structure to each organ. Thus function (faculty of soul) came first and was not the secondary but primary principle of life. Within this framework he developed a dynamic system of psychological physiology.[38]

The Romans through Galen accepted the Hippocratic model. Although Hippocrates did offer a classification of mental disease, Ackerknecht, mindful of the paucity of information available from humoural theorists, turned to Soranus of Ephesus (c. 100 A.D.) as the best source from which to gain an understanding of the concepts of the Greco-Roman period.[39] Ackerknecht says:

According to Soranus, phrenitis is so called because the mind (phren, originally the diaphragm), that is, thinking is affected. Soranus begins with a critical review of the definitions of phrenitis. . .then presents his own definition: an acute disease of the mind accompanied by acute fever, foolish gesticulations and a small, full pulse. We are thus obviously dealing with febrile delirium. . .He then turns to consider the differential diagnosis of phrenitis, mania, melancholia, pleurisy, pneumonia and mandrake and henbane poisoning. . . .He suggests instead a subdivision into phrenitis on the basis of status strictus (tension) and phrenitis on the basis of status laxus (relaxation). Some writers, he says, look for the seat of phrenitis in the brain, others in the head or in the aorta. Each in fact looks for it in the place which he believes to be the seat of the soul. . . .In the treatment of phrenitis Soranus recommends isolation in a moderately lit, warm and airy room, with high windows so that the patient cannot jump out. . .phrenitis due to tension should be nursed in a dark room. . . .If insufficient attendants are available, the patient should be carefully fettered in order to keep him quiet. . .warm poultices of oil, to be applied particularly to the head, and also careful blood-letting. On the third or fourth day the head should be shaved and treated with cupping, leeches and scarification. Passive exercises. . .careful diet are indicated. Wine should not be allowed. . . .One should maintain a serious attitude towards abnormally cheerful patients and a friendly one towards those who are downcast. . . .[40]

Mania, insanity, or moving madness Soranus defined as: a disturbance of reason without fever. . . .Its manifestations were fury, gaiety, sadness, silliness or anxiety, such as for example, a persistent fear of falling into ditches. . .and the causes of mania may be latent or, over-exertion, licentiousness, alcoholism and absence of the relief afforded by bleeding from haemorrhoids or by menstruation.[41] Treatment is similar to that for phrenitis and may include listening to dripping water in cases of insomnia, massage, walks, strengthening the patient's reason by discussion or reading, attending proper plays, delivering speeches, chess, travel and emetics.[42]

Ackerknecht adds that to Soranus melancholia is not seen

as black bile but as black rage. . .caused by digestive upsets, drugs, fear and grief. The main symptoms are depression, mutism, death wishes, marked suspiciousness, weeping, muttering and occasional joviality. . . .Melancholia is a disease of the esophagus. Treatment is the same as for mania. . . .[43]

Thus Soranus viewed phrenitis, mania, and melancholia as the chief mental diseases, but he viewed them as if they were physical illnesses. Soranus did not mention hysteria, and he considered homosexuality a disease of the psyche.[44] Although these descriptions of mania and melancholia are not the same descriptions that are in use today and the term phrenitis has entirely disappeared from psychiatric terminology these early concepts continued to influence psychiatric thinking for 1700 years.

Galen influenced western medicine for over 1400 years. He elaborated, expanded, and developed his own system based on the living organism as a dynamic interplay of naturalistic forces. Because of the functional and structural relationships that he described, many of his observations are still valid.[45]

When Galen died imperial Rome was still at the height of power, but the superstition and mysticism of new religious cults influenced and beclouded the Roman mentality. For this reason and others—a top-heavy bureaucracy, a slave system that had outlived itself, numerous barbarians—Rome became decadent, declined, and by the fifth century fell to the barbarians. With the ascendancy of Christianity to power, thought in all aspects of life was controlled by Church dogma. Change in the theory and practice of medicine and psychiatry became rigidly petrified in a Galenic and theological mold.

THE MIDDLE AGES AND THE RENAISSANCE

The Church revived and reformulated Platonic and Neoplatonic thinking. And in St. Augustine (354-430) these ideas reached a pinnacle. Augustine's theology and philosophy of soul did the most to shape the doctrines of the Catholic Church. Of the soul, he said:

> I believe that the soul's proper abode, to put it that way, and its homeland is God Himself by whom it has been created. But its essence I cannot properly identify for I do not think it comes from these common and familiar natures with which we come in contact by means of these our bodily senses. I do not think, for example, that the soul consists of earth, or of water, of air, or fire, or of all things together, or of any combination of them. . . .Again, should you ask me about the body, I shall fall back upon those four elements. But when you ask about the soul, since it seems to be something simple and to have an essence all its own, I shall be no less embarrassed then if you ask, as I said, what earth comes from.[46]

Further, he said:

> But if you want a definition of the soul, and ask me—what is soul? I have a ready answer. It seems to me to be a special substance, endowed with reason, adapted to rule the body.[47]

Thus to Augustine the soul comes to man primarily through reason and not through the senses.

Debates over the seat of the soul persisted throughout the medieval period. For centuries those who followed Galen localized the seat not, as he did, in the substance but rather in the ventricles of the brain and they also suggested a relationship between the shape of the head and the character of the mind. At first the soul localized in two ventricles, then three, until finally the Arabian physicians developed a fourfold and even a fivefold localization hypothesis. To the anterior ventricles medieval physicians assigned a sensory or imagination function; to the middle ventricle—reason, intellect, and understanding; to the posterior ventricle—memory. Arguments and disagreements were endless since the relation between ventricle and its function varied depending on the authority.[48]

In later medieval times Augustine's theology of the soul came under attack by some scholastics. The leading protagonist was St. Thomas Aquinas (1226-1274) who revived and modified Aristotle's concept of the soul. From a commentary by St. Thomas of Aristotle's *De Anima*, Percival Bailey quotes:

> By "soul" we understand that by which a living thing is alive. . . .We must not think of the soul and the body as though the body had its own form, making it a body, to which a soul is superadded, making it a living body; but rather that the body gets both its being and its life from the soul. . . .By the powers of the soul we mean the vegetative, the sensitive, the intellectual. . . .[49]

In effect the soul is the last judgment, the source of all mental activities and is simple, substantive, and spiritual. Furthermore, Aquinas placed emphasis on experience gained through the senses as a basis of knowledge.

Throughout the medieval period demonology, witchcraft, and supernaturalism were widespread. The body was considered evil and flagellation was the applied remedy. Man was tortured by demons and spirits, and exorcism was administered. People were miraculously cured by visiting sacred places; vampires appeared; demons assuming femal forms had intercourse with sleeping men (succubi); demons in the male form had intercourse with sleeping women (incubi); humans assumed the traits of animals (lycanthropy); and other forms of demonology also took hold of the people. Their outlook became fanatical and mad.[50]

During the Renaissance the priests were still exorcizing and executing individuals possessed by the devil. It was thought that demons caused both mental illness and sin. The remedy was codified and prescribed by priests. The danger of suggesting another approach was to be labeled a heretic.[51] But in the sixteenth century Paracelsus (1493-1541) and others, opposed to the inhuman practice of exorcism and execution, denied that devils or witches caused mental disease. Paracelsus explicitly stated: " 'nature is the sole origin of all diseases.' "[52]

In another area of activity—psychiatric classification—Paracelsus, who was also a physician, broke somewhat with the Galenic triadic system that classified diseases proceeding from the head down (mania, melancholia, phrenitis).[53] He created a system with five divisions:

   I.   Epilepsy
   II.   Mania (acute, violent mental disorders)
   III. Vitus chorea
   IV.   Suffocation of the intellect (all kinds of paroxysmic accidents, except epilepsy)
   V.   Waynsinn ("insanity"), with five subforms
         1. Lunacy (periodic disorders, rhythmed by phases of the moon)
         2. Insanity (hereditary mental disease)
         3. Vesania (mental conditions caused by poisons)

4. Melancholia (emotional disorders)
5. Preternatural diseases (demoniacal possessions and
   obsessions)[54]

Paracelsus meant: epilepsy was a disturbance of the vital spirit; mania, a disturbance of reason and not sense, arose from the vital spirits; vitus chorea (St. Vitus dance, dancing mania) was caused by vital spirits precipitating certain salts in the veins of laughter; suffocation of the intellect (a combination of epilepsy and hysteria) was due to intestinal worms, intrauterine events, overeating or excessive sleeping; insanity was caused by the stars or moon, heredity, poisons, or emotional disorder.[55]

Paracelsus introduced chemistry into medicine. For epilepsy he used camphor, powdered unicorn, and a special substance manufactured by alchemists called Arcana. For mania, he used scarification of the toes, fingers, and head to allow the air (vapors) to escape; and cooling and astringents to fight the disease vapors. For lunacy he developed a system of treatment in which he could counteract the magnetic forces of the moon. He treated hereditary insanity by "artificial coitus" and drugs. The other mental illnesses were treated more or less in the same manner—a combination of drugs, scarification, ducking in cold water, confinement to a dark cell, and astrological methods. Psychotherapy was conspicuously lacking.[56] Paracelsus did not entirely break with Galenic or medieval tradition which contributed, in part, to his failure in constructing a new system of classification, etiology, and treatment.

Other systems came and went during the sixteenth and seventeenth centuries. If these systems were based on one or more closed systems—be they theological, psychological, philosophical, biological—they were doomed to failure. But some advances were made in introducing new terms and concepts. Felix Platter (1536-1614) developed a classification system based on observation. His categories interpreted into modern terminology included mental deficiency and dementia, disturbances of consciousness, psychosis, and mental exhaustion. Subsumed under these categories were such entities as idiocy, imbecility, feeblemindedness, coma, catalepsy, silly behavior, inebriety and other intoxications, violent emotions and passions, melancholia, hypochondriasis, mania, acute delirium with fever, mental exhaustion, and so forth. These categories are remarkably similar to our present classification.[57] Thomas Sydenham (1624-1663) disregarded all metaphysical speculation. He advocated careful observation and thought that disease was neither purely physical nor psychological. "He believed in diseases rather than in a single kind of disorder at the root of all ailments."[58] Thomas Willis (1621-1675), the father of neurology, laid the foundation for the concepts of cerebrocortical functioning and cerebral localization.[59] Whereas physicians were seeking a medical explanation of mental illness, theologians and philosophers insisted upon their prerogatives of the past: theologians claimed that they were the physicians of the soul while philosophers asserted themselves to be the judges of abnormal states of mind. Despite the negative attitude of theologians and philosophers toward a strictly medical approach to mental illness, the roots of modern psychiatry were planted.

THE MODERN AGE

Over the years philosophy gradually freed itself from medieval impositions. During the seventeenth century René Descartes (1596-1650) dared to imply openly that philosophers rather than theologians were the most qualified to delve into speculations on man's nature. Robert Watson noted that to Descartes:

> The rational soul and the mind are synonymous. . . .In fact, as he used the term, thought includes all that we are conscious of. . . .Self is known through consciousness. . . .Understanding is the basic instrument of thought; imagination, memory, and sense are aids to understanding. . . .[60]

Prior to Descartes the mind was subsumed under other terms, i.e., psyche, soul, or spirit. The modern concept of mind began with the assumption by Descartes that soul, mind, psyche, consciousness, and self were interchangeable terms and had the same meaning. Descartes further postulated that all knowledge was derived from consciousness, i.e., a thinking subject, which he summed up in his famous statement: *cogito ergo sum* (I think, therefore I am).

Descartes assumed that the mind and body were distinct and separate substances. These two substances of the organism (the incorporeal mind and the corporeal body) met in the pineal gland* and interacted with each other. This was merely one form of the mind-body dualism, e.g., psychophysical parallelism. Descartes also theorized that there were two types of thought: acquired (the result of experience) and innate (the result of heredity).[61]   Thus two new dualisms were introduced: mind-body and environmental-hereditary.

Cartesian thought centered in man's psychical life and permeated the age that followed. But the Age of Enlightenment was powered by the philosophical and literary movements that emerged in England during the last half of the seventeenth century. Alexander Pope (1688-1744) expressed the new age well with these words: "The proper study of mankind is man."

John Locke (1632-1704), who studied medicine but did not take a degree, became the leading figure in philosophy. His doctrine of empiricism provided the antithesis to Cartesian rationalism. Locke denied that the starting point of knowledge originated with "innate ideas" in the human mind. This led him to posit the mind at birth as a "white paper, void of all characters, without any

---

Note: Descartes did not consider the pineal gland to be the seat of the soul; for the soul, he thought, was not entirely within the pineal gland.

ideas." Experience, he asserted, furnished the mind with the raw materials from which knowledge was built. Experience meant perception of sensations (observations of external, sensible objects) and reflection (observations of internal operations of the mind). Briefly put, sense-experience was the ultimate source of all knowledge.[62]

Modern empirical psychology began with Locke. Subsequent generations of psychologists were influenced by his approach to psychological problems and rightly called him the father of psychology. The structure of his psychology rested on his concept of personal identity, of which he wrote:

> For I presume it is not the idea of a thinking or rational being alone that makes the *idea of a man* in most people's sense: but of a body, so and so shaped, joined to it;. . .This being premised, to find wherein personal identity consists, we must consider what *person* stands for;—which, I think, is a thinking intelligent being, that has reason and reflection, and can consider itself as itself, the same thinking thing, in different times and places; which it does only by that consciousness which is inseparable from thinking. . .it being impossible for any one to perceive without *perceiving* that he does perceive. . . . Thus it is always as to our present sensations and perceptions: and by this every one is to himself that which he calls *self*. . . .Self is that conscious thinking thing. . . .This may show us wherein personal identity consists: not in the identity of substance, but as I have said, in the identity of consciousness. . . .[63]

Locke made the point here that personal identity consisted of self-consciousness which distinguished man, self, or person from all other forms of life or beings.

More or less free from the fetters of theology, psychiatry, aided by scientific advances in medical and nonmedical areas and based on rationalism and empiricism, entered the eighteenth century. Body and brain could be studied on a scientific basis. To put it another way, it was now "possible to give up a purely somatic viewpoint and to introduce psychology deliberately into psychiatry.[64]

The impetus for the psychological etiology of mental disease came from Georg Ernst Stahl (1660-1734). Stahl believed that "the chemical and physical reactions of the body are kept going by means of the soul (anima) and disease was a fight between the anima and harmful influences."[65] He divided the causation of mental illness into diseases of organs and diseases in which no organic basis could be found.[66] Over a hundred years later, in 1855, Littré and Robin were the first to use the term "Functional" to describe a disturbance without a structural lesion.[67] Thus Stahl foresaw the possibility that mental illness could, in certain cases, be a purely psychological disease. Yet the organicists predominated until the twentieth century.

William Cullen, founded and headed the organicist school. He believed that disturbances of the nervous system caused mental illness. In addition to coining the term neuroses, he introduced hydrotherapy with quick changes of temperature, and he treated his patients in conformity with the practice of his time: restraints or chastisement, drugs, bloodletting, diet, etc. Cullen's monographs were standard texts in medicine for more than a century.[68] Starting with Cullen and Stahl two major conflicting schools of thought emerged—organicists and functionalists.

Rationalists and humanists opposed a classification according to class, order, genera, and species. The preeminent rationalist philosopher Immanuel Kant (1724-1804) proposed a classification with two major categories of mental illness: weakness of the soul related to cognitive faculties and sickness of the soul. Kant extrapolated from his analysis of the faculties of mind to build a classification system, in which the intellectual faculties rather than the emotional or the volitional were dominant.[69]

Franz Joseph Gall (1757-1828) introduced the terms *cranioscopy* and *organology* and initiated a new approach to the relationship of brain to mind based on cerebral anatomical studies. He thought that mental faculties could be localized in specific areas of the cerebral cortex. His followers, J.C. Spurzheim (1776-1832) and others, elaborated Gall's work into systems called *craniology, physiognomy,* and *phrenology.* Gall did not anticipate the misguided direction his followers would take. Phrenology disintegrated into a mystical and magical cult flourishing primarily with students of the occult and with faith healers.

In the early part of the nineteenth century the prevailing opinion was that the brain was the organ of the mind. It was simple. The brain was thought to operate as a whole with no localization of function. Gall and Spurzheim opposed this view. In 1810 they published a theory which stated that the faculties were innate with each faculty having a definite place on the surface of the brain. The size of the area that each faculty occupied measured the degree to which each contributed to the total character of the individual. They also saw a relationship between the outer surface of the skull and the contour of the brain surface. Thus by examination of the head, immediate determination of the relative sizes of the faculties could be made. This was a system of cerebral localization and personality diagnosis. Even Gall, the one true scientist involved with the doctrine, believed that he had located 27 distinct psychological faculties in the brain. From these speculations scientific investigations of the relationship between mind and brain began.[70]

In 1865 Pierre Paul Broca (1824-1889), a medical practitioner, made the first substantive advance on the problem of cerebral localization. He concluded, albeit on incorrect evidence, that injury to the third frontal convolution of the left cerebral hemisphere resulted in disordered speech (aphasia). Broca's demonstration stimulated scientific study of cerebral localization.[71] Knowledge of the brain increased and most authorities now agree on the areas where impulses, i.e., visual, auditory and tactile reach the cortex and where motor activity arises. But diverse opinions prevail concerning feeling, memory, intelligence, and other higher functions of the mind.[72]

The search for the seat of consciousness was conducted by neurophysiologists, anatomists, and neurosurgeons. They followed consciousness from the cerebral cortex through the basal ganglia, hypothalamus, midbrain, brain stem, and found that consciousness could not be localized. Recent evidence, however, indicates that consciousness and mind arise as a consequence of the total organization of the cerebral hemispheres and not its parts. Each hemisphere behaves as though it has a mind with a consciousness all its own. But it is not known how thoughts lead to action nor how chemical and electrical activity of the billions of nerve cells receive, store, and use information; express emotion; or explain mechanisms of learning, memory, and reasoning. How the nervous system generates consciousness, mind, and behavior is for the most part still unknown, but the search continues.[73]

The humanists—Philippe Pinel (1745-1826), Vincenzo Chiarugi (1759-1820), Benjamin Rush (1745-1813), and William Tuke (1732-1819)—initiated reforms for the treatment of the mentally ill in France, Italy, the United States, and England. They opposed physical force, restraints, chains, and cruelty; instead they proposed hygienic and safety methods, manual work, proper diet, and kindness. Their efforts resulted in changes within mental institutions and provided the basis of an enlightened attitude toward the mentally ill.[74]

Pinel followed Cullen's classification and developed his own. But unlike Cullen, he did not consider neuroses as physical diseases. Pinel thought neuroses were functional, organic, or a combination of both.* He referred to the functional as moral and the organic as physical neuroses. Moral neurosis (which became known as moral insanity) was treated by "moral treatment," a precursor to modern day psychotherapy.[75] Moral insanity resembled what was later included under psychopathic personality.[76] (Today it is called personality disorder.) In addition, Pinel offered several classification systems, from very complex nosologies to a classification system that consisted of only four categories: mania, melancholia, dementia, and idiotism. For Pinel, these were concepts and not mere descriptions; they were categories of functions that advanced knowledge.[77] Consequently, Pinel not only advanced treatment (community and individual) and proposed descriptions and classifications but also revived the debate between the organicists and functionalists.

Classification proceeded along several lines in the first half of the nineteenth century: descriptive or symptomatic (Linnaean model); etiological (physiopathological model); faculty psychological model; cause, course, outcome

---

*Menninger (p. 443) credits Pinel as the first to use the term "functional." Riese credits Littré and Robin. See texts for references.

or a combination of these. Others considered mental illness a disease of the whole being; hence, not classifiable.[78]

Jean É-D. Esquirol (1772-1840) continued the humanistic and academic tradition of Pinel. Esquirol incorporated statistics and studied the cause, course, and prognosis of mental disease. He also redefined and introduced terms such as hallucination, illusion, remission, intermission, dementia, idiocy, and divided mental illness into the five following categories: lypemania (depressive states), monomania (paranoid states), mania, dementia, imbecility and idiocy. He also expanded the concept of partial insanity (psychopathy) and wrote the first scientific textbook of psychiatry.[79,80] Esquirol searched for psychological causes in the etiology of mental illness. Alcoholism and masturbation, to him, were symptoms and not causes.

Ackerknecht says:

> He saw much more clearly the roles that social upheavals and the isolation of modern man play in the genesis of mental illness. . . .It is not a coincidence that one of the French terms for mental disease is 'alienation,' that is, estrangement.[81]

In addition Esquirol related prognosis to body weight: a loss of weight in acute psychoses and a gain during recovery dictates a good prognosis; a gain in weight during the acute phase indicates a bad prognosis.[82] He contributed to every area of psychiatric activity—classification, diagnosis, treatment, etiology, law, teaching, and so forth.

Psychiatry during this period (first half of the nineteenth century) was mainly free from religious influences. But one vestige remained, Margetts writes, in the spiritualist Johann C. Heinroth (1773-1843):

> He regarded the body and soul as one, madness as a disease of the entire being. Mental health was harmony of thought and desire, disease a loss of this balance. The soul was a free force, excited by stimulation and through provocation, and endowed with the power of choice between good and evil. The body was the external part of the ego, the organ of the soul, and the senses were the intermediary; 'the witness that body and soul are one.' Madness was a wild destroying activity of the will, an unfree state of the soul, and all unfree states of the soul were due to sin and evil passions i.e. fall from grace.[83]

Heinroth thought that Christianity was the prophylaxis and treatment for insanity. Yet he developed a classification system based on faculty psychology and coined the term psychosomatic in 1818. He was regarded by some as a competent physician whose approach was truly psychosomatic.[84]

Heinroth's influence lasted until Wilhelm Griesinger (1817-1868) published the first modern textbook of psychiatry (1845). Griesinger stated that mental illness was a disorder of the brain whether a lesion was or was not demonstrable.

Consequently, since a one-to-one correlation between brain function and mental process was unknown, classifications developed based on a reflex arc model; hence, they were considered physiological.[85] Perhaps an illustration from the work of one of Griesinger's most brilliant followers, Carl Wernicke (1848-1905), will clarify this point.

Wernicke's basic model was one of psycho-physical parallelism, i.e., a change in function of the nervous system leads to a change in the psychological phenomena. He based his thinking on the work of Wundt* and on the theory of aphasia. Jaspers says:

> Griesinger's statement 'mental illnesses are cerebral illnesses' was now to find its concrete fulfilment. The basic view seemed to have won through successfully when *Wernicke* took it up. This genius fell into the trap of his own teaching on aphasia. He discovered sensory aphasia and its localization in the left temporal lobe. He devised a schema based on association psychology in which an analysis of speech performance and speech comprehension was to coincide with a topographical distribution in the cortex of the left temporal lobe (1874: 'The syndrome of aphasia'). What he denoted as the 'psychic reflex arc,' 'the psychic focal lesion,' appeared to be demonstrated in the field of aphasia. . . .'The analysis of aphasia provides us with a paradigm for all other psychic events.' With this statement, the schema became the starting-point for basing the whole of psychiatry on principles of cerebral localization.[86]

The following diagram, taken from Adolf Meyer, might aid the reader in following Wernicke's system.

Psychosensory Sphere	Intrapsychic Sphere	Psychomotor Sphere
Anesthesia	Afunction	Akinesis
Hyperesthesia	Hyperfunction	Hyperkinesis
Paresthesia	Parafunction	Parakinesis[87]

Although his classification system did not succeed, he did endow "psychopathology with a number of concepts that today we take for granted, such as power of registration, perplexity, explanatory delusions, overvalued ideas, etc. . . ."[88]

Classification based on the cause, course, and outcome of illness concerned many in the middle of the nineteenth century. Benedict A. Morel (1809-1873) proposed the degeneration hypothesis. Ackerknecht said that it

---

*Wilhelm Wundt (1832-1920), father of modern experimental psychology, established the first experimental laboratory in Europe in 1879. William James (1842-1910) established his laboratory at Harvard University in the same year.

held out hopes of establishing unequivocal physical signs of mental illness, more tangible than the variable changes hitherto demonstrated in the brain, and hopes too of synthesizing all known facts and finally arriving at an aetiological rather than a symptomatic classification of mental disorders.[89]

Morel thought that degeneration was caused by intoxication, social milieu, pathological temperament, moral sickness, inborn or acquired damage, and heredity. He developed an etiological classification of the insane that stipulated a hereditary predisposition as the cause of insanity and criminality.[90] In 1852, he coined the term dementia praecox using dementia to mean deterioration and praecox (precocious) to mean rapid.[91] Morel's concepts of deterioration and dementia praecox flourished for years but were eventually discarded.

Another group of workers from the French school, however, also concerned with cause, course, and outcome of mental disease, arrived at other conclusions. After Pinel and Esquirol pruned the Linnean classification to several basic entities, Jean-Pierre Falret (1794-1870) and Jules Baillarger (1809-1890) began to form concepts of the manic-depressive entity. In 1851 Falret emphasized that psychiatry was following the symptom picture and not the clinical course. He described *folie circulaire*, a condition where mania and melancholia follow each other in successive periods. That, he thought, constituted a distinct clinical entity in which the depressive period lasts longer than the mania period. In 1854 Baillarger described *folie à double form* which Falret thought was the same as his *folie circulaire*—not a double but a single entity of disease with two phases. From 1851 until 1882 the French were debating the problem of mania and melancholia—building up the entities, changing names, and so forth. The Germans—W. Griesinger, (1817-1868), R. Von Krafft-Ebing (1840-1903), Ewald Hecker (1843-1909), Karl Ludwig Kahlbaum (1828-1899)—were also working on concepts of melancholia. Hecker described a mild form of *folie circulaire* and called it cyclothymia. Kahlbaum formulated the disease entity or symptom complex concept around 1865, i.e., a group of signs and symptoms with no known etiology. In 1869 Kahlbaum described catatonia and two years later Hecker described hebephrenia. In effect, dementia praecox and melancholia became separate entities. The stage was now set for the greatest systematizer of them all, Emil Kraepelin (1856-1926).[92]

Before considering Kraepelin's contributions, the meaning of several terms and concepts that have extreme importance to psychiatry need to be clarified. Confusion over the meaning of the word insanity in its medical usage has existed since the time of the early Greeks. Aristophanes used the word melancholia to mean "mad, out of one's mind, without any lowness of spirit."[93] Hippocrates, on the other hand, equated melancholia with fear (phobos) or distress that lasts for a long time.[94] By the time of Esquirol, the definition of the term melancholia became so diffused that it lacked real meaning. Esquirol tried to correct this problem. He divided melancholia into two entities: (1) melancholia with delirium was called lypemania (depression); (2) melancholia with paranoid ideation was called monomania. He further separated lypemania from dementia, mania, and hypochondria.[95]

Joseph Guislain (1797-1860) assumed that all mental disorders were preceded by an early stage of depression.[96] M. Allen considered mania and melancholia as the same phenomena but overactive in different directions. Both, he thought, were followed by a stage of exhaustion.[97] Flemming, referring to the vesaniae (insanities), divided them into mania and melancholia.[98] Zeller, divided the vesaniae into two different groups: those characterized by abnormality in affective life and those characterized by disorders of ideas and will. The latter group, Zeller thought, represented *psychic weakness*, an allusion to a view expressed by Berze.[99] Zeller believed that the affective disorders preceded the disorders of thinking and will. Thus in 1840, he regarded "insanity as showing in its different forms different stages of one disease process which may be modified, interrupted, changed by all sorts of intercurrent pathological happenings, but which, on the whole, keeps to a steady successive course which can go on to complete disintegration of psychic life—the Einheitspsychose."[100] Einheitspsychose meant a singular state (derangement) of the mind. Thus the term psychosis was born.

Some other advances involved the psychosomatic controversy of the day. Baron Ernst von Feuchtersleben (1806-1849) stressed the mind-body relationship and the role of the mind in producing physical illness.[101] Although Heinroth coined the term psychosomatic, von Feuchtersleben is considered the father of psychosomatic medicine because he stressed the total personality and the psychological elements in disease.[102] New nomenclature and further advances followed. George Miller Beard (1840-1883), an American, first published the term neurasthenia in 1871. The term comes from the Greek neuro (nerve) and asthenia (weakness).[103] Cesare Lombroso (1836-1909) used Morel's concept of degeneration to relate to criminals, originated criminal anthropology, and coined the term criminal degenerate.[104] In 1899 Dugas introduced the term depersonalization.[105] S. Weir Mitchell (1830-1914) devised the famous rest cure for nervous patients: rest, isolation, overfeeding, and massage.[106]

Emil Kraepelin exerted his influence through his textbook which was first published in 1883; it reached the ninth edition by 1927. In each succeeding edition Kraepelin modified his categories.[107] Adolf Meyer (1866-1950) says:

Without going into detail I ask you to glance at what happened to Kraepelin and his school with regard to paresis and dementia praecox. In his zeal to identify lesion types with symptoms specific to a special 'disease process,' he did not have enough regard for the total picture. Among annual admissions from the same territorial region, with the population presumably living under the same conditions, he gave three times the number of diagnoses of paresis as proved to prevail when accurate diagnostic methods became available. In keeping with his conception of cause, course, outcome which had been shaped by general paresis, Kraepelin next ventured on a simplification of psychiatry which has been accepted the world over—the separation of the so-called functional psychoses into the manic-depressive group and the, to him, essentially organic or, at any rate, deteriorating, dementia praecox. At first, with his overemphasis on the deteriorating features, he diagnosed up to 51% of all his admissions as dementia praecox, whereas the figures dropped to about 18% with the collapse of what among ourselves we should call the boom. With the most praiseworthy candor Kraepelin published the fluctuation of diagnostic judgment, most marked with regard to his understanding of the two foremost nosological entities.[108]

These words, written in 1903 when Kraepelin's ideas were most renowned, clearly depict the weaknesses in the Kraepelin's system. Years later, in 1963, Menninger, analyzing the basis of Kraepelin's system, says:

He was by no means the first nosologist to recognize the need for longitudinal study of mental illness, nor the first to associate certain forms of disturbance with age periods, nor the first to classify diseases in terms of outcome. Yet his system provided within itself an explanation of the concepts utilized, and effected a synthesis which showed their interrelationship. This fact was, as we shall see, both the strength and the weakness of his nosology. As it developed through the nine editions of his textbook, the classification became not the product of a theory but a theory itself, and one which exercised a retarding effect upon new theory and new classification demanded by new facts.[109]

Kraepelin's influence dominated psychiatry throughout the world for nearly 50 years. Kraepelin brought psychiatry closer to medicine; did significant studies on memory and alcoholism; introduced modern research methods into psychiatry; emphasized prognosis in diagnosis; differentiated manic-depressive psychoses, paranoia, dementia praecox; and presented a system that had worldwide acceptance.[110]   Today we are again striving for clear-cut definitions of the different types of mental illness; a classification system not based on symptoms or prognosis alone but on the underlying process or processes of disease; as well as a rational form of treatment.

The late nineteenth and early twentieth centuries ushered in a group of antagonists to Kraepelin—the dynamic school. There was, however, an intermediary between the systematizers and the dynamic schools—Eugen Bleuler (1857-1939), a Swiss psychiatrist who developed the concept of schizophrenia, a term he coined in 1911. The term indicates a "splitting" of consciousness and Bleuler thought the splitting could occur not only during puberty but either before or after puberty. He also thought that remissions occur in schizophrenia. Bleuler's position challenged and destroyed Kraepelin's criteria for dementia praecox. Kraepelin combined catatonia, hebephrenia, and paranoia into a single disease entity subsumed under dementia praecox, which he thought was a chronic disease with an unfavorable prognosis as the inevitable outcome; thereby, distinguishing it from manic-depressive psychoses. Bleuler accepted Kraepelin's subtypes but added a fourth one, simple schizophrenia. Bleuler did not think that the prognosis was always unfavorable—there were remissions—but he did believe that patients with schizophrenia never completely recovered (healing with a scar). He divided schizophrenia into fundamental and accessory symptoms. The fundamental symptoms—those common to all types of schizophrenia—were autism, inappropriate affect, ambivalence, and a disturbance in thought associations. The accessory symptoms included hallucinations, delusions, ideas of reference, catatonia, deficient insight into self and external reality, and so forth. Therefore, Bleuler referred not to schizophrenia but to the group of schizophrenias or syndromes. He thought each member of the syndrome probably had different etiologies. He further broadened Kraepelin's concept of dementia praecox but Bleuler's definitions of fundamental symptoms were not clear and the resuting uncertainties provoked subsequent controversy and disagreement.[111,112] Bleuler presented a balanced and organized viewpoint on schizophrenia: his diagnosis was based on symptomatology, not prognosis; he eliminated the term dementia praecox from psychiatric nosology; he included somatic, organic, as well as dynamic psychological observations; and he synthesized his view in such a manner as to open the possibility that schizophrenia could be an intrapsychic or interpersonal disease, or a reaction of the biological organism to internal and external stresses. In this way he was a link between Kraepelin and the members of the dynamic school—Adolf Meyer, Pierre Janet (1859-1947), Sigmund Freud (1856-1939), and Carl Jung (1875-1961).[113]

Adolf Meyer advanced American psychiatric education and research during the first half of this century, and developed a system of diagnosis and treatment—psychobiology or ergasiology. Meyer proposed that behavior was a vector of all forces acting upon the individual. He attempted to abolish Kraepelin's static terminology and to replace it with dynamic psychobiology.

Meyer replaced the terms disease and illness with the term reaction type—an idea first proposed by Alfred Hoche.[114] The theory centered around the notion of energy (erg) and he used the term ergasia to denote the totality of the individual's response. Energasia denotes normal adaptation. By substituting the appropriate prefix, Meyer then developed a nomenclature: meregasia (neuroses); parergasia (psychoses); thymergasia (affective states); anergasia (organic brain disease); oligergasia (constitutional mental subnormality); etc. His system did not gain wide acceptance; however, Meyer's emphasis upon the importance of considering the total person—man in his environment—has had great influence on modern psychiatric thought. Meyer viewed each individual as unique, assessed diverse factors that led to illness, evaluated the factors necessary for adjustment, and based treatment upon these considerations.[115]

Adolf Meyer maintained a middle course between dynamic (introspective) and behavioristic schools of psychiatry. Dynamics, a term adapted from mechanistic sciences, explains or describes the changing interplay either within a body system or between one system and another. That interplay involves homeostatic mechanisms at various levels of organization—anatomical, biochemical, physiological, psychological, and socio-cultural levels. A disturbance at one level changes not only the equilibrium at that level but at the other levels as well. Hence, signs and symptoms indicate a disturbance in the body's balance.[116]

Théodule A. Ribot (1839-1916) established the French school of dynamic psychiatry and scientific psychology. He translated Herbert Spencer's *Principles of Psychology* into French and applied Hughlings Jackson's (1835-1911) physiological theories on the hierarchy of nervous functions—an application of Darwin's theory of evolution—to the understanding of normal and pathological psychology. Ribot was the first to state that memory loss is due to a progressive dissolution (opposite of evolution) in organic brain disease. The new, complex, poorly organized memories are lost before the old, simple, well-organized ones. Ribot believed that regression in affects may be due to psychological and unconscious causes and that affects were rooted in instincts. To him, there existed a dynamic unconscious, stored with energy and divided into three layers: an inherited collective unconscious, a personal unconscious derived from brain structure, and an individual unconscious developed from life experiences. Ribot insisted that mental dissociation was the basic mechanism of psychopathology.[117,118]

Pierre Janet (1859-1947), a student of Ribot, believed in the principle of split consciousness or dissociation and elaborated a dynamic system of mind centered around psychic energy, tension, or force. The push, pull, weakness and strength of available energy produce an integration or a dissociation of psychic functioning. He introduced the term psychasthenia to describe individuals whose ideas have low energy levels which are found in those with phobias, anxiety, and obsessive compulsive states. Janet recognized that there is a portion of self called the subconscious in which mental activities and events occur outside of personal awareness. He devised a psychology of conduct based on a hierarchy of tendencies: the superior self is rational, experimental, and progressive; the intermediate is intellectual, assertive, reflective; the inferior is reflex, perceptive, social. The self functions at these various levels: some levels are available for introspective consciousness and some are not; but all levels have as real an influence on our thought, action, and conduct as conscious introspection. Janet published this work before 1893 as part of his doctoral thesis on hysteria.

To him, the "fixed ideas" of hysteria developed below consciousness (subconscious) and reflected a high energy level, and hysteria was a psychological sickness.[119]

Another influence on Janet was his teacher Jean-Martin Charcot (1825-1893). Besides making innumerable contributions to medicine and neurology, Charcot also investigated hypnosis and hysteria and thereby helped develop the modern concept of neuroses.   Charcot believed that an idea was capable of producing hysterical manifestations and that hypnotism could influence these symptoms.   He thought that hysteria was responsive to suggestion;   however, he emphasized that hysteria was an organic disease due to a brain defect or pathology.[120]

Hypnotism of course did not begin with Charcot. Paracelsus in the sixteenth century taught that the mumia, a vital force contained in a vehicle, when magnetically extracted from the body during disease produced a cure.   Thus the notion of the curative power of magnetism began.   One hundred and fifty years later this concept arose as a means of explaining the cause and treatment of mental disease.   Franz Anton Mesmer (1734-1815) believed that disease was influenced by stars and planets, and that "the *fluidum* described by Paracelsus had curative properties and that the magnet could be an agent to induce the *fluidum* into the body."[121]   Mesmer conducted séances around a wooden tub, whose bottom was covered with iron filings, glass, and bottles, and iron rods extended from its trough.   People surrounded the tub; those closest touched the rods; those in the surrounding circles were connected with the inner-circle people by silk cords and interlaced hands.   Mesmer appeared lavishly dressed in a bishop's garments, carrying "magnetic" iron rods. Treatment consisted of the patient being touched or stroked by the wand. Mesmer claimed he restored the balance of fluid in the patient's body, thereby reestablishing the necessary equilibrium between the person and the heavenly bodies thus producing a cure. This system, called mesmerism or animal magnetism, contained within it—although unknown to Mesmer—the seeds of hypnotism.[122]

Mesmer had followers whose discoveries contributed to changes in the practices of medicine, religion, and psychiatry.   John Elliotson (1791-1868) in 1843 described surgery without pain in patients who were mesmerized. That was probably the beginning of hypnotism for surgery.[123]   James Esdaile (1808-1859) operated on hypnotized Hindu convicts and[124] pioneered hypnotic anesthesia.[125]   Phineas P. Quimby, an American clockmaker, in 1848 attended the lectures of Charles Poyen, a French hypnotist.   These lectures impressed Quimby and over a period of years he practiced hypnotism and eventually developed a reputation as a healer.   He wrote ten bound volumes of manuscripts describing his treatment and he named his discovery the "Science of Health" or the "Science of Christ."   In 1862 Mary Baker Eddy (1821-1910) was successfully treated by Quimby for spinal weakness and lack of vitality.[126]   Zilboorg, claiming that Mrs. Eddy was suffering from hysterical paralysis said, "The direct historical and inner psychological continuity from Mesmer to Christian Science is both telling and striking."[127]   James Braid (1795-1860) believed mesmerism was a subjective state and not due to a mysterious fluid. He disregarded Mesmer's methods and terminology and in 1843 introduced the term hypnotism, a phenomenon he ultimately thought was due to suggestion.[128]   These developments are some of the precursors to psychoanalysis and the Christian Science religion.

Mesmer's terminology disappeared as Charcot's work in Paris progressed and hypnotism gained in popularity. A.A. Liébeault (1823-1904) treated patients with suggestion during periods of hypnotic sleep.   He had been working in Nancy, France since 1864.   Hippolyte-Marie Bernheim (1840-1919), after studying with Liébeault, published their work in 1884 claiming the curative power of suggestion.   They noticed that many people—not only hysterics—tended to accept authoritative statements without proof and even contrary to reason and that others besides hysterics could be hypnotized.   These men interpreted hypnotic phenomena and the symptoms of hysteria as the result of suggestion; hence, hypnotism cured hysterical symptoms by suggestion and differed from suggestion only in degree. In fact suggestion without hypnotism worked in hysteria. Charcot rejected this explanation. As a consequence two conflicting schools of thought developed: the Paris school believed in the organic etiology of hysteria and followed Charcot; the Nancy school believed in the psychological etiology of hysteria and followed Liébeault and Bernheim.[129]   Bernheim introduced the term psychoneurosis for hysteria and allied conditions.[130]   The bridge from Paracelsus to Freud was complete since Freud studied with Charcot in 1885 and with Liébeault and Bernheim in 1889.[131]

Freud combined an emphasis of psychological causes for mental illness with the then prevalent mechanistic scientific thinking. His school of dynamic psychiatry, psychoanalysis, maintains that there is a cause and effect relationship among psychic processes, symptomatology, and observable behavior.   The assumption, using a machine analogy, is that a knowable cause (usually psychological) is underneath each feeling, thought, or act. As previously noted, all past efforts to reduce human thought, feeling, and behavior to absolute elements or essences had been futile and had ended in failure. Nevertheless, Freud's theory of dynamic psychiatry did exactly this. It offered explanations of normal and abnormal mentation, affect, behavior, as well as a theory of stages of development.   Freudian psychopathologists, using their psychological understanding, assumed "scientific" connections in which one psychic state or phenomenon emerged from another and inferred that by introspective investigation and patient verification these connections could be ascertained.   They further assumed that by explaining these connections to the patient, both in the present and past, a curative process was initiated. Insight, understanding, and explanation produced the cure. Freud offered a complete system—a method of investigation, etiological explanations, and therapy. This was equally true for those who broke with Freud but persisted in "explaining" man in psychological terms—Jung, Adler, Horney, Sullivan, Erikson, etc.

Freud collaborated with Joseph Breuer (1841-1925) in studying hysteria. Breuer had been treating patients using hypnosis since 1880, and in 1895 he and Freud published *Studies on Hysteria* in which they proposed catharsis as an adjunctive method of treatment in patients who were under hypnosis.[132] Later Freud discarded hypnosis and catharsis and developed psychoanalysis. He proposed that unconscious conflicts caused neuroses, not anatomical lesions or physiochemical disturbances, and developed an elaborate system of psychology. Freud and his successors constantly changed and modified their concepts. Some of Freud's more important concepts include: the concept of the unconscious and of defense mechanisms, the development of an instinct theory and its relationship to anxiety, a theory of ego psychology, a model of mind (ego, id, superego), interpretation of dreams, a theory of libido development and neuroses, and a technique and method of treatment.[133] The following outline of the classification of neuroses is based upon Freudian theory.

THE NEUROSES
    A.   Actual Neuroses
            I.   Anxiety Neurosis
          II.   Neurasthenia
       III.   Hypochondria
       IV.   (Traumatic Neuroses?)
    B.   Psychoneuroses: Regression or Fixation Neuroses
            I.   Transference Neuroses
                a. Hysteria
                    1. Conversion hysteria
                    2. Anxiety
                b. Compulsion Neurosis (Obsession)
          II.   Narcissistic Neuroses (Psychoses)
                a. Paraphrenia
                b. Schizophrenia
                c. Manic-depressive
                d. Paranoia
        III.   Other Regression Neuroses
                a. Perversions
                b. Neurotic Character
                    1. Introvert, schizoid
                    2. Extrovert, cycloid
    C.   Mixed Neuroses
    D.   Borderline Cases[134]

The preceding outline represents some of the earlier work of Freud and his followers in developing a classification system; however, for the most part Freudians have tended to avoid classification in favor of structural, dynamic, economic, and genetic formulations of various mental disturbances. Their concern was not with the symptoms or classification systems but with the underlying etiological dynamic processes. The Freudian school enjoyed tremendous popularity in the United States until the mid-1950s and only within the past ten years has its acceptance and popularity declined.

Freud, as the outline has shown, divided neuroses into actual neuroses, psychoneuroses, mixed neuroses, and borderline cases. The actual neuroses consisted of neurasthenia, anxiety neurosis, and hypochondria. Freud thought that these entities could not exist in a person who had a normal sexual life. In essence, then, the actual neuroses were physical diseases. He writes:

> Now I must point out to you the decisive difference between the symptoms of the *actual neuroses* and those of the *psychoneuroses*, with the first group of which (the transference neuroses) we have hitherto been so much occupied. In both the actual neuroses and the psychoneuroses the symptoms proceed from the libido; that is, they are abnormal ways of using it, substitutes for satisfaction of it. But the symptoms of an actual neurosis—headache, sensation of pain, an irritable condition of some organ, the weakening or inhibition of some function—have no 'meaning,' no signification in the mind. Not merely are they manifested principally in the body, as also happens, for instance with hysterical symptoms, but they are in themselves purely and simply physical processes; they arise without any of the complicated mental mechanisms we have been learning about. They really are, therefore, what psychoneurotic symptoms were so long held to be....Having learnt that the symptoms of the psychoneuroses express the mental consequences of some disturbance in this function, we shall not be surprised to find that the actual neuroses represent the direct somatic consequences of sexual disturbance.[135]

Freud stated the above in a series of lectures during the winter sessions of 1916-1917 at the University of Vienna. The division into actual neuroses with an organic etiology and psychoneuroses with a psychological etiology eventually led most psychiatrists to discard the term neuroses in favor of psychoneuroses.

Simultaneously with the progress in dynamic psychiatry, Ivan Petrovich Pavlov (1849-1936), a Russian physiologist, developed the principles of conditioned reflex. His work was originally based on studies of the digestive and salivary secretions in animals and later extended to neuroses and certain psychotic symptoms in humans. The conditioned reflex is a reaction to a stimulus that ordinarily would not produce that response. A primary or unconditioned stimulus provokes an expected response, i.e., food causes salivation. Presenting food and at the same time ringing a bell (the secondary or conditioned stimulus) will also result in salivation; ultimately however, ringing a bell without presenting food will result in salivation. The conditioning stimulus (i.e., bell) produces a response referred to as a conditioned reflex (i.e., salivation). Not only can vegetative and motor responses be conditioned but so can complex behavior patterns. Conversely, by associating a painful secondary stimulus with a primary stimulus it is possible to inhibit the unconditioned reflex. Pavlov reasoned that normal and abnormal behavior could be interpreted and explained on the basis of the conditioned reflex. Disease is an imbalance and health a balance between excitation and inhibition of nervous system activity. Hence, by various techniques involving reflexology Pavlovian's thought a scientific basis for treating the mentally ill could be established.[136]

Pavlov won the 1903 Nobel Prize for his experiments on digestion but his methods were disputed. Vladimir Bechterev (1857-1927), a Russian clinician and experimental psychologist, studied around 1884 with Wundt, Charcot, and other leading European teachers. He organized the first psychophysiological laboratory and brain institute in his country and founded the Russian school of neurology. He criticized Pavlov's experimental methods and conclusions. Bechterev in 1910 published his theory of associative reflexes. He thought that learning and habits were acquired responses to social or collective experiences and that the mechanisms for these actions were located in the cerebral cortex. Bechterev considered the role of the cerebral cortex as primarily a synthesizer of responses of more complex behavioral patterns, while Pavlov considered the cortex an analyzer of stimuli. Further, Bechterev thought that the somatic motor response was a truer measure of behavior than the vegetative visceral responses. Bechterev devised an objective psychology in which he discarded the word psychology and replaced it with the word reflexology. He considered only behavior not subjective experience as the legitimate object of science.[137]

Russian reflexology became the basis for behaviorism which John B. Watson (1878-1958) introduced into the United States in 1912. Watson criticized those who believed consciousness to be the proper study of psychology:

Behaviorism, on the contrary, holds that the subject matter of human psychology *is the behavior of the human being.* Behaviorism claims that consciousness is neither a definite nor a usable concept. The behaviorist, who has been trained always as an experimentalist, holds, further, that belief in the existence of consciousness goes back to the ancient days of superstition and magic.[138]

Conscious and unconscious behavior become obsolete terms for behaviorists—introspection a meaningless exercise in futility. All that exists is human adjustment, the activity of the whole organism in its daily functioning, the stimulus and response, the conditional or unconditional reflex, and the controlled experiment.[139] From these experimental beginnings behavior or conditioning therapy, a term coined by B.F. Skinner (1904-   ) and D.R. Lindsley in 1954, arose.[140]

A historical background such as this should have particular value for the psychiatrist. To trace the mystery of the seat of man's mind is to trace the evolution of reason. To study the attempts of the early priest/philosopher/scientist to understand self and the interaction of the self with the environment illuminates the problems that psychiatrists face. For it aids the psychiatrist in putting his own work in the perspective of time.

This completes an overview of the changes in psychiatric thinking up to the last 40 or 50 years. Historical sections in the succeeding chapters will fill in some of the details and recent developments. It should be apparent that through the first quarter of the twentieth century the problems of classification, diagnosis, etiology, and treatment of mental illness were far from settled. Yet if psychiatry is ever to become a science, classification and diagnosis are essential. Owsei Tempkin, after reviewing past classification systems in general medicine, concluded:

Only when the medical categories of health and disease and the conceptual tools for grasping them, viz., diagnosis, prognosis, indication, and therapy are brought to bear upon a science does it acquire the nature of a medical science. And diagnosis, by definition, includes classification of the things to be discerned. This seems to be the moral taught by the history of classification in the medical sciences, and this may also explain why classification in medicine is older than the medical sciences.[141]

Once etiology, diagnosis, and classification are known, treatment becomes more rational. For example, paresis and pellegra with psychosis were two diseases whose diagnosis baffled physicians. Until bacteriologists identified *Treponema pallidum*—the organism responsible for paresis—and biochemists discovered the deficiency in the vitamin niacin that caused pellagra, there was no satisfactory treatment for either disease. When etiology and diagnosis are specifically connected, the same situation could exist regarding other diseases that are now called mental.

As long as diagnosis is in doubt, course and treatment are guesswork; hence the variety of treatment approaches—prayer, magic, mysticism, psychotherapy, hypnosis, drugs, surgery, behavior therapy, and so forth. Past history should have taught us not to put faith in one type of treatment, unless definitive etiological and diagnostic criteria are scientifically established and to beware of any treatments that may cause irreversible damage.

Psychiatry now seems to be freeing itself from the dogmatic assertions of the dynamic introspectionists. Yet the recent advances in drug treatment foster a new group of faith healers. Until the categories of depression and schizophrenia are more clearly defined, correlations with such substances as norepinephrine, dopamine, or other drugs are open to serious doubt. Behavior therapists who view man as a complex series of reflexes without consciousness must know that humans are not machines; neither are dogs nor any other living organism. If the errors of history are not learned, they are bound to be repeated.

Strides have been made in methods of observation, data collecting, diagnosis, etiology, and treatment. The criteria for diagnosis are getting tighter. Categories are becoming more limited; hence, reliability and validity are bound to increase. Psychiatrists should be aware that changing categories too frequently, or on the other hand, applying criteria that are too loose or too rigid can also lead to difficulties. More aspects of etiology are taken into consideration than in past years and should yield results. Treatments are now more diverse than ever and increase the psychiatrist's flexibility of therapeutic approaches. Outpatient delivery care systems are becoming more available and the inpatient census is constantly being lowered. These are good signs. But now as before the basis of psychiatry should rest on observation of the patient and on a nondogmatic comprehensive orientation—man in his total environment.

Finally, man has speculated about mind from the supernatural origins of soul to the metaphysical and metapsychological explanations of mind and behavior and still remains unsatisfied. Man has shackled himself with one classification system after another. The most sensible rule, therefore, for a psychiatrist to follow in his daily practice is to rid himself of speculations about philosophy and overly rigid nosology. In sum, the psychiatrist should base his judgment about each particular patient on observation, knowledge of psychopathology, a comprehensive concept of diagnosis, disease, and treatment, and his own common sense.

REFERENCES

1. Editorial, *J. Amer. Med. Assoc.* 188(4): 388–389 (1964).
2. Zilboorg, G., *A History of Medical Psychology.* New York: Norton, 1941, p. 307.
3. Garrison, F. H., *An Introduction to the History of Medicine,* 4th ed. reprinted. Philadelphia: Saunders, 1929, p. 358.
4. Bromberg, W., *Man Above Humanity—A History of Psychotherapy.* Philadelphia: Lippincott, 1954, pp. 74–76.
5. Editorial, op. cit., p. 389.
6. Riese, W., "The pre-Freudian origins of psychoanalysis," in *Science and Psychoanalysis* (Integrative Studies), vol. 1 (edited by Masserman, J.H.). New York: Grune & Stratton, 1958, pp. 66–69.
7. Ackerknecht, E.H., Psychopathology, primitive medicine and primitive culture. *Bull. Hist. Med.* 14:30 (1942).
8. Bowle, J., *Man Through The Ages.* Boston: Little, Brown, 1962, pp. 15–24.
9. Zilboorg, G., op. cit., pp. 27–28.

10. Castiglioni, A., *A History of Medicine* (transl. by Krumbhaar, E.B.).   New York: Knopf, 1958, pp. 18–30.
11. Jacobson, T., "Mesopotamia," in *Before Philosophy* (edited by Frankfort, H., Frankfort, H.A., Wilson, J., and Jacobson, T.).   Baltimore: Penguin, 1963, pp. 142–148.
12. Major, R., *A History of Medicine*, vol. I.   Springfield, Ill.:   Charles C. Thomas, 1954, pp. 26–33.
13. Wilson, J., "Egypt," in *Before Philosophy,* op. cit., pp. 55–70.
14. Garrison, F.H., op. cit., pp. 53–59.
15. Shaffer, J.A., *Philosophy of Mind.*   Englewood Cliffs, N.J.: Prentice-Hall, 1968, p. 2.
16. Venzmer, G., *5000 Years of Medicine* (transl. by Koenig, M.).   New York: Taplinger, 1972, pp. 65–67.
17. Zilboorg, G., op. cit., pp. 28–30.
18. Major, R., op. cit., pp. 56–65.
19. Simon, B., Models of mind and mental illness in ancient Greece: II.   The Platonic model.   *J. Hist. Behav. Sci.* 8:392 (1972).
20. Frankfort, H. and Frankfort, H.A., "The emancipation of thought from myth," in *Before Philosophy,* op. cit., pp. 256–260.
21. Ibid., p. 257.
22. Aristotle, "De Anima," in *Introduction to Aristotle* (transl. by Smith, J.A.).   New York: The Modern Library, 1947, p. 153.
23. Frankfort, H. and Frankfort, H.A., op. cit., pp. 259–260.
24. De Witt, N.W., *Epicurus and His Philosophy.*   Cleveland and New York: The World Publishing Co. (A Meridian Book), 1967, pp. 65–66.
25. Aristotle, op. cit., pp. 150–153.
26. Jaspers, K., *The Great Philosophers.*   New York: Harcourt, 1962, pp. 139–140.
27. Plato, "Timaeus," in *The Works of Plato* (transl. by Jowett, B.).   New York: Random House, 1937, pp. 25–66.
28. Aristotle, op. cit., p. 174.
29. Ibid., pp. 171–235.
30. Garrison, F.H., op. cit., pp. 83–84.
31. Brock, A.J., *Greek Medicine* (reprinted from 1929 ed.).   London: Dent, 1972, p. 5.
32. Garrison, F.H., op. cit., pp. 92–100.
33. Ibid., p. 99.
34. Singer, C., *A History of Biology.*   New York: Abelard-Schuman, 1959, pp. 7–9.
35. Ibid., p. 40.
36. Menninger, K., *The Vital Balance.*   New York: Viking, 1963, p. 420.
37. Veith, I., *Hysteria: The History of a Disease.*   Chicago: Univ. Chicago Press, 1965, p. 15.
38. Riese, W., *A History of Neurology.*   New York: M.D. Publications, 1959, pp. 79–85.
39. Ackerknecht, E.H., *A Short History of Psychiatry*, 2nd revised ed. (transl. by Wolff, S.).   New York: Hafner, 1968, p. 11.
40. Ibid., pp. 12–13.
41. Ibid., pp. 13-14.
42. Ibid., p. 14.
43. Ibid., pp. 14–15.
44. Ibid., p. 15.
45. Singer, C. and Underwood, E.A., *A Short History of Medicine,* 2nd ed.   New York: Oxford University Press, 1962, pp. 59–60.
46. St. Augustine, "De Quantitate," in *Body, Mind and Death* (edited by Flew, A.).   New York: Macmillan, 1973, p. 75.

47. Ibid., p. 97.
48. Magoun, H.W., "Early development of ideas relating the mind with the brain," in *Neurological Basis of Behaviour* (edited by Wolstenholme, G.E.W. and O'Connor, C.M.). Boston: Little, Brown, 1968, pp. 4-27.
49. Bailey, P., The seat of the soul. *Persp. Biol. Med.* 2(4): 417 (1959).
50. Galdston, I., "Psyche and soul: psychiatry in the Middle Ages," in *Historic Derivations of Modern Psychiatry* (edited by Galdston, I.). New York: McGraw-Hill, 1967, pp. 19-22.
51. Ackerknecht, E.H., *A Short History of Psychiatry,* op. cit., p. 19.
52. Pachter, H.M., *Paracelsus.* New York: Henry Schuman, 1951, p. 234.
53. Menninger, K., op. cit., p. 427.
54. Ibid.
55. Ackerknecht, E.H., *A Short History of Psychiatry,* op. cit., pp. 22-25.
56. Ibid., pp. 24-26.
57. Jelliffe, S.E., Some historical phases of the manic-depressive synthesis. *Assoc. Res. Ner. Ment. Health* 2:23-27 (1929).
58. Menninger, K., op. cit., p. 431.
59. Ackerknecht, E.H., *A Short History of Psychiatry,* op. cit., p. 32.
60. Watson, R.I., *The Great Psychologists.* Philadelphia: Lippincott, 1971, pp. 155-157.
61. Ibid., pp. 160-164.
62. Locke, J., *An Essay Concerning Human Understanding,* vol. I, Book 2. New York: Dover, 1959, pp. 121-124.
63. Ibid., pp. 448-460.
64. Ackerknecht, E.H., *A Short History of Psychiatry,* op. cit., p. 34.
65. Ibid. p. 36.
66. Ibid.
67. Riese, W., *A History of Neurology,* op. cit., p. 31.
68. Editorial, op. cit., 388-389.
69. Menninger, K., op. cit., pp. 441-442.
70. Bailey, P., op. cit., pp. 419-425.
71. Ibid., p. 425.
72. Ibid., p. 431.
73. Sperry, R.W., *Mental Phenomena as Causal Determinants in Brain Function, in Consciousness and the Brain: A Scientific and Philosophical Inquiry* (edited by Globus, G.G., Maxwell, G., Savodnik, I.). New York: Planum Press, 1976, pp. 170-174.
74. Freedman, A., Kaplan, H.I., and Sadock, B.J., *Modern Synopsis of Comprehensive Textbook of Psychiatry/II,* 2nd ed. Baltimore: Williams and Wilkins, 1976, pp. 18-22.
75. Veith, I., op. cit., p. 179.
76. Kavka, J., Pinel's conception of the psychopathic state. *Bull. Hist. Med.* 23(5):461-468 (1949).
77. Menninger, K., op. cit., p. 444.
78. Ibid., p. 445.
79. Ibid., pp. 446, 448-449.
80. Hunter, R. and Macalpine, I., *Three Hundred Years of Psychiatry 1535-1860.* New York: Oxford University Press, 1963, pp. 732-733.
81. Ackerknecht, E.H., *A Short History of Psychiatry,* op. cit., p. 49.
82. Jaspers, K., *General Psychopathology* (transl. by Honig, J. and Hamilton, M.). Chicago: Univ. Chicago Press, 1963, p. 849.
83. Margetts, E.L., The early history of the word "psychosomatic." *Can. Med. Assoc. J.* 63:403 (1950).
84. Ibid., pp. 403-404.

85. Marx, O., Wilhelm Griesinger and the history of psychiatry: A reassessment. *Bull. Hist. Med.* 49:519–544 (1972).

86. Jaspers, K., op. cit., p. 482.

87. Meyer, A., *The Collected Papers of Adolf Meyer,* vol. 2, Psychiatry (edited by Winters, E.). Baltimore: The Johns Hopkins Press, 1951, p. 337.

88. Jaspers, K., op. cit., p. 852.

89. Ackerknecht, E.H., *A Short History of Psychiatry,* op. cit., p. 54.

90. Ibid., pp. 55–59.

91. Menninger, K., op. cit., p. 449.

92. Jelliffe, S.E., op. cit., pp. 38–42.

93. Lewis, A.J., Melancholia: A historical review. *J. Mental Sci.* 80:13 (1934).

94. Ibid., p. 1.

95. Ibid., p. 13.

96. Ibid.

97. Ibid., p. 14.

98. Ibid., p. 15.

99. Ibid.

100. Ibid.

101. Stainbrook, E., Psychosomatic medicine in the nineteenth century. *Psychosom. Med.* 14(3):212 (1952).

102. Roback, A.A., *History of Psychology and Psychiatry.* New York: Greenwood Press, 1961, p. 282.

103. Altschule, M.D., *Roots of Modern Psychiatry.* New York: Grune & Stratton, 1965, p. 163.

104. Ackerknecht, E.H., *A Short History of Psychiatry,* op. cit., pp. 57–58.

105. Shorvon, M.B., Depersonalization syndrome. *Proc. Roy. Soc. Med.* 39:779 (1946).

106. Zilboorg, G., op. cit., p. 443.

107. Menninger, K., op. cit., p. 457.

108. Meyer, A., *Psychobiology: A Science of Man* (compiled and edited by Winters, E.E. and Bowers, A.M.). Springfield, Ill.: Charles C Thomas, 1957, pp. 148–151.

109. Menninger, K., op. cit., p. 457.

110. Ibid., p. 463.

111. Bleuler, E., *Dementia Praecox or the Group of Schizophrenias* (transl. by Zinkin, E.). New York: International University Press, 1950.

112. Carpenter, W.T., Current diagnostic concepts in schizophrenia. *Amer. J. Psychiatry* 133(2):172–176 (1976).

113. Hoch, P., *Differential Diagnosis in Clinical Psychiatry* (edited by Strohl, M.D. and Lewis, N.D.C.). New York: Science House, 1972, pp. 603–606.

114. Ibid., p. 604.

115. Meyer, A., *The Commonsense Psychiatry of Dr. Adolf Meyer* (edited by Lief, A.). New York: McGraw-Hill, 1948.

116. Gray, M., Principles of the comprehensive examination. *Arch. Gen. Psychiatry* 10:380 (1964).

117. Delay, J., Jacksonism and the works of Ribot (transl. by Bailey, P.). *Arch. Neuro. Psychiatry* 78:505–515 (1957).

118. Ribot, T., *The Diseases of Personality,* 2nd revised ed. (authorized transl.). Chicago: Open Court, 1895, pp. 1–17.

119. Bailey, P., The psychology of conduct: A review. *Amer. J. Psychiatry* 8:209–234 (1928).

120. Zilboorg, G., op. cit., pp. 361–364.

121. Marks, R.W. (Ed.), *Great Ideas in Psychology*. New York: Bantam, 1966, p. 2.
122. Ibid., pp. 4-5.
123. Ibid., pp. 15-18.
124. Ibid., pp. 18-19.
125. Ibid., p. 20.
126. Dakin, E.F., *Mrs. Eddy: The Biography of a Virginal Mind*. New York: Scribner, 1929, pp. 38-44.
127. Zilboorg, G., op. cit., p. 347.
128. Marks, R.W., op. cit., pp. 21-22.
129. Ibid., pp. 22-27.
130. Noyes, A.P., *Modern Clinical Psychiatry*, 2nd ed., rewritten and enlarged. Philadelphia: Saunders, 1939, pp. 334-335.
131. Veith, I., op. cit., pp. 259-263.
132. Breuer, J. and Freud, S., *Studies on Hysteria. The Standard Edition of the Complete Psychological Works of Sigmund Freud*, vol. 2. London: Hogarth, 1957.
133. Freedman, A., Kaplan, H.I., and Sadock, B.J., op. cit., pp. 227-270.
134. Wechsler, I.S., *The Neuroses*. New York: Saunders, 1929, p. 127.
135. Freud, S., *A General Introduction to Psychoanalysis* (transl. of revised ed. by Riviere, J.). New York: Garden City Publ. Co., 1943, pp. 336-337.
136. Pavlov, I.P., "The conditioned reflex," in Marks, R.W. (Ed.), op. cit., pp. 344-352.
137. Yakovlev, P.I., "Bechterev," in *Brazier MAB: The Central Nervous System and Behavior*. Madison, N.J.: Madison Printing Co., 1959, pp. 187-210.
138. Watson, J.B., "What is behaviorism?" in Marks, R.W. (Ed.), op. cit., p. 384.
139. Ibid., pp. 383-399.
140. Wolpe, J., *The Practice of Behavior Therapy*, 2nd ed. New York: Pergamon, 1973, p. xi.
141. Tempkin, O., "The history of classification in the medical sciences," in *The Role and Methodology of Classification in Psychiatry and Psychopathology* (edited by Katz, M.M., Cole, J.O., and Barton, W.E.). Chevy Chase: Md.: National Institute of Mental Health, 1965, p. 19.

2
CLASSIFICATION

In psychiatry, as in all of medicine, it is essential to name, define, and arrange phenomena into entities, groups, clusters, or categories. Diagnosis, the label or name given to related phenomena, identifies and distinguishes one specific group from others. Classification, nosology, taxonomy, nomenclature, terminology, or systematics are terms that refer to the organization of groups into systems. Without classification there can be no science.

Unfortunately, classification systems of psychiatry generate confusion, misunderstanding, and controversy. Some psychiatrists disregard classification altogether. Others create systems out of hybrid fusions of psychological theories, physiological concepts, biochemical and pathological data, clinical symptomatology, or combinations thereof. Without a standardized classification system diagnosis depends upon the viewpoint of each psychiatrist. An arbitrary choice at best! The same phenomena can be capriciously placed within various categories or systems of classification depending on the psychiatrist's orientation. Unless limits of psychiatric terminology are acknowledged, confusion will be perpetuated and little progress can be made toward determining the cause, course, prevention, outcome, or treatment of mental illness.

Indeed, psychiatrists must agree on national as well as international classification systems. Communication and cooperation in various regions of the world would be facilitated if some sort of agreement on a classification system could be reached. Yet due to unique social and cultural environments, each region should retain portions of its classification. The complexity of the problem cannot be simplified by directives from an international body, loose generalities, minute groupings, or conversely, denying the need for a classification system.[1]

A weakness found in every nosology is the fallacy that disease entities have a known etiology, course, prognosis, and treatment. That lineal notion, if it persists, will perpetuate erroneous classification systems and static concepts of disease entities. Hence, the need for a multifactorial system is apparent.[2] Until more knowledge is acquired it is best to recognize the shortcomings and regard all existing systems as tentative and open to change. For purposes of uniformity, at the present time, the official nomenclature of the American Psychiatric Association as described in the *Diagnostic and Statistical Manual: Mental Disorders*, second edition, in short the DSMII, should be followed.[3]

Although neuroses are only one of the categories of mental illness, an overview of classification is necessary to identify neuroses as one part of total nosology. In this way the relationship of neuroses to the whole system and of each neurosis to one another can be clarified and understood. The DSMII is not a consistent system of classification. It is based on several criteria, i.e., diseases of brain, mind, and behavior.[4] For instance, cerebral arteriosclerosis is considered an organic brain syndrome, neuroses a functional psychological disorder of the mind, and exhibitionism a behavioral disturbance. To include these diverse categories as distinct groups in one system is illogical since each category is determined on a different basis. Yet that is what the DSMII does. It forces the psychiatrist to think in minute categories and lineal diagnosis and disregards the relationships of the various levels of organization. To avoid this error, systems theory and operational methods become necessary.

The operational approach recognizes the homeostatic mechanisms involved within the organism and its relationship to the environment outside of the organism. Genetic, biological, developmental, psychological, sociological, and other factors are integral for all diagnoses and the artificial separation of brain, mind, and behavior is discarded. Thus neuroses and all other forms of mental illness are studied and viewed in a similar manner. But the DSMII differentiates the various neuroses according to symptoms, signs, and behavior while denoting a psychological etiology. This is a false assumption and should be understood and considered wherever and whenever the neuroses are discussed. Furthermore, neuroses and classification systems are concepts—abstractions not things—and operational methods of evaluation would be closer approximations to scientific investigation. Tart writes:

> Operationalism is a way of rigorously defining some concept by describing the actual operations required to produce it. Thus an operational definition of the concept of "nailing" is defined by the operations (1) pick up a hammer in your right hand; (2) pick up a nail in your left hand; (3) put the point of the nail on a wood surface and hold the nail perpendicular to the wood surface; (4) strike the head of the nail with the hammer and then lift the hammer again; and (5) repeat step 4 until the head of the nail is flush with the surface of the wood. An operational definition is a precise definition, allowing total reproducibility.
>
> Some claim that whatever cannot be defined operationally is not a legitimate subject for scientific investigation. That is silly. No one can precisely specify all the steps necessary to experience "being in love," but that is

hardly justification for ignoring the state of being in love as an important human situation worthy of study. A further problem is that in psychology, operationalism implicitly means *physical* operationalism, specifying the overt, physically observable steps in a process in order to define it. In the search for an objectivity like that of the physical sciences, psychologists emphasize aspects of their discipline that can be physically measured, but often at the cost of irrelevant studies.[5]

Operationalism not only describes the method of observation but also the conditions under which the observation occurs. Since psychiatric classification involves the innumerable variables of the total person in an environment as well as a human observer, a rigid operational approach becomes impossible. Hence, within the boundaries of today's knowledge, attempts can be made to approximate the operational approach but none can be considered on the same scientific basis as those of the physical sciences.

PURPOSES AND METHODS

Classification is a prerequisite for all science and serves many purposes. First, it attempts to describe individuals, phenomena, or processes to reveal their true nature and relationships. In this way certain laws may be derived. Second, classification aims to achieve an economy of memory by grouping certain traits and characteristics under convenient labels; thereby facilitating communication. Third, nosology provides a system of studying the relationship between various groups. By using quantitive methods (testing), classification permits statistical analysis. Fourth, it aids in relating phenomena occurring within the individual to other phenomena within the same individual. Fifth, it defines and clarifies transition states. The cluster models will often clearly define boundaries, whereas a diffusion model best describes the transition between clusters. Finally, classification should generate interest, hypotheses, and investigative studies.[6]

Classification in medicine and psychiatry has unique purposes. The most obvious is to help predict cause, course, prognosis, prevention, and treatment. It also serves certain social needs of society. The following are some examples of situations for which psychiatrists use nosology to influence patients and even nonpatients: in public mental hospitals to justify retention or discharge; in private sanatoria and outpatient facilities to explain the disorder and to indicate proper treatment; in child-guidance clinics to understand the child-parent relationship and facilitate treatment; in military service to aid in actions that the service may take toward the soldier; in a court of law to establish and convince others that the defendant is morally right or wrong, guilty or innocent, etc.; in research to seek the underlying truth; and in prison to aid with administrative duties.[7] It is impossible to devise one psychiatric classification system or an investigative methodology that can be used for all these purposes with any degree of validity. Under certain conditions such as prisons, courts of law, or research, distinct classifications are needed. For the everyday work of the vast majority of psychiatrists, however, a system that helps them take care of patients will suffice.

Clinical psychiatrists resort to several methods to collect data: observing the patient's behavior, interviewing the patient and his relatives, discussing and sharing information about the patient with other professionals; and studying the reports of psychological tests.

Several interrelated components are involved in constructing a classification system. Precise definitions of terms are the first step. Psychiatric terms are difficult to define explicitly (denotation) or implicitly (connotation). Then follows the organization of data into similar groups. Here the major questions are: to determine what constitutes a similar group and what is the relationship between the abstract label given to the group and the individual under study. Is the psychiatrist discerning the essential or core elements of a group or is he selecting peripheral data? Grinker describes his mental processes as he makes a diagnosis as follows:

> I first hear and recognize the largest integrated component derived from observation and description of behavior and verbalization. This is like a center piece of a jig-saw puzzle. I then attempt to fit the smaller not incorporated pieces into this central component. I do not expect that all will fit in and those that do not are extraneous to the essential diagnosis. However, if several large chunks do not fit and seem diametrically in opposition to one I have chosen, I then switch to another one as the central piece and attempt to fit the smaller components into it. I may have to do this several times to get the maximum fit from the available bits of information. There can be no unified whole as the tyro would want, but bits of information related to the individual's personal life and defenses may have to be discarded in order to achieve an ultimate diagnosis. . . .[8]

The next component in constructing a system involves general principles and procedures and taxonomy (the science of classification). Psychiatric classificatory systems can be devised by observation (building a typology) or by a priori principles, in which the individual fits. To date, neither one has produced a satisfactory system. An ideal system would allocate all data into only one group. That would ensure a minimum of uncertainty and ambiguity.[9]

A classification system should be based on a specific method. Shindell suggests that examiners question the

> . . .specific source from which information might be obtained, question what might constitute a manageable portion which we could examine, question the

method by which our observation could be made, question the manner in which our observational results might be translated into precise and manipulatable symbols, and finally question whether the symbols we used constituted an accurate presentation of our findings.[10]

Following that one must even question the possibility of chance variations before drawing a conclusion. This can serve as a safeguard against imprecision and errors of personal bias. After arriving at a conclusion it is necessary to investigate alternate methods of classification. It is most important not to arbitrarily push one alternative system in preference to another and to adhere reasonably close to scientific method while establishing a system.

Classification must not be so rigidly applied in practice as to require a pigeonhole for each and every form and mode of human behavior. Judgment, nuance, and common sense must not be sacrificed in order to adhere to the rigid confines of science.

There are qualitative and quantitive differences in traits or characteristics that do not easily fit into one group or another. For instance, each individual experiences anxiety. When does the psychiatrist decide that a patient has an abnormal amount of anxiety, that is to say, is an anxiety neurotic? Similarly all people are at times depressed or are concerned about somatic complaints. When does the psychiatrist diagnose depressive neurosis, when hypochondriasis? It is the same with all the neuroses. Are there transitions from normal to neurotic to psychotic? Are there transitions within a range and not a definite point? Borderline states are being defined and many patients today are placed in these categories.[11]

Computers in the past 20 years have played an ever-increasing role in classification and diagnosis. They offer a sophisticated method of dealing with data and carry out complicated computations in a short time. The computer has also stimulated the development of algorithms (procedures) for classification, which have led to attempts to objectify the classificatory process. Programs for psychiatric diagnosis have been proposed but to date none is acceptable. A major problem is that data fed into the computer are limited to a set number of answers which the patient gives to questions. Another problem is that the computer's answers are preprogrammed. Besides, mechanical interpretations leave no room for intuition or nuances of meaning. The most common test for computer analysis is the Minnesota Multiphasic Personality Inventory (MMPI). It allows an easy, inexpensive, quick method for patient evaluation. But for developing a classification system a cerebral cortex is first needed that can supply the computer with the proper algorithm.[12-14]

PROS AND CONS

Those in favor of a classification system say that if all classifications were abolished each case would have to be described in detail. There would be no general principles for communication between student, teacher, or practicing physicians. Education would be made considerably more difficult, research and administration would bog down in endless verbiage. These protagonists believe that existing classification systems, despite many shortcomings, do contribute a degree of organization and orderliness to psychiatry, reduce the number of variables by noticing similarities and grouping, and help facilitate communication. Furthermore, classifications do aid in offering some knowledge of cause, course and prognosis, and in planning treatment.

An argument against classification cites overlapping conditions. Many patients suffering from hysterical neurosis have obsessive traits and are subject to depression. But the existence of multiple or borderline states is in itself no reason to do away with classification. Can severe obsessive compulsive neurosis lead to schizophrenia? Present criteria are just not delineated enough to fit a case into one category or another. Even the degree of disability is questionable since mild, moderate, or severe are arbitrary determinations. By analogy nature in its infinite variety has transitional or borderline states. Is it dark or light during dusk and dawn? Does the existence of dusk or dawn necessitate the elimination of the terms day and night?

Other objections are that the number of diagnostic entities are either too small or too large for a proper nosology and differ in name and number from country to country. Is the lack of a universally acceptable classification system sufficient reason to do away with the whole system? The whole system should not be thrown out simply because agreement has not been reached. The system can expand or contract when necessary to accommodate changing disease manifestations or newly acquired knowledge, and to fit regional conditions. Clinical manifestations change with the social and cultural situation and are often expressions thereof. It was once normal for young girls in western societies to faint. Today fainting is rare. But other conditions have now become common among young girls, e.g., confusion of social roles, drug addiction, and the like. Again, flexibility is necessary for proper classification.

Another argument against nosology is that it serves no useful purpose because as much data as possible must be collected anyway. This is true, but as noted, factual material acquires meaning when arranged into a definite frame of reference and only what is relevant for evaluation need be collected. Insight is the goal and not a mass of material. Insight is attained by relating theories or hypotheses to the material and searching for cause, course, outcome, prevention, and therapeutic correlations. When a patient is called a compulsive neurotic, it is only a partial description. Even such a limited diagnosis, however, has more significance and value than a vast mass of assorted facts.

Some claim that the major consideration is psychodynamics not diagnostic labels. For them classification is unimportant. Yet innumerable schools of dynamic psychology exist. Can it be proven which school reveals the relevant and essential psychodynamic variables? Although the first steps to diagnosis must be definition, observation, and description, this does not preclude dynamic formulations from also being of value. These formulations can be immensely valuable in understanding patients but should be submitted to rigorous criticism and proof. The psychiatrist should be ready to abandon those formulations that do not fit the clinical evidence. Psychodynamic considerations are a complement and supplement to the nosological diagnosis. Diagnosis, in its broadest sense, includes predictions (prognosis), course, etiology, prevention, and therapy. The label is a valuable symbol and not a rigid category.[15]

DEFINITIONS

Prediction and explanation are workable terms for psychiatry but are, indeed, of a low order of probability. In the living organism, innumerable variable factors are constantly relating to one another. The variable factors inside relate the inner balance of the individual—atom, molecule, cell, organ systems, biological organism. The factors outside relate the balance of the individual with the social and physical environment, politics, economics, and so forth. The mind mediates between the inside and outside environments. Prediction depends on probability (what may happen). To predict, then, one needs correlations between present and future events or processes. Explanation, on the other hand, tells what has happened and requires correlations between present and past events or processes. Thus it is possible at times to explain (evolution) and not to predict; at other times to predict (barometric pressure drops prior to a storm) and not to explain. Scientific explanation is possible without prediction; conversely, scientific prediction is possible without explanation. Clinical psychiatry cannot approach scientific explanation or prediction until an appropriate classification system is devised.

Prediction and explanation rely on four factors: time, space, matter, and certain events or processes. If the relationship among these factors is such that both explanation and prediction are consistent at all times, one can formulate a law of causality. If not, laws or rather rules other than causal ones are formulated, i.e.: rules of logic—the relations of things existing at the same time; rules of parallelism—the relationship of parallel phenomena existing at the same time, e.g., "psychic" phenomena and parallel brain and sense organ phenomena; and rules of systems—the correlations between various levels of integration. These rules, whether merely consequences or complications of the causal law, remain unknown. Since there are so many variables within the individual and his environment, prediction and explanation are not possible; hence, there are no causal laws that apply to the work of psychiatrists but only to rules of logic, parallelism, and systems.[16]

Psychiatrists use terms such as reliability, homogeneous, heterogeneous, and validity. These terms relate to evaluating and constructing classification systems.

Reliability of a system involves the examiners. It is the percentage of agreement among psychiatrists that a patient fits into a specific diagnostic category. How often will two separate examiners make the same diagnosis? Reliability infers specific characteristic traits or symptoms that constitute a diagnosis, namely, the hardcore manifestations or clues that lead to diagnosing one individual as a schizophrenic and another as a hysteric. In further evaluating traits, or groups of traits, we must consider whether these traits fit into only one category (homogeneous) or into many categories (heterogeneous). Validity infers the correlations or connections of the core diagnosis, namely, the peripheral knowledge or correlations (etiology, course, prognosis, treatment, and prevention).[17-21]

Some of the questions which should be asked in evaluating a classification system are: (1) Is it comprehensive, that is, does it include all possible diagnostic considerations? (2) What is the theoretical basis of the system? Is it consistent throughout? (3) How reliable is the system? Are the classes divided in such a way as to allow single traits, signs, or symptoms (or clusters thereof) to fit into one diagnostic category (homogeneous) or many (heterogeneous)? Are the diagnostic terms clear and concise or are they confused, misleading, and vague? (4) How valid is the system? How correct are the correlations or connections?

HISTORY

In comparison with the principles upon which past classifications were based, modern day psychiatrists classify according to organic brain disease (organic brain syndrome), bodily dysfunctions (psychophysiological disorders), symptomatology (neuroses and psychoses), intelligence (mental retardation), and deviant personality types. With the exception of the more specific breakdown with organic brain syndrome it is difficult to discern any real change.[22]

Since all current classification systems lead back to Kraepelin, his ideas deserve special study. Before examining his ideas specifically, a word about those who were major influences upon his thinking is in order. Immanuel Kant was a proponent of faculty psychology and his classification of mental illness was based on disturbances of perception, cognition, feeling, intelligence, and will. Pathology in these faculties was labeled hypochondria, mania, melancholia, amentia, dementia, and so on.[23] Kahlbaum and Morel contributed to Kraepelin's thinking. Kahlbaum developed the concept of disease entities and attempted to correlate these entities with various stages in an individual's life (childhood, adolescence, maturity, etc.). Morel classified disease according to both etiology and outcome. Kraepelin studied with Wilhelm Wundt and was influenced by the methods of experimental psychology. Kraepelin differentiated entities into various subgroups, and delineated disorders of perception, thinking, judgment, reasoning, intelligence, emotions, action, and volition. These he fitted into categories of mental disease: insanities due to external sources, dementias, organic dementias, emotional disorders, senility, psychogenic neuroses, psychopathy, and defective intellectual development. This was a complete integrated system of diagnosis with groups, subgroups, an underlying explanation, and a "predictable" course and prognosis.[24]

In the United States Kraepelin's system was followed in almost the original form until World War II, when in the military services its diagnostic inadequacies led to serious difficulties. In the late 1920s, each medical center used its own system of nosology. These private nosological systems spread throughout the country only by psychiatrists who were trained in one center and then moved to another area. This resulted in blocking effective communication and statistical studies between geographical areas. To combat this confusion the New York Academy of Medicine conducted a series of conferences from 1927 to 1932 and published a proposed nomenclature for the United States. In 1933 the first standard official classification appeared, and by 1942 it had two revisions. As World War II progressed only 10% of the psychiatric patients in the military services fit into the categories of the standard classification which was based on patients in public psychiatric hospitals and not outpatients, and 90% of the military cases could not be properly classified. To correct this situation, the navy, and later the army under the direction of William Menninger and his staff, devised a new classification. It listed five major categories: transient personality reactions to acute or special stress; psychoneurotic disorders; character and behavior disorders; disorders of intelligence; and psychotic disorders. After the war, problems in classification again appeared. By 1948 a confused situation existed similar to the one in the 1920s. There were at least three nomenclatures in use (standard, armed forces, and Veterans Administration) and none of these agreed with the International Classification System. Eventually a committee was formed by the American Psychiatric Association and in 1952 they published the first *Diagnostic and Statistical Manual* (DSMI). For the first time a system was devised that was more or less accepted and used throughout the United States.[25,26]

Prior to publication of the DSMI a very muddled situation existed regarding the terms neuroses and psychoneuroses. Since Freud distinguished between actual neuroses and psychoneuroses, the term neuroses was gradually replaced by psychoneuroses. The psychoneuroses were substitutive reactions or psychological illnesses.[27] By 1939 the Committee on Statistics of the American Psychiatric Association recognized the following subtypes of psychoneuroses:

1. hysteria (anxiety hysteria, conversion hysteria)
2. psychasthenia or compulsive states
3. hypochondriasis
4. anxiety state

5. neurasthenia
6. reactive depression (simple situational reaction)
7. mixed psychoneuroses[28]

The American Medical Association published in 1942 the following classification of the psychoneuroses:

A.   Anxiety Hysteria
B.   Conversion Hysteria
   1. Anesthetic type
   2. Paralytic type
   3. Hyperkinetic type
   4. Paresthetic type
   5. Automatic type
   6. Amnesic type
   7. Mixed hysterical psychoneurosis
C.   Psychasthenic States, or Obsessive Compulsive States
   1. Obsession
   2. Compulsive tics and spasms
   3. Phobias
   4. Mixed compulsive states
D.   Neurasthenia
E.   Hypochondriasis
F.   Anxiety State
G.   Reactive Depression
H.   Anorexia Nervosa
I.   Mixed Psychoneurosis[29]

In the DSMI, psychoneurotic reactions were subsumed under Psychoneurotic Disorders and the following subtypes were listed:

1.   Anxiety reaction
2.   Dissociative reaction
3.   Conversion reaction
4.   Phobic reaction
5.   Obsessive compulsive reaction
6.   Depressive reaction
7.   Psychoneurotic reaction, other[30]

The DSMII, in 1968, reintroduces the term neuroses and discards psychoneuroses. The subtypes are:

1.   Anxiety neurosis
2.   Hysterical neurosis
   a. Hysterical neurosis, conversion type
   b. Hysterical neurosis, dissociative type

3. Phobic neurosis
4. Obsessive compulsive neurosis
5. Depressive neurosis
6. Neurasthenic neurosis (Neurasthenia)
7. Depersonalization neurosis (Depersonalization Syndrome)
8. Hypochondriacal neurosis
9. Other neurosis
10. Unspecified neurosis[31]

The DSMI did of course arouse controversy. By 1968 the American Psychiatric Association published the DSMII. In that edition over 100 specific diagnostic entities were included under ten categories: mental retardation; organic brain syndromes; psychoses not attributed to physical conditions listed previously; neuroses; personality disorders and certain nonpsychotic mental disorders; psychophysiologic disorders; special symptoms; transient situational disturbances; behavior disorders of childhood and adolescence; and conditions without manifest psychiatric disorder and nonspecific conditions. Despite all this a satisfactory classification has not been found. Work is now under way on the third edition of the *Diagnostic and Statistical Manual: Mental Disorders* (DSMIII) for publication in January 1979. The hope is that this revision will improve the reliability and validity of psychiatric diagnosis, facilitate testing of etiologic hypotheses, aid in comparing various types of treatments, and bring about a closer liaison with the ninth revision of the *International Classification of Diseases* (ICD9) also to be published in 1979.[32]

DSMIII changes, although not finalized, were proposed in the draft version on March 30, 1977. There are approximately 20 categories, each with various subtypes; however, the terms neuroses, psychoses, neurasthenia, psychophysiological, and hypochondriasis are not mentioned. DSMII subgroups of neuroses are included under Dissociative, Affective, Anxiety, Factitious, and Somatoform Disorders. It proposes extensive descriptions of each entity including operational definitions with inclusive and exclusive criteria, a glossary, and a multiaxial classification system. The axes proposed are:

Axis I   Clinical Psychiatric Syndrome(s) and Other Conditions
Axis II   Personality Disorders (adults) and Specific Developmental Disorders (children and adolescents)
Axis III   Non-mental Medical Disorders
Axis IV   Severity of Psychosocial Stressors
Axis V   Highest Level of Adaptive Functioning Past Year[33]*

If these changes remain as proposed will they be more satisfactory than the DSMII?

*Provisional classification: Published as a looseleaf manual entitled *DSM-III Draft, 4/15/77.* Chapter 2, page 3 drawn up as of March 30, 1977.

NORMALITY AND HEALTH

Normality and health are not things but concepts; likewise, disease is not a thing but a concept. Engelhardt says:

> Health is a normative concept but not in the sense of a moral virtue. Though health is a good, and though it may be morally praiseworthy to try to be healthy and to advance the health of others, still, all things being equal, it is a misfortune, not a misdeed, to lack health. Health is more an aesthetic than an ethical term; it is more beauty than virtue. Thus, one does not condemn someone for no longer being healthy, though one may sympathize with him over the loss of a good. Further, it is not clear exactly what is lost when one loses health.[34]

Health, in this sense, becomes a value—something that is good, beautiful, and desirable. This leads to ambiguity since "good" is a relative term whether used esthetically, morally, or ethically. Health becomes a matter of judgment and carried to an extreme could lead to absurdity. In perspective, however, judgment as one factor in a consideration of health could be very helpful.

Although the DSMII does not define normal or health, physicians need some guidelines. The word normal is used in many ways. A person is said to be of normal height when his height approximates the statistical average. A dentist refers to normal teeth as teeth which are perfect; this definition implies only perfect and imperfect states. Normal can indicate an absence of abnormal findings—anatomical, biochemical, or physiological. Psychiatry uses the term normal in all these ways; however, psychiatry has additional criteria. Normality is judged as adaptation. Normality or abnormality comes to depend on adaptation to a specific environment.[35] Society thus becomes a major variable. Because of the vast differences between individuals as well as societies, defining normal, in which the role of value is added, leads to endless complexity. For example, are homosexuals, masturbators, alcoholics, drug addicts normal or abnormal? Value judgments cannot and should not be avoided.[36]

Consequently, we know little about normal psychology and even less about abnormal. Behavior that passes as normal in the near northside of Chicago may not be considered normal in Cicero. A wide range is allowed of what falls within normal limits, and care is taken not to label as pathological that which conflicts with one's own standards. Since normal shades into abnormal by gradual degrees, the diagnostic criteria cannot be exact. In brief, normal people can manifest unusual behavior. This in itself is not sufficient evidence of mental illness. Statistically abnormal or eccentric persons are not necessarily ill. In contrast unusual behavior may be considered a psychiatric illness if there is a failure of adaptation. A firm conclusion for diagnosis requires additional measures so that a psychiatrist can *reasonably* regard a condition as either normal or abnormal. But what criteria can be used? There are no easy solutions. True, psychiatry cannot afford to stand still until this fundamental problem is solved; yet it may be in the paradoxical position where it has no choice until these basic questions are answered.[37]

NEUROSES

Over the centuries many names for mental illness have developed: insanity (not sound); lunacy (influenced by the moon); possession (controlled by the devil); madness (wild conduct); mania (excitement); psychosis (a state of mind); neurosis (weakness of the nerves). Each term was defined in accord with the prevalent precepts of the day, and as time passed each took on new meanings. The social implications of these psychiatric terms invariably stigmatized those to whom they were applied. Today the words psychoses and neuroses are still used by the medical profession and insanity is used by the legal profession. Menninger feels that both neuroses and psychoses should be discarded from our vocabulary.[38] And in discussing psychoses Diethelm says, "An acceptable definition of psychoses is lacking in modern literature because one deals with a generalization which is not definable."[39] Oberndorf says, "Definitions of neurosis differ almost as widely as the clinical manifestations which we call neurotic."[40] Yet he, as many others, proceeds to use the term after giving his own definition. Chrzanowski says, "The use of the term 'neurosis' to denote mechanical malfunctioning as well as distorted life patterns representing restrictions in the overall growth of the whole individual is confusing."[41] These myriad conflicts in definition lead to the conclusion that some general agreement in terminology must be reached before real advancement can be made.

The diagnosis in the DSMII classification could indeed leave the false impression that these are syndromes or "illnesses" (a concurrence of signs and symptoms), "diseases" (concurrence of signs and symptoms with related pathologic causal factor or factors, course, and prognosis), or "sicknesses" (society's definition of abnormal behavior).[42] This is far from true. The diagnostic terms are used as rough estimates of the predominant patterns of behavior or symptomatology and differ from each other and from normal in the ways they relate to adaptation. Names such as illness, disease, or sickness reflect various schools of labeling and have created semantic difficulties. A resolution of this difficulty would be to refer to all of these conditions as disease and thereby avoid false dichotomies.

Anxiety in the DSMII is:

> . . .the chief characteristic of the neuroses. It may be felt and expressed directly, or it may be controlled unconsciously and automatically by conversion,

displacement and various other psychological mechanisms. Generally, these mechanisms produce symptoms experienced as subjective distress from which the patient desires relief.

The neuroses, as contrasted to the psychoses, manifest neither gross distortion or misinterpretation of external reality, nor gross personality disorganization. A possible exception to this is hysterical neurosis, which some believe may occasionally be accompanied by hallucinations and other symptoms encountered in psychoses.

Traditionally, neurotic patients, however, severely handicapped by their symptoms, are not classified as psychotic because they are aware that their mental functioning is disturbed.*

Although one may question the DSMII's emphasis on anxiety, there is no doubt that the diagnosis of neuroses is dependent on signs and symptoms and that each neurosis has an exclusive cluster which differentiates it from all others. In addition, the individual's adaptive capacity, and attitudes and behavior are important since neuroses can produce either self deprivation and personal difficulties or cause pain to others. The term neuroses has four connotations: it refers to combinations of symptoms and signs; it implies imbalances among constitutional, physical, psychological, or current life stresses; it reflects explanatory and evaluatory systems (dynamic psychopathology); and it may have implications for prognosis, course, and treatment. All four connotations must be considered with each case. Mere description without looking for meaning is slogan hunting and blind; conversely, dynamics without description is equally meaningless as it leads to broad and trite formulations that tend to become dogma or religion. Therefore, neuroses must be viewed as a comprehensive disease and not from a purely psychological perspective.

Our present classification system has obvious shortcomings but without it psychiatrists could not communicate with each another. Hence, it is not accepted at face value or as a dogma but for what it is—a method of communication. Even so there is the overwhelming belief by the general public, some psychiatrists, and other professionals in the mental health field that neuroses (and some even say psychoses) are psychological and sociological diseases.[43-45] They deny the genetic, biochemical, and physiological factors in mental illness but stress society and culture.[46,47] For this reason, among others, it is vital that psychiatrists clearly understand the various diagnostic models and how these models influence practice, research, and education. Using certain methods of study and thinking can lead to scientific advancement whereas other methods can lead to politicizing and dogmatic irrationalities.

*DSMII, p. 39.

DIAGNOSTIC MODELS

Completely satisfactory models for diagnosis are impossible so long as there is no one known etiology. This places the psychiatrist in the position of doing the next best thing: constructing models. Psychiatry uses the medical, disease, typological, dimensional, psychological, behavioral, and comprehensive models.

In the medical model psychiatric illness is conceptualized on the same basis as all other medical illnesses.[48] This model does not presuppose that the patient is ill but gives a systematic, thorough method of evaluating him. Kety writes:

> It should be pointed out that according to the medical model, a human illness does not become a specific disease all at once and is not equivalent to it. The medical model is an evolving intellectual process, consonant with the scientific method, which involves long periods of observation and description, increasingly sharper differentiation, and research rather than wishful thinking.
>
> The medical model of an illness is a process that moves from the recognition and palliation of symptoms to the characterization of a specific disease. . . .That progress depends upon the acquisition of knowledge and may often take many years or centuries. Numerous medical disorders and one or two mental illnesses have moved to the final stages of understanding, but many are still at various points along the way. After the recognition of symptoms, there comes the realization that some symptoms occur in fairly regular clusters, which are then described as syndromes. These may ultimately turn out to represent one or several etiological and pathogenetic components, the nature of which may be obscure at earlier stages of knowledge.[49]

The medical model predominates because it has proven its usefulness over a long period of time. No other model has been more effective. The medical model is a process that begins by recognition of symptoms, moves to a specific syndrome, then progresses to become a disease model with known etiology, course, and prognosis. With such data a rational specific treatment can be administered. The process is not static and begets a constant increase of knowledge. The major disadvantage of the medical and the disease models is that they imply one lesion, that can be demonstrated in structural, chemical, or functional abnormalities. Besides the medical/disease models do not allow for the proper evaluation of the causal relationships among the various levels of organization and limit etiological considerations to the biological level. Today not many psychiatrists regard diseases as a distinct entity with one cause. The disease model will be discussed in more detail in the next chapter.

The typological model describes discrete categories. In reality a type is a fictitious construct. It assesses a particular case and extrapolates it as an ideal, or collects many cases and presents them as a statistical mean. The value of a typology varies with the closeness in which a category approximates the reality of a particular case. Since the basis for a typology is derived from clinical manifestations, profile studies, and cluster or factor analysis, it is apparent that types, although often helpful in assessing an individual, do not convey the reality of that person as a total human being. Hence typological classification does not represent what really exists. In fact, it may miss the major problems of a suffering patient, may lack reliability and validity, and may emphasize certain manifestations while neglecting others which could be far more important. Yet this model is used for all standard psychiatric diagnosis, including the DSMII. The advances through this method were made in not becoming involved with unnecessary assumptions. However, a particular symptom can indicate a number of different mental illnesses (depersonalization exists as a discrete neurotic illness, or as part of an agoraphobic neurosis, schizophrenia, or organic brain disease) and the repeated appearance of clusters is justification for establishing an empirical category or syndrome. The major disadvantages of this method are: it can place too much emphasis on clusters, syndromes or types, and not enough on the underlying meaning of the phenomena; and the borderlines between typologies may not be clearly drawn. Hence, if this method is rigidly applied, psychiatry can in the name of "science" become dehumanized and if many patients fall between the types, the reliability may be very low.[50]

The dimensional model involves measurement and is a quantitative system of evaluating an individual along an axis or axes. A dimension can be a trait, symptom, concept, sign, or some other parameter. The problem is to determine the extent to which any of these are present in a particular individual. Theoretically, the dimension may have a 0% representation or a 100% representation in a particular individual. The implication is that all individuals are similar qualitatively by possessing the dimension but differ quantitatively. For example, dimensions measure the amount or degree of thought disorder, depression, social competence, psychological disorganization, psychoses, psychoticism, neuroticism, introversion or extroversion, etc. In effect, mental illness becomes an exaggeration of normal. Those psychiatrists who subscribe to the dimensional concept consider the qualitative differences as defined in typologies to be inappropriate, inadequate, and artificial. In the dimensional model, only the point along the continuum as determined by psychological testing measures is essential. This method works with highly sophisticated mathematical formulas. The advantage of the dimensional model is that all information is used which allows for a flexibility not possible with types. In typologies, overlapping and transitional data are frequently lost. For example, an I.Q. with its specific number reveals more than the categories of idiot, moron, normal, or superior intelligence. Another advantage of dimensions is the extensive consideration and evaluation given to borderline and atypical cases. This would be expected since it avoids categories or clusters and thereby has special value in situations where several variables are investigated for quantitative relationships. Thus, if variable A is reduced or increased, what effect does it have on variable B? This may indicate how much a dimension is contributing to the clinical manifestations. The disadvantage is that before the dimensional system can be utilized practically, it must be translated into typologies. To illustrate, at what point along the axis A-B, in studying the degree of depression in a patient, does the psychiatrist use drugs or electro-convulsive treatment? In fact, once such a point is determined, it automatically becomes a category. Another disadvantage occurs in situations where only dimension is used, for much information gets lost regarding the other aspects of the person. Perhaps the most important criticism is that the dimensions, like typologies, whether one or many, can look only at a limited number of parameters and miss the essence of the individual. Accordingly, dimensional models have many of the problems of typologies and, except as a research tool seem to offer few practical advantages. Also, the theoretical basis of the dimensional model as a spectrum or continuum of normal to abnormal is questionable. Finally, if a dimension is merely a method of quantifying faculties, history should have taught us how wrong the faculty psychologists have been in the past, i.e., substitution of fancy mathematical techniques for phrenological ones in no way corrects the basic fallacy inherent in studying mind as a collection of faculties.[51-53]

The psychological model subscribes to the notion that psychiatric illness results from a faulty psychic apparatus, and that classification should not be based on symptoms but should be replaced by data of an entirely different kind. The data can be scores on psychological tests, underlying intrapsychic psycho-dynamic mechanisms, interpersonal relationship patterns or styles of behavior, and social role functioning and attitudes. These are all considered part of the psychological model since all act through the mental apparatus—intrapsychic or social. Within each of these frameworks many splinter movements exist. Some of the popular movements in the interpersonal schools consist of the followers of Alfred Adler, Karen Horney, Harry Stack Sullivan, Erich Fromm, Eric Berne, etc. None of the proposed classification models of these groups has received wide-spread usage. All possess low reliability because they are based on inferential judgments (explanation and evaluation) and the prognostic usefulness is probably lower than any of the other models discussed above.[54]

The behavioral model developed from the work of Pavlov. Essentially it replaces concepts such as consciousness, sensation, and emotion with those of conditioning and reflexology. It deals with stimulus, response, learning, habit, and receptor and effector functions. Personality and abnormal behavior become a system of responses, viz., the sum total of an individual's reactions and tendencies to reactions. Classification systems are built on this premise and for the most part are traits or single symptom descriptions. The model has, for example, the affectionate, assertive, and oppositional categories of behavioral and other psychological categories, but its main concern is with learning and unlearning behavior.[55]

The comprehensive model for psychiatric diagnosis attempts to combine in one system attributes of all the above models while attempting to eliminate some of the disadvantages. It selects variables for diagnosis that are best suited for explanation and prediction. It includes variables for diagnosis that go chronologically backward and forward from a starting point in the here and now. Therefore, essential data are sought in the biography which relate to cause, symptomatology, course, and outcome of the disease. The here and now data relate to the current life situation and stresses, and the forward data relate to prognosis and therapy. Diagnostic labels should provide a readily available method of determining these parameters with a maximum degree of reliability and validity. The major disadvantages of this model are that it takes a great deal of time to elicit the necessary information, it encompasses value judgments, and reliance must be placed on typology for reliability and validity.[56] The comprehensive approach begins with observation and description to establish a nosological diagnosis, progresses to the collection of essential data which leads to evaluation and explanations, and then presents this material in an organized fashion. A word of caution at this point: the data can be interpreted by the various schools of thought in various jargons and this can be misleading and confusing; therefore, it is suggested that psychopathology be described in terms which are dynamic but not formal. For the most part, the comprehensive approach attempts to avoid psychiatric theories or hypotheses of behavior. The distinction between the two is important and recognizing this can prevent presenting a theory or hypothesis as if it were an established scientific law.[57]

Further consideration of the variables is necessary. First, the nosological diagnoses should be multiaxial wherever possible. The three major areas could be personality, symptomatology, and organic. Second, the current life situation and ordinary stresses should be considered: sleep, work, diet, interpersonal relationships, finances, etc. Difficulties in any of these areas can have relevance for etiology, course, prognosis, and treatment, as can unusual stresses—accidents, wars, serious physical illness, and the loss of loved ones. Third, from this interplay of forces the dynamics can be approximated. Fourth, a biography can trace the past course of the disease and help us to have better understanding of the patient. Genetic, dynamic, and biographic data all relating to the current life situation (work, social relationships, etc.) not only help in explaining but also in predicting the outcome of the disease. From a biography one can also get clues as to treatment: what worked and what did not work in the past, not only for the patient but for his family as well can be valuable information. The clinical psychiatrist needs all the information he can get to arrive at rational decisions. The researcher may attempt to quantitate these relationships.[58]

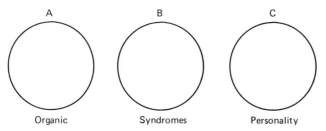

Fig. 2-1. Each circle represents a pure diagnostic parameter, a situation which is never seen in life, hence overlapping is used to represent a situation closer to reality.

The Venn diagrams (Figs. 2-1 and 2-2) can help to organize and summarize our thinking. Organic conditions are represented by circle A, symptomatic syndromes by B, personality disorders by C, and current life situation and stressors by the large broken-line circle. The area within the large, broken-line circle represents the more immediate relationships such as family, relatives, social and working contacts. The area surrounding the broken-line circle includes the relationships within a society which effect the individual's life such as mores, folkways, ethics, taxes, economic conditions, political systems, climatic conditions, etc. Thus a comprehensive diagnosis would include all of the above plus the proximate and distant forces that influence the individual. For example, a typical diagnosis would be an acute anxiety neurosis in an obsessive personality who recently lost his job, or an acute organic brain disease with a conversion hysterical neurosis and a hypomanic personality.[59]

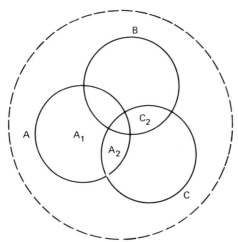

Fig. 2-2. The area A_1 would represent an organic condition in almost pure form; A_2 an organic condition with personality problems; C_2 a mixed picture with personality problems being primary and syndromes secondary. Other combinations can easily be detected.

REFERENCES

1. Satorius, N., Classification: An international perspective. *Psychiatric Ann.* 6(8):361–367 (1976).
2. Grinker, Sr., R.R., unpublished manuscript.
3. *American Psychiatric Association: Diagnostic and Statistical Manual of Mental Disease,* 2nd ed., American Psychiatric Association, Washington, D.C., 1968.
4. Szasz, T., *The Classification of "Mental Illness": A Situational Analysis of Psychiatric Operations.* Utica, N.Y.: State Hospital Press. [Reprinted from *Psychiatric Quart.* 1:2-3 (1959).]
5. Tart, C.T., *States of Consciousness.* New York: Dutton, 1975, p. 175.
6. Sokal, R.R., Classification: purposes, principles, progress, prospects. *Science* 185(4157): 1115-1123 (1974).
7. Szasz, T., op. cit., pp. 4-25.
8. Grinker, Sr., R.R., op. cit.
9. Wing, J.K., The uses of classification in psychiatry. *Psychiatric Ann.* 6(8):355 (1976).
10. Shindell, S., Statistics, science, and sense: part 5: hypotheses and conclusion. *J. Amer. Med. Assoc.* 186:849 (1963).
11. Mack, J.E. (Ed.), *Borderline States in Psychiatry.* New York: Grune and Stratton, 1975.
12. Spitzer, R. and Endicott, J., Diagno II: Further developments in a computer program for psychiatric diagnosis. *Amer. J. Psychiatry* 125 (7):12-21 (1969) Suppl.
13. Fowler, R.D., Automated psychological test interpretation: The status in 1972. *Psychiatric Ann.* 2(12):10-28 (1972).
14. Stroebel, C.F. and Glueck, B.C., The diagnostic process in psychiatry: Computer approaches. *Psychiatric Ann.* 2(12):58-77 (1972).
15. Kety, S., From rationalization to reason. *Amer. J. Psychiatry* 131:957–963 (1974).
16. Rensch, B., "The laws of evolution," in *The Evolution of Life: Its Origin, History and Future,* vol. 1 (edited by Tax, S.). Chicago: Univ. Chicago Press, 1960, pp. 97-101.
17. Stengel, E., Classification of mental disorders. *Bull. WHO* 21:601-605 (1959).
18. Zigler, E. and Phillips, L., Psychiatric diagnosis: A critique. *J. Abnorm. Soc. Psychol.* 63:607-618 (1961).
19. Beck, A.T., Reliability of psychiatric diagnosis: A critique of systematic studies. *Amer. J. Psychiatry* 119:210-216 (1962).
20. King, L., The meaning of medical diagnosis. *ETC: A Review of General Semantics* 8(3):202-211 (1951).
21. Tarter, R., Templer, D., and Hardy, C., Reliability of the psychiatric diagnosis. *Dis. Nerv. Syst.* 36:29-31 (1975).
22. Menninger, K., Mayman, M., and Pruyser, P.L., *The Vital Balance.* New York: Viking, 1963.
23. Kant, I., *The Classification of Mental Disorders.* Doylestown, Pa.: Doylestown Fund, 1964.
24. Kraepelin, E., *Text-book of Psychiatry,* 8th ed. (edited by Robertson, G. and transl. by Barclay, R.M.). Edinburgh: E. & S. Livingstone, 1921.
25. Menninger, W. *et al.,* Technical Medical Bulletin, Washington, D.C., U.S. Gov. Printing Office, No. 23, October 19, 1945.
26. *American Psychiatric Association: Diagnostic and Statistical Manual of Mental Disorders,* 1st ed., American Psychiatric Association, Washington, D.C., 1952.

27. Noyes, A.P., *Modern Clinical Psychiatry,* 2nd ed., rewritten and enlarged. Philadelphia: Saunders, 1939, p. 331.
28. Ibid., p. 340.
29. Strecker, E.A., Ebaugh, F.G., Ewalt, J.R., *Practical Clinical Psychiatry,* 7th ed. New York: Blakiston, 1951, p. 375.
30. *American Psychiatric Association,* 1st ed., op. cit., p. 9.
31. *American Psychiatric Association,* 2nd ed., op. cit., p. 9.
32. Spitzer, R., Endicott, J., and Robins, E., Clinical criteria for psychiatric diagnosis and DSMIII. *Amer. J. Psychiatry* **132**:1187-1192 (1975).
33. Spitzer, R. and Sheehy, M., DSMIII: A classification system in development. *Psychiatric Ann.* **6**(90):102-109 (1976).
34. Engelhardt, Jr., H.T., "The concepts of health and disease," in *Evaluation and Explanation in the Biomedical Sciences* (edited by Engelhardt, Jr., H.T. and Spicker, S.F.). Dordrecht, Holland and Boston: Reidel, 1975, p. 125.
35. Murphy, J.M., Psychiatric labeling in cross-cultural perspective. *Science* **191**:1019-1028 (1976).
36. Engelhardt, Jr., H.T., The disease of masturbation: Values and the concept of disease. *Bull. Hist. Med.* **48**:234-248 (Summer 1974).
37. Engelhardt, Jr., H.T., Explanatory models in medicine: Facts, theories, and values. *Tex. Rep. Biol. Med.* **32**(1):225-239 (Spring 1974).
38. Menninger, K., Mayman, M., and Pruyser, P., op. cit., p. 9.
39. Diethelm, O., "The fallacy of the concept psychosis," in *Current Problems in Psychiatric Diagnosis* (edited by Hoch, P.H. and Zubin, J.). New York: Grune & Stratton, 1953, p. 25.
40. Oberndorf, C.P., "Diagnostic and etiological concepts in the neuroses," in *Current Problems in Psychiatric Diagnosis* (edited by Hoch, P.H., and Zubin, J.). New York: Grune & Stratton, 1953, pp. 81-83.
41. Chrzanowski, G., "Neurasthenia and hypochondriasis," in *American Handbook of Psychiatry,* vol. 1 (edited by Arieti, S.). New York: Basic Books, 1959, p. 263.
42. Satorius, N., op. cit., p. 360.
43. Sloman, L., The role of neurosis in phylogenetic adaptation, with particular reference to early man. *Amer. J. Psychiatry* **133**(5):543-547 (1976).
44. Rosenhan, D.L., On being sane in insane places. *Science* **179**:250-258 (1973).
45. Szasz, T.S., "Repudiation of the medical model," in *Psychopathology Today* (edited by Sahakian, W.S.). Itasca, Ill.: Placock, 1970, pp. 47-53.
46. Dunham, H.W., Society, culture, and mental disorder. *Arch. Gen. Psychiatry* **33**: 147-156 (1976).
47. Kety, S., op. cit., pp. 960-962.
48. Gray, M., Principles of the comprehensive examination. *Arch. Gen. Psychiatry* **10**:370-381 (1964).
49. Kety, S., op. cit., p. 959.
50. Kendell, R.E., *The Role of Diagnosis in Psychiatry.* Oxford: Blackwell, 1975, pp. 130-131.
51. Strauss, J., Diagnostic models on the nature of psychiatric disorders. *Arch. Gen. Psychiatry* **29**:445-449 (1973).
52. Hine, F.R., Dimensional diagnosis and the medical student's grasp of psychiatry. *Arch. Gen. Psychiatry* **32**:525-528 (1975).
53. Kendell, R.E., op. cit., pp. 119-136.
54. Horwitz, L., *Clinical Prediction in Psychotherapy.* New York: Jason Aronson, 1974.

55. Wolpe, J., *The Practice of Behavior Therapy,* 2nd ed.   New York: Pergamon, 1973, p. 89.
56. Strauss, J., A comprehensive approach to psychiatric diagnosis. *Amer. J. Psychiatry* **132**:1193–1197 (1975).
57. Gray, M., op. cit., pp. 378–380.
58. Elstein, A.S., Clinical judgment: Psychological research and medical practice. *Science* **194**(4266):696–700 (1976).
59. Feinstein, A., *Clinical Judgment.*   Baltimore.   Williams & Wilkins, 1967, pp. 164–172.

3
ETIOLOGY

Medical history is constantly evolving. Theories of disease, classification systems, methods of collecting data, and treatments are always changing. Terms need constant clarification because they too change in meaning. What are the basic assumptions of current day medical and psychiatric practice regarding the causation of disease? The terms causation and disease might appear at first glance to be simple, everyday words—clear and unambiguous. Yet in actuality, these terms are among the most confusing, nebulous, and difficult to define in medicine. What meaning and relevance do they have for the study of psychiatry and neuroses?

The meaning of "cause" has always been debated among philosophers and to this day differences in meaning exist. Bertrand Russell writes:

> The atomists, unlike Socrates, Plato, and Aristotle, sought to explain the world without introducing the notion of *purpose or final cause.* The "final cause" of an occurrence is an event in the future for the sake of which the occurrence takes place. . . .Why does the baker make bread? Because people will be hungry. Why are railways built? Because people will wish to travel. In such cases, things are explained by the purpose they serve. When we ask "why?" concerning an event, we may mean either of two things. We may mean: "What purpose did this event serve?" or we may mean: "What earlier circumstances caused this event?" The answer to the former question is a teleological explanation, or an explanation by final causes; the answer to the latter question is a mechanistic explanation. . . .experience has shown that the mechanistic question leads to scientific knowledge, while the teleological question does not. . . .[1]

And Russell warns about carrying mechanistic explanations too far.

> One event is caused by another, the other by a third, and so on. But if we ask for a cause of the whole, we are driven again to the Creator, who must

Himself be uncaused. All causal explanations, therefore, must have an arbitrary beginning.[2]

Scientific explanation, therefore, involves the complexities of cause and effect. One definition of cause is to explain a specific event or process in terms of some necessary antecedent or concomitant event or condition.[3] Events or processes can depend for their functioning on past causes: some in the recent past (adequate nutrition), others in the distant past (genetic material), and still others in the remote past (scientific "final causes" pertain to the essential conditions on earth for the appearance of life).

Biological processes involve antecedents and events that are related to one another and form patterns or Gestalts. Dwight Ingle, a biologist, writes:

> The concept of Gestalt includes the organismic concept—recognizing the exquisite complexity of living things. The living organism is a dynamic system which incorporates many directive causes within its boundaries. Analytical methods are necessary to discover individual factors causing natural events but are likely to alter the process under study. Man tends to conceptualize particulars as independent systems and processes so that some concepts are likely to represent artifacts of analysis. When two or more entities are integrated into a new whole, not all the properties of the new system can be predicted from knowledge of the parts; the whole is more than the sum of its parts. Science needs both the analytical and organismic approach applied at all levels of organization to gain knowledge of events and systems.[4]

The scientific method can be applied in part to anatomy, biochemistry, physiology, pathology, psychopharmacology, reflexology, etc. This method, however, cannot explain human behavior. For behavior, no known method is refined enough to meet the requirements for proof of causal connections.[5] Psychiatry, therefore, must resort to other methods that are flexible enough to deal with subtleties and at the same time have relevant explanations of data for rational patient treatment.   Perhaps the medical historian's approach, combined with appropriate scientific method, can offer a viable basis for exploring the causes of mental illness.

The medical historian tries to discover how past thinkers explained disease and whether they were proven right or wrong by time. Historians analyze the internal and external factors that led past writers to formulate particular explanatory theories. This is similar to the psychiatric approach. But the psychiatrist applies his method to one patient, family, or group. One significant difference is that historians do not deal with the intrinsic truth or errors of the cause or causes of disease but are concerned with exposing the ideas of past thinkers on disease. Psychiatrists, on the other hand, must constantly probe for errors and fallacies in their own thinking as it applies to causality in patients. The psychiatrist must stick close to the patient's material and then offer an explanation. The advantage to the psychiatrist of using both the historical and scientific methods is that it allows room for flexibility. Scientific method can be used wherever applicable and helps avoid pitfalls, e.g., of explaining neuroses as the result of either biological or environmental factors alone. With scientific method research can be conducted and reasonable conclusions drawn while the historical method imposes a caution, an uncertainty in the psychiatrist's mind that lessens his tendency for dogmatic assertions. Further, judgment interpretations are inherent in the historian's method. All explanations are not equal; some are good, some bad, others awful, and still others can be downright foolish. Once these considerations are planted in the psychiatrist's mind, he will explain disease in a manner which is closer to the realities of his patient's existence.[6]

In medicine the term cause is sometimes included in the definition of a disease. With typhoid fever for example, a definition would include the clinical manifestations plus the cause, *S. typhosa*. This definition implies that one essential feature must be present for the diagnosis of the disease, *S. typhosa*. There are, however, other diseases that are not infectious for which one cause cannot be determined, i.e., metabolic, degenerative, etc. Hence, in diseases where there is more than one cause, in other words, multiple causes (factors), the term etiology is applied. This means that when one specific "cause" is known a positive disease is identified and separated, and when multiple causes are determined no such positive identification is postulated. That distinction is fallacious.[7]

Lester King, medical historian, clearly illuminates the concept:

In regard to diseases, for example, we often find to our dismay that we cannot separate one from another as sharply as we might like. First, we must determine what factors are relevant to a given disease. Then we must evaluate them, to decide the significance of each, especially under changing circumstances. In the search for precision we lump together a great many relevant factors into a scrap-bag called "etiology." Some of these factors are more significant than others. Whenever we light on one that seems particularly sharp and particularly important, we tend to call this specific factor *the* cause. In so doing we can provide a sharp criterion or definition. Then we can make a diagnosis with complete assurance—the assurance that can come only from definition. But if we study causation in its broader aspects, we realize that so-called monocausation is a myth, that all diseases are a complex interaction of various factors, and that diseases do not occur without the coordination of many discrete events.[8]

DISEASE CONCEPTS

Even in medicine today some consider that disease exists in morphological, chemical, physiological, and other impersonal terms, and illness is designated in terms of the interaction of disease and host (person), and environment.[9] Psychiatrists do not make such distinctions between man and his environment or between illness, sickness, and disease. The problem is one of definition and concept. Like normal and abnormal, definitions of health and disease change with time and circumstances.[10]

It would be nice to define disease in a clear, nontautological, unambiguous manner. To say that disease is sickness, absence of health, or disturbed function is not good enough; other considerations are necessary to help clarify the situation. Let us review them:

(1) Traditionally the word "dis-ease" suggests a lack of "ease" and represents pain, discomfort, distress, or functional deficiency. These manifestations, usually called symptoms and signs, are expressed as complaints of the patient, the physician, or other individuals.

A complaint can be within or beyond a patient's awareness. Patients verbalize their complaints to varying degrees, depending upon personality structure and pain threshold level. Some patients with an open, draining, raw, infected wound would not complain at all and others with a similar wound would be screaming. Those who do not complain may not experience any symptoms or may stoically ignore the pain. Some individuals do not consider loose watery stools or severe chest pain as a complaint even though well aware of what is taking place. Then there are the complaints (problems) of which the individual may be unaware. Innumerable processes are constantly occurring in the body that do not reach consciousness and, if pathologic, may have serious consequences. Examples are silent nonpainful coronary infarcts; personality changes with certain brain tumors; and distorted thinking or misinterpretation of reality with schizophrenia and manic episodes. Therefore, the patient's complaints cannot be the only criteria for a definition of disease.

The physician may say that a patient has an illness. He bases his opinion on signs and laboratory tests. This assumes that the doctor knows all about disease or at least a great deal about what constitutes disease and health. If a physician cannot find a disease it does not mean a disease is absent; nor does it mean that his diagnosis is correct if he diagnoses a disease. At what range or point is a patient normotensive or hypertensive? At what range or point is an alcoholic an alcoholic? Is homosexuality a disease or is it normal? Is deviant behavior illness? The fact that the doctor treats such conditions does not in itself warrant the name disease. Accordingly, the physician cannot be the sole determiner of what constitutes disease.

Persons complain about each other. They may be relatives, friends, or society. This can mean that the person's behavior is disapproved of by someone else and he is "called" sick. It is known that mores change as do fashions. Does this mean that the woman who wore pants in 1890 was ill and in 1976 is healthy? Another consideration is that health in one society or culture may be sickness in another. Therefore, to use the complaints of the patient, physician, or the general public as criteria for disease is unacceptable.[11]

(2) Disease involves structural abnormality in the cell, organ, biochemical alterations, chromosomal and genetic peculiarities, physiological abnormalities or other demonstrable bodily functions. This level of description, at first glance, seems objective. It does not rely on the complaint of the patient, physician, or society, and provides observable criteria. It assumes that structural and functional standards exist, however, and deviations constitute disease. This is not true. Structures vary in size, shape, composition, and functional efficiency. There is no clear division of what constitutes abnormal structure or function.[12] Again, where does normal end and abnormal begin? What about complaints, symptoms, and conditions with no demonstrable structural or functional abnormality? Are they to be written off as "no disease"? Are most major categories treated by psychiatrists not disease but myths?[13,14] The absence of a demonstrable lesion either ignores the person as having no "disease" or separates him from others with real "disease." This type of separation is unacceptable.

(3) Disease is a reaction of the organism to the environment and is the result of each individual's inability to adapt. This definition emphasizes the differences or uniqueness of individuals rather than similarities. In so doing it offers no criterion to distinguish health from disease and makes reasonable classification impossible. Furthermore, no provision is made for distinguishing temporary disturbances such as tachycardia or metabolic acidosis secondary to exercise from a paroxysmal tachycardia or metabolic acidosis secondary to diabetes. It also assumes that there is a valid statistical normal either in the structure, function, or in the environment of that organism. Statistical deviations can be harmful or advantageous to the individual. Statistics are no more helpful in defining disease than in defining normal.[15]

The adaptation definition raises the question of perfect versus imperfect. If disease is imperfect adaptation then health is perfect adaptation. Dimensions are implied. What is the degree of sickness or health? If the extent of sickness is known, the extent of health should then be known. Psychoanalysis is a major conceptual framework, however, which subscribes to the theory that deviations from perfect are regarded as forms of illness. In the words of Kendall:

> According to this theory, the unavoidable vicissitudes of early life activate morbid psychological mechanisms which impair personality development and functioning in everyone to a greater or lesser extent. Although these

handicaps are regarded as potentially reversible if appropriate treatment is provided, this implicitly reduces health to an idealized state of complete normality, an almost hypothetical state to which man can only aspire, and some degree of sickness becomes his universal lot. There is, to be sure, nothing inherently absurd or illogical in this, but it does carry profound implications for society's attitudes towards the sick, for individuals' attitudes to themselves, and not least for the staffing and financing of medical services. On all these counts, a more restricted concept of sickness seems preferable.[16]

The adaptation definition distinguishes disease from health on the basis of whether or not the characteristics under consideration place the individual at a biological disadvantage. For an individual to be ill, statistical deviation from the norm, whether too little or too much, must place him at a biological disadvantage. In effect this says that characteristics that are usually considered advantages or disadvantages are only so depending upon whether or not they totally contribute to the person's ability to adapt biologically. This eliminates dependence upon the primacy of one characteristic or group of characteristics and emphasizes the relationship of the total organism's adaptive capacity. As long as it is not to one's biological disadvantage, it is not sickness.[17-19]

Certain questions arise. Does biological disadvantage apply to the individual or to the group? Who is to make this value judgment—individual, researcher, or group? What about situations where in one environment a trait is an advantage and in another a disadvantage? Even though the adaptation definition has many defects, it does help clarify ideas about health and disease and brings a relationship between medicine and psychiatry closer.

Yet for sickness to exist, it is essential that certain phenomena, either alone or in groups, be present. Medical workers in fields such as cancer or coronary artery disease are well aware that these diseases are the result of complex pattern-relations or interactions occurring at various levels: work, diet, genetic, social, psychological, etc. These workers are involved with risk factors and the relationship among the factors and not with cause or causes. Thus in general medicine, as in psychiatry, the considerations are the same.[20,21]

Disease models are ambiguities that go back to Plato's idea of disease entities as things, logical entities, or both. The Platonists searched for a true classification of disease while the Aristotelians and the Hippocratic school concentrated on observation. "Subsequently, various names have been given to these two schools—rationalists/empirical, nominalist/realist, ontological/biographic—but the controversy remains the same."[22] Are diseases things or functions? Are diseases contextual or substantial? Are diseases entities or deviations from normal? Or are diseases viewed both ways? That is, from the viewpoint of a medical (typological) and a dimensional (psychological) model.[23] H. Tristram Engelhardt, Jr. attempts to answer these questions:

The concept of disease is an attempt to correlate constellations of signs and symptoms for the purposes of explanation, prediction, and control. . . Diseases involve patterns of causes correlated with clusters of signs and symptoms which constitute the illnesses at hand. Disease models, as nomological patterns, are interpretable in larger patterns in a way not readily apparent if those models modeled disease things or independent disease types. Thus, one can concomitantly have a medical and a psychological account of the etiology of coronary artery disease, which are not incompatible, but mutually completing. . . .The variables are chosen for the purpose of speaking about and altering that illness. They are relationships structured for particular diagnostic, prognostic, and therapeutic goals. . . .The issue of the medical versus the psychological model of disease is thus a rehearsal of the mind-body problem. . . .The identification of objectivity with physical descriptions suggests that if diseases are things, then they have nothing to do with the subjective world of values and social relations often imported into concepts of mental illness. Under such a view, mental illnesses could be diseases only if they described the malfunctioning of a mental thing (e.g., a *res cogitans*).[24]

In sum, disease is a concept and it can be characterized by clinical manifestations, with or without supporting laboratory data, and the result of many interrelated causes. Disease can neither be viewed as a thing nor as a point along a spectrum (e.g., good or evil, better or worse, perfect or imperfect, etc.) but as a combination of both. Ideally a disease concept should aid the physician to predict course and outcome of the disease, to prevent its occurrence, and to treat the patient. Last, inherent in any disease concept is a value system, i.e., comparing what exists (disease?) to what should exist (health).

PSYCHIATRIC DISEASE CONCEPTS

The foregoing concepts of disease are as applicable to psychiatry as they are to general medicine. In psychiatry, however, they are applied as follows.

(1) The Aristotelian concept is called the *unitary theory of disease*. It proposes a variety of mental illnesses with fluid boundaries or transitions that merge into each other. The forms of illness have a natural history and follow a course with a sequence that begins with depression or anxiety and progresses to panic → delusion → dementia. All mental diseases would fit somewhere along this spectrum. The dimensional and psychological diagnostic models are represented here.

Although all concepts of health and disease have value judgments, the unitary concept is particularly susceptible to this type of analysis. For instance health is what ought to be, slight anxiety is a deviation, severe anxiety is a further deviation, hence less desirable, and panic is the least desirable form of anxiety.

If the anxiety becomes chronic, an anxiety neurosis may develop; or if it progresses it may lead to delusions (psychoses) and ultimately dementia. With all illnesses, therefore, value judgments are involved. In psychiatry, neuroses, psychoses, personality disorders, sexual perversions, alchoholism, drug dependence, and so forth involve value systems (what ought to be) of both the individual and society. If by consensus any of these conditions exist within a patient it is defined as a disease. In somatic illnesses as well, value systems are involved. For example, diseases caused by an environmental pollutant are blamed on society at which point laws are enacted that attempt to keep the air clean and the water pure. Similarly coronary artery disease is attributed to many factors including warnings on cigarette packages regarding the smoking hazard, preferring low fat and cholesterol diets, recommending proper exercise, and the like. Thus health and disease are determined by the relationship and value system of organism and environment.[25]

The value system implied in the unitary theory involves a health edict and it becomes the responsibility of the physician and society to maintain the patient in a state of health. Thus there are government mandates in such areas as community mental health centers, commitment to mental institutions, right to treatment, immunization policies, chlorination and fluoridation of water supplies, etc. The physician, it follows, "is confronted with an imperative to change the patient, alter him, and bring him into accord with norms of health that society has accepted."[26] Likewise the patient under such circumstances can be forced to accept treatment against his will or desires. This highly complex situation involves intermingling of law, medicine, psychiatry, politics, and morals.

(2) The Platonic concept is called the *natural disease-entity theory*. Each entity differs from the other and has its own characteristic symptoms, etiology, course, and prognosis. There are no transitions. The disease-entity theory accepts as entities or diseases: delusions, hallucinations, obsessions, abnormal behavior, kleptomania, and the like. Each symptom can be the basis for a diagnostic label. It can also have groups of symptoms (syndromes) or use biographical data as a criterion for a diagnostic category (e.g., manic-depressive disease). The term "entity" leaves the impression that a disease is a thing, not a concept. The medical, disease, behavioral, and typological diagnostic models can fit this category.

The disease entity theory considers disease as an episodic invasion, resulting in a type of health care program which differs from the health care program of the unitary theory model. To quote Engelhardt:

> . . . .Under such a model, medicine reacts to particular causes, identified as the specific bearers of the signs and symptoms of diseases; disease appears as a discontinuity in health; and medicine as the means for plugging the gaps. Such gap-medicine focuses on health restoration rather than health maintenance.[27]

(3) The pattern relation analysis or relation identification model is called the *comprehensive or multiaxial theory of disease*. This combines in one system attributes of both unitary and entity theories of disease. It analyzes the relationship between variables and selects those variables that are best suited to explain the patterns of the signs and symptoms. The comprehensive theory accepts a broad framework in which heredity and environment are aspects of nature which are as inseparable as body and mind. Heredity represents the influence of past experience on the organism. Environment represents the external stimuli on a growing and evolving receptive or nonreceptive organism and either results or fails to result in stimulating inherent potentialities. This implies a dynamic organism in a continually changing environment.[28-30]

The basic position of this theory is that by differentiating the variables knowledge can be more readily attained. Furthermore, the clinical manifestations are the result of not one but many connected or interrelated causes. Hence, the individual patient is studied from four different aspects. Each aspect or factor is analyzed with regard to its role in producing a disease. The following factors are delineated. First, constitutional factors which refer to the totality of a person at any given time or moment are viewed as a dynamic process rather than as something static.[31] The two components subsumed under constitution are personality and heredity. Second, physical factors consist of somatic size, type, and physical illness. Third, psychological factors include social, political, economic, and cultural aspects. Fourth, current life situation and stress involve the here and now circumstances under which the patient is living. All factors must be weighed and balanced in any consideration of disease. The totality of these four factors either gives rise to or fails to give rise to the clinical picture of a disease. To explain, if there is a strong constitutional factor, it takes more of the other factors to result in a disease; conversely, a weak constitutional factor takes less of the other factors to result in a disease. This analogy of quantity also holds true for the physical, psychological, and stress factors. Strong stress on a strong constitution can lead to disease; excessive psychological factors on a strong constitution may not lead to disease and so forth. It is the combination of variables that is important. In each case all the factors have to be weighed. A disease, then, becomes equivalent to the final common pathway as understood from neurophysiology.[32] It can be summarized:

$$A + B + C + D = disease$$

A = heredity and personality (constitutional)
B = somatic and pathological (physical)
C = all-inclusive term (psychological)
D = effect of stresses and current life situation (interrelationships)

The disease-entity and the unitary theories are descriptive and provide useful information. They include the individual case method which is based on observation and description and can help with pertinent connections or insights; however, a disease does not always follow the course as outlined in the unitary theory, and dividing diseases into clusters or entities as in the disease-entity theory is an artificial separation which can be misleading. The same clinical manifestations may arise from different etiologies. The comprehensive theory is the most inclusive since it includes aspects of the other theories, avoids dogmatic positions, recognizes its limitations, and is open to change. For these reasons the comprehensive theory is preferred to all others. The major disadvantages are the long time needed and the hard work involved to make a comprehensive evaluation.

CONSTITUTIONAL FACTORS

The role of heredity in producing mental disorders should not be minimized. Intellectual deficiencies are present from birth in Down's syndrome and phenylketonuria and develop later in life in Huntington's chorea. Schizophrenia and manic-depressive disease (bipolar) seem to have a genetic factor. Behavior is dependent to a certain extent on the structure of an inherited nervous system. Hence intellectual subnormality, mental illness, and behavioral abnormalities lead us to suspect that genetics is important for our study of neuroses.[33]

Each ovum contains 46 chromosomes. There are 22 identical pairs of chromosomes and one pair that is not identical. The similar chromosomes are called autosomes, the remaining pair is the sex chromosomes. Males possess an XY pair in which the X chromosome is longer than the Y. Females possess two X chromosomes. An ordinary microscope can easily detect the difference between the X and Y chromosome. One member of each pair comes from the mother and the other member from the father. Chromosomes are composed of desoxyribonucleic acid (DNA) molecules. Segments of the DNA molecules comprise the genes, the determinants of hereditary traits. It is estimated that each chromosome contains 20,000 to 40,000 different gene pairs. The genes are located in specific positions on specific chromosomes and are subject to variation. Consequently, when the fertilized ovum or zygote combines these two random sets of chromosomes, it seems highly unlikely that any two persons could ever have exactly the same heredity.[34]

Identical twins develop from the first cell division of the fertilized egg. After the cell division, separate organisms begin to grow. The separation can occur more than once and result in identical triplets, quadruplets, and the rest. This is the only way that two or more persons can be genetically identical. Fraternal twins develop from two fertilized ova. Since two sperms and ova are involved, these twins are no more genetically similar than ordinary siblings. Fraternal twins, like ordinary siblings, may be of the same or opposite sex. Because of their genetic equivalence identical twins are more valuable for psychiatric studies than either fraternal twins or siblings.

Genes are responsible for traits or certain characteristics. Possessing a gene, however, does not mean that the trait will develop. Expressivity is the extent to which a gene shows its effect clinically and this can vary from mild to severe. Expressivity is subject to the influence of other genes as well as the environment. Thus it is possible for the possessor of an abnormal gene or genes to be clinically (phenotype) normal or abnormal. This depends on how completely the gene (genotype) is expressed.[35]

There appear to be two main modes of genetic transmission: single-factor inheritance, where the presence of one gene determines, more or less completely, the trait or character; and the multifactor (polygenic) inheritance, where the interaction of many genes determines the trait or character. Most gross abnormalities and defects in inheritance are probably due to the action of single genes. These genes are either dominant or recessive, and can be associated with either autosomes or sex chromosomes. The dominant gene is expressed whether it is present in one or both chromosomes of the pair concerned, viz., homozygous or heterozygous. Eye color, curly or straight hair, color blindness, and Huntington's chorea are dominant traits. The recessive gene is expressed only in the presence of a similar contrasting gene, viz., in the homozygous form. Recessive inheritance is the most common type of transmission of human abnormalities and recessively inherited disorders usually have less variation and are more severe than those inherited as dominants. An example of recessive inheritance is phenylketonuria.[36]

Sex-linked inheritance is carried on the X chromosome. A woman who is the heterozygous carrier of the abnormal gene does not herself manifest the abnormal trait, but there is a risk that she will transmit the trait to a son or that her daughter will be a carrier. An affected man cannot transmit the abnormal trait to a son, but his daughter will be heterozygous and liable to transmit the trait to her offspring. An example of sex-linked inheritance is hemophilia.[37] In multifactor inheritance many genes are involved. Their individual effect is small, nonspecific, and additive but these genes combine to produce, in part, those traits that distinguish normal people. It is believed that the greater part of the variability in stature and intelligence has its source in multifactor or polygenic inheritance. Qualities of temperament and personality have, probably also to a marked degree, their source multifactorially determined, but our knowledge in this area is scanty.[38]

Chromosomal abnormalities are observed in number, structure, and arrangement. Down's syndrome (trisomy 21) is autosomal while XYY and Klinefelter's syndrome (XXY, XXXY, etc.) are sex chromosomal abnormalities. XYY is possibly associated with criminal behavior and in Klinefelter's syndrome the greater the number of X chromosomes the greater the degree of mental deficiency. Thus aberrations in either type of chromosome can produce alterations in physique, intelligence, behavior, personality, and the ability for successful adaptation.[39]

Twin and family studies on intelligence, personality, temperament, behavior, and neuroses demonstrate the problems of research on heredity as a cause of mental disease. A study of monozygotic (MZ) twins (separated in early life), compared with dizygotic (DZ) twins (reared together), found that the MZ twins, whether reared apart or together, had a greater similarity in personality than the DZ twins. Other studies found separated MZ twins no less alike in physique, temperament, or intelligence than twins not separated; and MZ twins resembled one another closely in the type of neurotic reaction they experienced but differed in the degree to which they suffered from the illness. The main factor in the latter study seems to be environmental. A study of twins of the same sex who were criminal—13 MZ pairs and 17 DZ pairs—found that in 10 out of 13 MZ pairs, one sibling within each pair committed crimes of a nature similar to that of his twin, e.g., one pair was repeatedly guilty of robbery and violence and another pair committed fraud. In the 17 binovular pairs, there were only two pairs of twins who showed a similarity in their criminal records. The conclusion was that criminal behavior is determined by genetic factors but that the environment brought out criminality. Work with 12 MZ and 12 DZ pairs of twins disclosed that where one twin had hysteria the other twin did not have the same diagnosis. The conclusion was that there is no genetic causal factor in hysteria. Family studies largely present conflicting evidence in the matter of genetic etiology, but it has been found that obsessional traits run in families and that there is a certain degree of genetic specificity in the neuroses.[40]

It is evident, then, that no definitive conclusions can be drawn with regard to the effect heredity has on neuroses. Yet there seems to be a hereditary component in intelligence, temperament, physique, personality, criminality, and obsessiveness. Since these factors may all be involved with neurotic disease, heredity deserves serious study and consideration.

Personality is the second component of the constitutional factor. At any given moment personality is defined as an expression of total experience from intrauterine life to the present. Personality traits include patterns of behavior that are unique to each individual. Personality is intimately connected with heredity and experience, and reflects elements of both. The term comes from the Latin *persona*: the mask through which an actor speaks. Perhaps, as the original definition implies, it really does express the roles an individual plays. But in psychiatric jargon personality has come to mean recurrent patterns or traits of behavior. These patterns are usually lifelong characteristics. Certain personality types seem to predispose individuals to specific types of neuroses.

PHYSICAL FACTORS

The physical factors are considered under two major headings: (1) somatic (body size and body type) and (2) pathology or physical illness. Body size was once thought to have an important relationship to psychiatric illness. We have since learned that in addition to heredity, size is probably more related to nutrition than to any other factor. In the past, studies were made comparing men on the basis of their body size. These studies, which have since been discredited, concluded that small men when compared to large men had lower intellectual capacity, lower educational attainment, poorer work records, and that a higher proportion did unskilled work. Other studies claimed that larger men tended toward rebelliousness and aggressiveness, whereas the smaller men tended toward dependent, anxious, and hypochondriacal traits. All of these claims, however, had one thing in common: no proof.[41]

The ancient conception of personality as dependent upon body type has been revitalized in the last 70 years by researchers as Sigaud, Viola, Kretschmer, Sheldon, Rees, Eysenck, and Lindegård. These researchers considered height, width, and depth of the body and correlated these bodily dimensions with personality. Kretschmer described pyknic individuals—those people with large body cavities, short neck, small extremities, and subcostal angle greater than 90°—to be warm, responsive, extroverted, and more susceptible to manic-depressive psychoses; asthenics—those people with narrow build, angular profile, and subcostal angle less than 90°—to be introverted, cold, aloof, and more prone to schizophrenia; athletic individuals—those people with broad shoulders, narrow hips, large bones, and well-developed musculature—to have a personality somewhere between the other two and to be associated with a higher proportion of criminality in adolescence. Sheldon used photography, physical measurements, psychological testing, and named the physical types as follows: endomorph, mesomorph, and ectomorph. He correlated these three types of physiques with three temperamental dimensions—viscerotonia, somatotonia, and cerebrotonia. Viscerotonia showed itself in relaxation, love of comfort, sociability; somatotonia—in vigor and assertiveness; cerebrotonia—in restraint and inhibition. Sheldon found high correlations (above +0.8) between measurements along the physical and psychological scales, but others have been unable to confirm these high values. He associated anxiety and obsessive compulsive neuroses with the ectomorph. Rees and Eysenck found hysteria in association with a eurymorphic (pyknic) pole, and depressive, obsessive compulsive, and anxiety characteristics with the leptomorphic pole. Each of these investigators found it necessary to coin a terminology, but enough exceptions to all of their correlations remain to question the validity of these studies. Yet for descriptive purposes they are helpful.[42]

Tanner proposed the term androgyny, i.e., a numerical index 3 X bi-acromial diameter minus the bi-iliac diameter expressed in centimeters. This index was found to have a normal distribution in each sex with a 90.1 ± 4.7 for men and a 78.9 ± 4.6 for women. It was found that psychiatric patients of both sexes had a lower androgyny and narrower bi-acromial diameter score than control groups. Going from masculine to feminine poles the distribution was: (1) normal; (2) homosexuals; (3) neurotics; (4) depressive; (5) schizophrenics. This index is not widely used and its value is seriously questioned.[43]

Organic pathology is the second component of the physical factors. It includes diseases that are usually studied in medicine and the psychological symptomatology associated with these physical diseases. The relationship between organic disease, which either directly or indirectly affects the central and autonomic nervous system, and the psychological symptoms which may occur as a result of organic disease, is a relevant consideration. These diseases fall under three headings.

(1) Brain structure changes which are permanent (irreversible): The factors that produce permanent change include any condition that affects the brain, e.g., degenerative diseases (arteriosclerosis, multiple sclerosis, space occupying lesions, senility), severe irreversible intoxications (poisoning by carbon monoxide, heavy metals, alcohol), traumatic injuries, etc. The cardinal features of chronic organic brain syndrome are a diminished control of affect and emotional lability, a relative failure of intellect with varying degrees of memory loss and impaired judgment, intermittent periods of confusion, and personality changes. These features may or may not be accompanied by neurological signs and neurotic symptomatology.

(2) Bodily structure and functional changes (usually reversible): This group has considerable variety. There are symptoms (not always the result of disease) that accompany emotion which are consistent with anxiety and mediated by the autonomic nervous system, e.g., palpitations, sweating, tremors, headaches, grogginess, respiratory and alimentary tract symptoms, frequent urination, and the like. Psychological symptoms occur in acute alcoholism, infections with high fever, thyrotoxicosis, drug intoxication, pheochromocytoma, hyperparathyroidism, porphyria, etc. These conditions have mental symptoms consistent with neuroses, psychoses, or acute organic brain syndrome. The latter can be characterized by disorientation, clouding of consciousness, and misinterpretation of external reality (illusions, delusions, and hallucinations). These conditions are of a temporary nature and are usually reversible once the basic problem is corrected.

(3) Psychological symptoms present (physical structural changes uncertain): Much of disordered mental functioning is never demonstrated on a histology slide. In brain biopsies of mentally ill patients, some researchers claim cellular pathology; however, most find nothing. This leads those committed to an organic etiology of mental illness to speculate that there is a functional disturbance based on structural changes which are not demonstrated. The

electroencephalogram (EEG) has value in studying the nature of consciousness, sleep, convulsive disorders, and other abnormalities; however, the relationship between brain waves and personality has given controversial results. Some researchers claim, while others deny, that the EEG patterns in uniovular twins are so constant that it is possible to match them from the EEG alone and that the dysrhythmia in epileptic patients exists in a high percentage of the relatives of these patients. If true, does this suggest a genetic basis for brain structure patterns? Another controversy surrounds the electroencephalographic changes that occur from childhood to adulthood and their correlation with psychological maturation. There are also claims that immaturity found in psychopaths is associated with anomalies of the EEG and that aggressive behavior can be correlated with EEG changes. Work remains to be done with EEG and behavior but its real importance today is still in the diagnosis of epilepsy and the localization of focal lesions in the brain.[44,45]

Autonomic, electrolyte, and endocrine systems influence metabolism and are indispensable for integrating the organism. The importance of this is well known, yet little precise knowledge of the mechanisms exists. For example, it is known that testosterone and estrogen influence the mind but it is not known how they do it. Other data equally unexplainable are: The high incidence of mental illness in adolescence and at the climacteric (early and late stages of the reproductive period); the marked degree of emotional disturbance that may accompany menstruation; and the occurrence of amenorrhea and altered sex drive with mental illness. In addition to the secretions of the gonads, other endocrine glands offer equally as challenging data regarding the mechanisms that affect the mind. In summary, the evidence suggests an intimate connection among mental states, biochemical, physiological, and endocrine systems. Further, the connections between hypothalamus, thalamus, pituitary, and cortex are such as to place the pituitary under the influence of the nervous system and this opens up endless possibilities of how an organism functions, and those details which are not known.[46-48]

The outbreak of epidemic encephalitis after World War I with the sequelae of postencephalitic personality and behavioral changes stimulated research correlating the brain with behavior. Recently, children who have problems with no demonstrable change in physical structure have received a great deal of study. These children may have learning difficulties, tics, behavioral and speech disturbances, psychiatric disorders, and the like, which leads to speculation that all personality and mental problems are the result of physical structural changes, even though these changes cannot be demonstrated. Caution must be exercised that etiological factors are not separated. All factors are related to one another. Curran writes: "Our knowledge, however, is at present so incomplete that the attribution of major mental illnesses, other than degenerative conditions and deliria, to physical factors, is at present no more than speculative."[49]

PSYCHOLOGICAL FACTORS

This all-inclusive term envelops the influences of environmental experience from intrauterine life to the present as well as intrapsychic experience. The roles of education, culture, tradition, religion, and parental attitudes are included as forces which mold psychological attitudes. It is far from settled, however, just how far personality is amenable to psychological influences. For this reason personality is arbitrarily included with constitutional factors although it could just as easily be considered under psychological factors. Again, emphasis should be placed on multifactorial pattern relations of disease rather than on isolated factors.[50] Dunham reviews the sociocultural factors and their relationship to personality and mental disorders and concludes that they are inconclusive:

> The findings from the epidemiological studies appear to be more substantive and concrete, but even here the solid findings fail to isolate any factors that show the influence of either the culture or the social structure in causing the psychoses. It is largely with the milder mental disturbances, the psychoneuroses and some character disorders, that one can make a case for the influence of culture. Certain maladaptive habits, attitudes, and behavior patterns that make for a precarious social existence have been learned from culture. But even here, the evidence falls short of proof and consists primarily of psychotherapeutic interviews where some prevailing theory already predetermines the interpretation of the verbal productions. With respect to the more severe disorders—the functional psychoses—I have indicated that the results appear to be more negative than positive.[51]

The major psychological theories in vogue today are behavioral, psychoanalytic, and descriptive. Each theory has its orthodox adherents as well as its splinter groups. To summarize the salient positions of these three may be helpful as a point of orientation. The behaviorists view neuroses as conditioned or learned responses and nothing more. The basic position is one of stimulus-response. As the child develops, habitual responses occur to recurring stimuli or groups of stimuli in a set manner. These responses become organized into Gestalts. In this manner the family's thoughts and attitudes condition the child. The assumption is that man is nothing more than a collection of responses to stimuli with no room for psychological explanation of behavior. The neuroses are learned conditioned responses or habits, and treatment consists of unconditioning the symptom.[52]

For clarity, the term psychodynamic is used here in preference to psychoanalytic. The term psychodynamic refers to all those theorists and therapists, from Freud and Janet until the present time, whose viewpoints of neuroses deal with unconscious or extraconscious concepts to explain mind, self, and society.

In brief, they deal with intrapsychic variables in addition to interpersonal relationships. These dynamicists relate neuroses to early development and consider anxiety in adulthood a reflection of the earliest anxieties experienced by the infant. We are left in the dark as to why one person develops one type of response and someone else another. Perhaps the psychoanalytic model is representative of all dynamic theories because in many ways it is the prototype of the others. The psychoanalytic theory of neuroses goes something like this: The patient finds himself in a conflict situation. This conflict may be intrapsychic or interpersonal. Solutions are sought to this problem. If a rational solution is found, there are no neuroses and anxiety diminishes. If a rational solution is not found and anxiety persists, the patient resorts to unconscious mechanisms to resolve the conflict. First regression occurs to earlier libidinal conflicts. This regression reactivates the original libido conflict which usually goes to a level where the libido is fixated. This in turn calls into operation early mechanisms of defense which lead to symptoms. Ergo, neuroses develop. The type of defense mechanism which predominates determines what name we give the neurosis, i.e., anxiety, hysteria, obsessive, etc. One can see that the end result is an irrational solution to a conflict. This solution in turn conflicts with the rational mind, so further conflict results which perpetuates the neurotic process. A vicious cycle develops.[53]

The disagreement between the behaviorist and the psychodynamic schools of thought is not merely semantic but real. The differences are on an observational and descriptive level. The behaviorist sees specific symptoms and anxiety. The psychodynamicist sees intrapersonal and interpersonal difficulties and more or less avoids the obvious: the symptoms which he considers not the real problem. Even in his descriptive presentation the dynamic psychiatrist may ignore specific symptoms or groups of symptoms, for he does not regard them as relevant and essential for understanding or treating the neuroses.[54]

The observational and descriptive method provides the major orientation for this book. One observes, describes, and attempts to make connections or interpretations as close to the data as possible. This is the biopsychosocial, the comprehensive approach. In terms of explaining or understanding, it uses the insights of all schools of thought insofar as the evidence will permit. Extensive psychologizing or philosophizing is discouraged.

CURRENT LIFE SITUATIONS AND STRESSES

This means evaluating the here and now situation to the extent that the present problems and stresses are etiological factors in illness. George Engel identifies five psychological characteristics that he considers essential precursors of physical illness. These psychological characteristics are correlated with life settings; either acute stresses (death, accidents, earthquakes, etc.) or chronic stresses (difficulties in relationships, slow loss of physical or mental prowess, failures in business, loss of standing in the family). The physical illness is preceded by the psychological state in which the patient feels that he is unable to cope with environmental changes. These are described as: (1) a feeling of helplessness or hopelessness; (2) a depreciated image of self; (3) a sense of loss of gratification from relationships or roles in life; (4) a disruption of the sense of continuity between past, present, and future; (5) and a reactivation of memories of earlier periods of giving-up. The author proposes that this psychological state predisposes the patient to biological reactions that decrease his capacity to deal with concurrent pathological processes. Engel refers to this condition as the giving-up—given-up complex and considers it as a contributing factor to physical illness.[55] Needless to say, similar considerations enter into the development of mental illness.

Generally, stress does not itself cause neuroses, but it can be a negative influence in disabling conditions such as deformity, physical illness, and pre-existing mental conditions. Neuroses may occur when the balance of etiological factors is so disturbed that the individual cannot compensate, adapt, or adequately cope.[56] The resistance to illness varies from person to person, but with enough stress even the most stoical will eventually have a breakdown. The most common stresses are death of a loved one, injury, illness, interpersonal difficulty, or loss of a job. Since changes do occur with aging the inability to accept the limitations imposed upon the individual as a result of age can precipitate mental illness. The key to understanding neurotic breakdown lies in the clinician's ability to separate the essential from the relatively inessential factors. It requires more faith than knowledge, more magic than realism, and more guts than brains for the psychiatrist to presume that he is capable of dealing with these complex variables. This challenge produces the agony and ecstasy that one suffers when one practices in this field.

REFERENCES

1. Russell, B., *A History of Western Philosophy,* 10th printing. New York: Simon and Schuster, 1945, pp. 66–67.
2. Ibid., p. 67.
3. Ingle, D.J., Causality. *Perspect. Biol. Med.* **14**(3):410 (1971).
4. Ibid., pp. 414–415.
5. Ibid., p. 416.
6. King, L.S., "Some basic explanations of disease: An historian's viewpoint," in *Evaluation and Explanation in the Biomedical Sciences* (edited by Engelhardt, Jr., H.T. and Spicker, S.F.). Dordrecht, Holland and Boston: Reidel, 1975, pp. 11–27.
7. King, L.S., Causation: A problem in medical philosophy. *Clio. Medica* **10**:95–109 (1975).

8. Ibid., p. 108.
9. Feinstein, A., *Clinical Judgment*. Baltimore: Williams & Wilkins, 1967, pp. 24–25.
10. King, L.S., *The Growth of Medical Thought*. Chicago: Univ. Chicago Press, 1963.
11. Gray, M., Principles of the comprehensive examination. *Arch. Gen. Psychiatry* **10**:371–372 (1964).
12. Kendell, R.E., *The Role of Diagnosis in Psychiatry*. Oxford: Blackwell, 1975, p. 1.
13. Szasz, T.S., The myth of mental illness. *Amer. Psychol.* **15**:113–118 (1960).
14. Moore, M.S., Some myths about "mental illness." *Arch. Gen. Psychiatry* **32**(12): 1483–1497 (1975).
15. Kendell, R.E., op. cit., pp. 12–13.
16. Ibid., p. 13.
17. Scadding, J.G., Meaning of diagnostic terms in broncho-pulmonary disease. *Brit. Med. J.* **2**:1425–1430 (1963).
18. Scadding, J.G., Diagnosis: The clinician and the computer. *Lancet* **2**:877–882 (1967).
19. Scadding, J.G., The semantics of medical diagnosis. *Biomed. Computing* **3**:83–90 (1972).
20. Kendell, R.E., op. cit., pp. 2–23.
21. Engelhardt, Jr., H.T., "The concepts of health and disease," in *Evaluation and Explanation in The Biomedical Sciences* (edited by Engelhardt, Jr., H.T. and Spicker, S.F.). Dordrecht, Holland and Boston: Reidel, 1975, pp. 125–141.
22. Satorius, N., Classification: An international perspective. *Psychiatric Ann.* **6**(8):359 (1976).
23. Engelhardt, Jr., H.T., op. cit., pp. 128–132.
24. Ibid., p. 135.
25. Engelhardt, Jr., H.T., Explanatory models in medicine: Facts, theories, and values. *Tex. Rep. Biol. Med.* **32**(1):235 (1974).
26. Ibid., 235.
27. Ibid., p. 236.
28. Gray, M., op. cit., p. 370.
29. Strauss, J.S., Diagnostic models and the nature of psychiatric disorders. *Arch. Gen. Psychiatry* **29**:445–449 (1973).
30. Strauss, J.S., A comprehensive approach to psychiatric diagnosis. *Amer. J. Psychiatry* **132**:1193–1195 (1975).
31. White, W.A., *Twentieth Century Psychiatry: Its Contribution to Man's Knowledge of Himself*. New York: Norton, 1936, pp. 53–56.
32. Curran, D., Partridge, M. and Storey, P., *Psychological Medicine: An Introduction to Psychiatry*, 7th ed. Edinburgh and London: Churchill Livingstone, 1972, pp. 16–47.
33. Guze, S.B., Hereditary transmission of psychiatric illness. *Amer. J. Psychiatry* **130**:1377–1378 (1973).
34. Stanbury, J.B., Wyngaarden, J.B., and Fredrickson, D.S., "Inherited variation and metabolic abnormality," in *The Metabolic Basis of Inherited Disease*, 3rd ed. (edited by Stanbury, J.B., Wyngaarden, J.B., and Fredrickson, D.S.). New York: McGraw-Hill, 1972, pp. 3–4.
35. Thompson, J. and Thompson, M., *Genetics in Medicine*. Philadelphia: Saunders, 1966, pp. 268–271.
36. Ibid., pp. 34–46.
37. Ibid., pp. 47–52.
38. Ibid., pp. 64–65.
39. Ibid., pp. 100–105, 122–123.

40. Slater, E. and Cowie, V., *The Genetics of Mental Disorders.* London: Oxford University Press, 1971, pp. 92–121.
41. Slater, E. and Roth, M., *Clinical Psychiatry,* 3rd ed. Baltimore: Williams & Wilkins, 1970, p. 69.
42. Ibid., pp. 69–70.
43. Ibid., p. 70.
44. Curran, D., Partridge, M. and Storey, P., op. cit., pp. 33–37.
45. Slater, E. and Roth, M., op. cit., pp. 71–72.
46. Mendels, J. (Ed.), *Biological Psychiatry.* New York: Wiley, 1973.
47. Kashiwagi, T., McClure, J.N. and Wetzel, R.D., Premenstrual affective syndrome and psychiatric disorder. *Dis. Nerv. Syst.* 37(3):116–119 (1976).
48. Curran, D., Partridge, M. and Storey, P., op. cit., pp. 36–37.
49. Ibid., p. 37.
50. Fabrega, Jr., H., The position of psychiatry in the understanding of human disease. *Arch. Gen. Psychiatry* 32(12):1500–1512 (1975).
51. Dunham, J.W., Society, culture, and mental disorder. *Arch. Gen. Psychiatry* 33:155 (1976).
52. Wolpe, J., *The Practice of Behavior Therapy,* 2nd ed. New York: Pergamon, 1973.
53. Nemiah, J.C., *Foundations of Psychopathology* (reprint 1971). New York: Oxford University Press, 1961.
54. Breger, L. and McGaugh, J., "Critique and reformulation of 'learning theory' approaches to psychotherapy and neurosis," in *Contemporary Abnormal Psychology,* edited by Maher, B. Baltimore: Penguin, 1973, pp. 307–347.
55. Engel, G.L., A life setting conducive to illness: The giving-up–given-up complex. *Ann. Int. Med.* 69:293–300 (1968).
56. Sloman, L., The role of neurosis in phylogenetic adaptation, with particular reference to early man. *Amer. J. Psychiatry* 133(5):543–547 (1976).

4
ANXIETY NEUROSIS

Feeling, affect, mood, passion, and emotion are diverse phenomena or processes that have never been satisfactorily defined, classified, or analyzed. These terms represent a variety of mental and physical states in which the basic element or elements are not known. Feeling is a general term that includes all undefinable, intangible psychic manifestations. One feels that something is not appropriate, that he belongs or does not belong, that taxes are too high, that the room is too small, or that he is angry, sad, glad, mad, joyous, tense, anxious, guilty, etc. Affect and mood, practically synonymous terms, are distinguished from one another by intensity and duration. Affects are intense feelings, usually short-lived and associated with bodily changes. Moods are not as intense as affects and last for longer periods. The term passion is not often used today except to indicate strong feelings such as love or hate. Emotion is a word that designates a combination of components including biochemical and physiological changes, behavioral or motor reactions, cognitive appraisal, affective or mood responses, and coping actions. Emotion, like disease, is a complex pattern relationship and not a thing.[1]

Although the components of emotion are poorly correlated, they are manifested on many levels. No one component is considered in isolation but in relation to the other components and to eliciting conditions. In effect, each component fits into a larger system and reflects only one part of the system. For example, the person's cognitive and mood components are part of his entire mental apparatus and reflect his interpretation or appraisal of the situation as well as his associated feeling state; biochemical and physiological responses are part of his biological system and reflect his type of bodily mobilizations; behavioral or motor responses are part of his total range of behavior and include expressive behavior (postural, facial, gestures, etc.) as well as autonomic and voluntary motor acts; coping actions are part of the person's ability to adapt and to protect himself and include avoidance, attack, submission, and so forth. Therefore, emotions, as defined above are consistent with a comprehensive model of diagnosis and disease.[2]

Feelings cannot be isolated from the totality of the individual's existence. To do so recalls the faculty psychologists' divisions of intellect, cognition, will, emotion, sensation, and perception. Yet until a terminology develops that allows the psychiatrist to think in a biopsychosocial context, he should be aware of this defect and recognize the limitations of his thinking processes. Feelings, no matter how strongly and sincerely felt, are often difficult to verbalize and leave the person frustrated with the inadequacies of our language to express and describe them. This can result in misunderstanding and erroneous conclusions. Lazarus aptly expresses the difficulty:

> The reason why there is so much apparent dissociation among components of an emotional syndrome is that each response element also has its own adaptive functions in relation to the person and the environment. Take self-reported affect, for example. It may reflect the picture the person (consciously or unconsciously) wishes to communicate as well as actual subjective experience. And, of course, any verbal expression is subject to a variety of constraints as part of a linguistic system which is not particularly well-suited to the expression of affect. Similarly, physiological changes reflect both internal homeostatic processes and externally created (emotional) demands; expressive reactions such as facial grimaces are governed partly by biological, species characteristics, and partly by the values which society or the particular person places on emotional expression; and instrumental acts are related not only to the achievement of emotionally relevant goals, but also to conflicting internal motives, social constraints against certain forms of behaviors, and so forth. Thus, each component reaction which enters into an emotional syndrome serves multiple functions, militating against a high correlation between them.[3]

Psychiatrists have proposed many methods of classifying emotions but the need is for a practical classification that evaluates emotions and circumstances. If the emotion is more or less reasonable, appropriate, and understandable, the patient's response is considered normal; if not, it is considered abnormal. Normal responses do not place the individual at a biological, psychological, or social disadvantage. Normal emotions are adaptive and promote a state of mind which enables the person to realize his potential. In this sense, emotions promote self-respect and dignity, and are protective. Abnormal emotions can be nonadaptive and nonprotective. Yet in some situations abnormal or morbid emotions can be either protective but not adaptive or adaptive but not protective. The patient who reacts to a chronic disabling neurological disease with anger and bitterness may be protecting himself against a complete loss of self-respect and pride while alienating himself from those who would take care of him. In contrast, the self-sacrificing, self-deprecating, submissive patient adapts because he pleases others;

but he does not protect himself because he curbs his freedom of thought and feeling. It is not always easy to draw the line between normal and pathological emotional states for they are ranges, not sharp lines, and complex phenomena. Emotions, thought, and behavior cannot be separated from each other. They are all interrelated and interdependent parts of a person in an environment. Yet for heuristic purposes they must be separated, defined, classified, and analyzed.[4]

ANXIETY AND FEAR, EMOTIONS

Anxiety has many definitions. Philosophers define it as uneasiness, malaise, dread, and anguish and are concerned with the underlying essential nature of the phenomena.[5] Psychiatrists and psychologists define anxiety as a complex emotional syndrome. Their concept can be based on the premise that the source of the anxiety is an unaware or at least an uncertain appraisal of threat. The appraisal of threat involves characteristics that have *symbolic, anticipatory, and uncertain elements*. Symbols are ideas, concepts, values, or systems of thought. Symbols are used by man as a means of giving meaning, both internally and externally, to his existence. When symbols are lost, anxiety may result. The second characteristic involves anticipation. An anticipatory appraisal of threat can result from either a conscious or unconscious conflict or an inability to comprehend the here and now in a meaningful manner. The third characteristic is uncertainty. Since the future is unknown and ambiguous, the person may appraise it as a threat and anxiety will result. These characteristics (symbolic, anticipatory, and uncertain) link the person's appraisal of a threat to himself (consciously and unconsciously), to his present and future circumstances, and to the appearance or nonappearance of anxiety.[6]

In addition to a cognitive appraisal of threat, anxiety has other manifestations. The biochemical, endocrine, metabolic, and physiological components are stress reactions. The behavior components are consistent with central nervous system arousal and consist of increased muscle tension and bodily movement, increased autonomic nervous system functions, and increased facial and bodily expressions, e.g., gestures, grimaces, tremors, some tics, etc. The affective or mood responses are verbalizations of feeling tense, irritable, nervous, insecure, jumpy, excited, talkative, apprehensive, etc. The coping component expresses itself in the patient's control of the anxiety in relationship to self (unconscious and conscious mechanisms of coping) and to environment (fight, flight, or submit, and so forth). These manifestations seen as a total pattern relationship constitute a specific distinct syndrome that is distinguished from all other emotions. It is referred to as anxiety.[7,8]

The emotions, anxiety and fear, should be differentiated. Distinguishing these two emotions is not a simple matter. There is no one criterion that by itself can differentiate fear and anxiety but rather a combination of criteria is needed. Both anxiety and fear are responses; however, the response varies depending on the person and the circumstance. In general, the frightened person reacts by flight, fight, or avoidance; the anxious one by intrapsychic coping mechanisms such as denial, repression, intellectuality, etc. Both respond to eliciting conditions or stimuli. Usually the source of fear is tangible and identifiable, but the source of anxiety is less clear. Both can be mediated through neural mechanisms such as stimulating the central nervous system with the use of drugs, electricity, or lesions. Thus anxiety and fear, like all emotions, have common as well as different elements, and clinically the two emotions can at times be difficult to distinguish.[9]

ANXIETY, A NEUROSIS

The morbid state of anxiety is called by the following synonymous terms: anxiety neurosis, anxiety state, panic, trait, or anxiety reaction. The predominant affect is anxiety, and the anxiety neurosis describes a variety of biological, psychological, behavioral, and coping responses. Each individual has his own unique patterns of response; therefore, the proportions of the above manifestations vary from person to person. The DSMII[*] loosely defines the anxiety neurosis with clinical manifestations, e.g., anxious overconcern that can extend to panic, frequently associated somatic complaints, and circumstances that are not restricted to a specific situation or object. This definition is not enough.

Anxiety neurosis is an emotional disease and as such has characteristics and manifestations that are similar to the emotion anxiety. It is, however, not an exaggerated state of normal anxiety but a clinical entity that can take several forms: acute (panic), subacute (trait), and chronic. All forms of anxiety neurosis may be manifested by episodic periods that last from a few minutes to days and can be interspersed with nonanxious intervals. Acute anxiety neurosis (panic) is an extreme form of anxiety that can include the expectation of the unknown in the form of dread of annihilation or doom.[10] Subacute anxiety neurosis (trait) is a relatively permanent and stable condition in which the person is characterized by a lifelong personality pattern of self deprecation, shyness, guilt proneness, and a tendency to respond with anxiety under a wide variety of stresses.[11] Chronic anxiety neurosis is a condition in which the variable components associated with anxiety (biological, psychological, behavioral, coping, stress) are sustained over a prolonged period of time.[12]

Anxiety can be associated with any mental or physical disease. The soundest individual may react with anxiety to a stressful situation, frustration, or conflict. With our present state of knowledge we do not know why one patient reacts one way and a second another. All forms of anxiety neurosis are diagnosed only when other illnesses are absent.[13]

*DSMII, p. 39.

HISTORY

Man has experienced anxiety throughout the ages. Yet anxiety, like fear, was not clearly defined or isolated as a separate entity by psychiatrists or psychologists until the nineteenth and twentieth centuries. This is the result of ever-persistent difficulties in classification and constant changes in terminology. Philosophers, however, did contribute toward an understanding of anxiety. In 1844 Søren A. Kierkegaard (1813-1855) wrote about anxiety. Other philosophers have since written on the topic but none defined anxiety in exactly the same sense as Kierkegaard. In addition, the term changes in meaning from German or French to English; exact synonyms cannot be found. Some of the terms that foreign philosophers used for anxiety could be translated to mean dread, anguish, uneasiness, or malaise.[14]

Psychiatrists and physicians used many names for disorders which could not be differentiated from anxiety neurosis. In 1863 Alfred Stillé (1813-1890), a Civil War surgeon, described "palpitations of the heart." Other expressions such as muscular exhaustion of the heart, cardiac neurosis, vasomotor neuroses, soldier's heart, neurocirculatory asthenia, and effort syndrome were once popular. In 1869 George M. Beard coined the term "neurasthenia" or "nervous exhaustion" which included anxiety. In 1871 Jacob DaCosta (1833-1900) described functional cardiac disorder as irritable heart disease (DaCosta's syndrome). In 1889 Hermann Oppenheim (1858-1919) coined the term "traumatic neurosis." In 1894 Sigmund Freud postulated that actual neurosis (anxiety, hypochondriasis, neurasthenia) was different from the psychoneurosis. In 1903 Pierre Janet coined the term "psychasthenia" (anxiety, phobia, obsessive compulsive) as distinct from neurasthenia. With the appearance of the standard classification systems, anxiety appeared as an entity in its own right. By 1952, in the DSMI, the anxiety reaction type was classified under psychoneurotic disorders. In the DSMII (1968), anxiety neurosis appeared.* Little agreement exists as to the number of distinct conditions described by the various diagnostic terms or how they relate or overlap.[15,16]

A historical perspective on anxiety cannot be separated from a history of thought regarding emotion. Attempts to clarify the what, why, and how of emotion had its modern roots in the thinking of Claude Bernard (1813-1878), the father of experimental medicine. In 1865 he published his greatest work, *An Introduction to the Study of Experimental Medicine*, in which he pointed out that the true medium in which an organism lives is the body fluids (plasma plus interstitial fluids). These fluids he called the internal environment to set

*DSMIII subsumes the following under Anxiety Disorders: Phobic Disorders (Agoraphobia with panic attacks, Agoraphobia without panic attacks, Social phobia, Simple phobia, Unspecified phobic); Panic disorder; Obsessive compulsive disorder; Generalized anxiety disorder; A typical anxiety disorder. From the: Provisional classification: Published as a looseleaf manual entitled *DSM-III Draft, 4/15/77.* DRAFT OF AXES I AND II OF DSM-III CLASSIFICATION as of March 30, 1977.

them off from the external environment or outside world. The organism achieves a free and independent life, physically and mentally, Bernard posited, because of the constant composition of the internal environment. Although he had meager insight into the nature of the internal environment, his generalization stands as a basic biochemical and physiological truth.[17]

In 1872 Charles Darwin (1809-1882) published *Expressions of Emotions in Man and Animals.* He thought that facial expressions and postural movements were evolutionary and originated in what were once useful actions. For example, he thought that showing the teeth in anger was a remnant of primitive combat tactics, derived from the time when man fought by clawing and biting. Further, Darwin postulated that anxiety reflects an expectation of suffering; depression, a loss of hope. He distinguished anxiety from fear by describing anxiety as a reaction to an unknown danger and fear as a reaction to a known danger. Darwin assumed that the psychic state of fear caused physiological responses such as heart pounding, increased breathing rate, changed facial expressions, and subsequent movement.[18]

In 1890 William James (1841-1910) and Karl G. Lange (1834-1900), a Danish physiologist, independently proposed an interpretation of emotion which became known as the James-Lange theory. Unlike Darwin's theory of emotion which assumed that the emotion caused the physiological response this theory postulated that bodily changes caused the emotional state. The James-Lange theory held that as a result of stimulating the motor and autonomic nervous systems, changes occurred which sent sensory impulses from receptors, particularly interoceptors, to the brain that are then appreciated as feelings. The kind of feeling depends upon the type of bodily response brought about by the stimulus. For example, fear arises from motor behavior and not from sense perceptions; a bear is frightened because he is running, and not running because he is frightened.[19] In its day this theory caused quite a controversy and once again seems to be creeping back into our thinking. Its revival is emphasized by biofeedback theorists.

John Dewey (1859-1952) started functionalism as a school of thought in 1896, the period in which he presented a conflict theory of emotion. Using the bear example of the James-Lange theory he said that we are afraid not because we run but because we are in conflict about what to do—whether to keep an eye on the bear to see if he is coming after us or to run away. Fear comes out of uncertainty, confusion, paralysis. This theory of emotion never caught on since it did not fit into the concept of adaptive behavior prevalent in his day.[20]

Sir Charles Sherrington (1857-1952) performed experiments which discredited the James-Lange theory. He cut the spinal cords of dogs in such a way that they had no sensations from viscera or skeletal muscles. These dogs still showed anger and affection. Though the evidence was inconclusive (since we do not really know how a dog feels) the outward expression resembled true emotion.[21]

Walter B. Cannon (1871-1945) in the early decades of this century extended Bernard's thesis in many directions. Cannon called Bernard's internal environment the fluid matrix of the body and coined the term "homeostasis." Cannon pointed out that the existence of a homeostatic state is evidence that mechanisms are acting or ready to act to maintain constancy and that these mechanisms are generally under automatic control. He introduced the notion of an emergency theory—fight or flight. Here the action of the sympathetic system is in general antagonistic to the parasympathetic system. With increased emotion, however, an overall stimulation in all autonomic nervous system functions occurs. Stimulation of the sympathetic nervous system accelerates heart rate, raises blood pressure, increases breathing rate, inhibits digestion, redistributes the blood, dilates bronchioles, increases blood sugar, and releases adrenalin. The result is that the skin gets pale and sweats, the mouth dries, muscular energy increases, more blood goes to the arm and leg muscles, and the blood-clotting mechanisms speed up. Cannon thought that these functions aided in dealing with emergencies by preparing the organism for intense effort; therefore, they had survival value. He thought that adrenalin was involved in adaptation to stress since adrenalin was secreted as part of an animal's response to rage or fear-producing stimuli. Further, the Cannon-Bard theory of emotion opposed the James-Lange theory. The Cannon-Bard theory proposed that a stimulus went to an integrative center in the thalamus or, perhaps, hypothalamus and proceeded to the cerebral cortex where the nature of the feeling was determined. Concurrently, motor impulses left the hypothalamic center and produced somatic and automatic behavior. Thus theoretically, feeling and behavior arose separately from an emotional center in the brain; whereas, in the James-Lange theory, feeling occurred as a result of behavior.[22,23] The beginnings of modern biological psychiatry were now established.

BIOLOGICAL BASIS FOR EMOTION

Since anxiety is a generalized condition that may occur with any psychiatric condition, its evaluation becomes very important. Incorrect evaluation of anxiety can lead to improper therapeutic measures.[24] Psychiatrists, psychologists, and researchers, therefore, have relentlessly searched for accurate definitions, mechanisms, and purposes for anxiety. One approach to the problem is by investigating the relationship between the biological organism and behavior.

Research with animals and man produced an extensive body of knowledge regarding anatomy, chemistry, and physiology of anxiety. This work assumes that behavior, thought, and feelings are manifestations of physical processes, particularly the endocrine and central nervous systems. If it were possible to describe the moment to moment physiological state of each cell in the nervous system, psychological phenomena would correspond to predictable changes in patterns of neural activity and molecular structure. With the present state of technology, however, even those who are most optimistic do not expect that such detailed analysis of neural function is possible in the foreseeable future.[25]

Perhaps as an introduction to the study of the brain, a review of its anatomy might be useful. Although the brain actually functions as a totality, for heuristic purposes it is divided into parts. The lower part or brain stem is a continuation of the spinal cord and merges into the hypothalamus, which connects the brain stem to the cerebral cortex, pituitary gland, and to the rest of the brain. Surrounding the brain stem and hypothalamus is the limbic system. The cerebellum looks like a separate part of the brain but is intimately connected with both the cerebral cortex and the brain stem.

Functionally, the cerebral cortex is the most advanced part of the brain. In this area sensations are received, interpreted, integrated, and action is controlled. The least advanced part, the spinal cord, is a reflex center and transmits information from the body and external environment to the cortex, or conversely from the higher centers to the body. The brain stem regulates vital body functions: respiration, pulse rate, blood pressure, etc. Besides this, the brain stem contains the reticular activating system that regulates the arousal or awareness level of the organism. The cerebellum is concerned with coordinated movements of the arms and legs and has feedback loops to modulate the commands of the cortex. The hypothalamus releases a hormone that controls the pituitary gland, is intimately involved with the emotions, and functions as pleasure, hunger, and satiety centers. The limbic system is concerned with memory and emotion; stimulation produces rage, ablation leads to docility, alterations can produce hypersexuality, asexuality, or perverted sexuality. The amygdaloid seems to have a relationship to aggressive behavior. Although it may appear that the brain has cerebral localization, there is no proof. The general consensus is that the brain functions in its totality.[26]

The basic unit of the brain like all other organs, is the cell. The nerve cells or neurons are connected by a series of dendrites that carry information to the cell body and axons that carry information from the cell body. Axons and dendrites meet at a gap, the synapse. Originally it was thought that the nerve impulse was transmitted electrically from the axon of one cell to the dendrite or body of another cell. But it is now known that in the majority of cases this is not so; instead, a chemical called a neurotransmitter diffuses across the space. Neurotransmitters are either excitatory or inhibitory to the succeeding neuron. It is thought that 10 or 12 different classes of neurotransmitters exist, each functioning with a specific neuron or group of neurons. Once a neurotransmitter is released from a nerve ending it can be destroyed by an enzyme or by re-uptake return to the nerve ending that released it. In brief, this describes the anatomical, physiological, and chemical relationships of the neuron.[27]

Neurotransmitters regulate emotions and seem to originate from amino acids. Catecholamines consist of norepinephrine and dopamine. Norepinephrine is more concentrated in the hypothalamus than anywhere else in the brain. Dopamine has the most cell bodies in the substantia nigra and in nerve endings of the corpus striatum. Catacholamine synthesis occurs in presynaptic noradrenergic neurons and starts with the amino acid tyrosine that is taken into the neuron from the bloodstream. Tyrosine is transformed by enzymatic substances as follows: tyrosine → dopamine → norepinephrine. Norepinephrine seems to be a major factor in psychic states which involve euphoria and excitement, and dopamine has something to do with the integration of fine body movements. In Parkinson's disease dopamine is severely depleted. The neurotransmitter serotonin is made from tryptophan and has its highest concentration in the hypothalamus, and its cell bodies are clustered in the raphe nuclei of the brain stem. Serotonin neurons function in the regulation of sleep and wakefulness. Histamine is also concentrated in the hypothalamus. It is implicated in urticarial and anaphylactic reactions, stimulating gastric secretion, and is released following a burn. Acetylcholine is the neurotransmitter that acts at the neuromuscular junction and in a major portion of the parasympathetic nervous system. The principal neurotransmitter of the sympathetic system is norepinephrine. The amino acids are the most numerous neurotransmitters in the brain, and glycine and gamma-aminobutyric acid (GABA) are the best known. They serve as inhibitors to nerve functioning.[28]

The endocrine system is the other important system involved with emotion. Cannon's notion of fight or flight can be related today to stimulation of the adrenal medulla by the posterior hypothalamus which releases epinephrine; and stimulation of the anterior hypothalamus which causes the adrenals to release norepinephrine. The physiological components of flight are similar to those of anxiety and fear; there is a stimulation of the autonomic nervous system and an increase in epinephrine. In the fight reaction norepinephrine increases. As a point of interest, rabbits that tend to be timid and frightened show a predominance of epinephrine and aggressive lions show a predominance of norepinephrine. It is established, however, that increased epinephrine with its physiological sequelae characterizes not only anxiety but other types of emotional arousal such as pleasure, enjoyment, anger, or sexual excitement.[29]

Anxiety is associated with an increase in the activity of the pituitary adrenocortical system. In situations that produce anxiety in monkeys the level of 17-hydroxycorticosteroid rises in urine and plasma. When the animals are left undisturbed, the 17 OHCS decreases.[30] Hans Selye has shown that under acute stress the adrenal glands of animals show striking changes; they become enlarged, produce more adrenalin, and discharge their steroids into the bloodstream; the adrenals also change their color from yellow to brown. When the animals are subjected to chronic stress (exposure to cold), the adrenals enlarge, then return to normal size; but after a period of time as the stress continues the adrenals again enlarge and lose their steroids, and eventually the animals die. Selye coined the term "general adaptation syndrome" for the bodily reactions to stress. For Selye, stress was not synonymous with anxiety. But anxiety can be one of the responses to stress. Stress can be anything that places the organism under pressure, and the general adaptation syndrome is a nonspecific response of the body to any demand made upon it. The response is concerned primarily with the action of the adrenal cortex and medulla. The adrenal medulla makes the catecholamines. The adrenal cortex makes the corticoid hormones which are released as a defense against the unfavorable manifestations of stress. The glucocorticoids (cortisol, cortisone, corticosterone) promote gluconeogenesis, regulate pituitary adrenocorticotropic (ACTH) and melanocyte-stimulating (MSH) hormones, effect salt and water metabolism, effect the central nervous system (promote normal psyche, lower electrical threshold), and effect the cardiovascular system (sensitize vessels to catecholamines, atherogenesis). They also effect the hematologic, gastrointestinal, and osseous systems, and promote body defenses (increase capacity for work, and inhibit inflammation, antibody production, and the effects of the antibody-antigen reaction). The androgens have androgenic, anabolic, and pyrogenic effects. They effect the growth of sexual hair, promote baldness, and growth of phallus, deepen voice, increase sebaceous secretion, increase protein synthesis, increase muscle mass and strength, promote bone growth and epiphyseal closure, promote calcium utilization, etc. The mineralocorticoids (e.g., aldosterone) promote conservation of sodium and water. Emotions are intimately connected with the adrenal glands.[31,32]

Corticoids are released by the adrenal cortex under stimulation of the adrenocorticotropic hormones of the pituitary gland, which in turn is stimulated to release that hormone by the releasing factor of the hypothalamus. The hypothalamus is stimulated by the cerebral cortex which perceives the stress from the environment. Thus a self-regulating biofeedback mechanism is set into motion: cerebral cortex → hypothalamus → pituitary → adrenocorticotropic hormone → adrenals → catacholamines and corticosteroids. This homeostatic mechanism can be diagrammatically illustrated.[33]

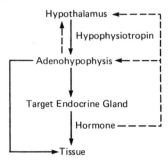

Corticosteroids when administered to patients frequently produce agitation and increase anxiety. The variety of changes that may accompany anxiety cannot all be traced to the effect of corticosteroids; hence, the mechanisms by which anxiety is produced under these conditions needs explaining. Anxiety may be the result of neurochemical changes. Evidence indicates that these changes, induced by the corticosteroids, modify the serotonin pathways in the tegmental region of the midbrain. This results in an increase in arousal which is part of the subjective sensation of anxiety.[34]

Under stress the face may flush or pale, the blood pressure rise or fall, the heart quicken or seem to stand still; there may be either increased or decreased colonic, renal, or bladder function. Any of these may be present and may occur singly or in combination. But the term stress has eluded earnest attempts at precise definition, and humans when challenged respond with all their bodily equipment, including any combination of visceral, somatic, or social behavior.

The type of breakdown—ulcers, asthma, hypertension, anxiety, etc.—depends on the vulnerable organ or system. The same principles of multifactorial etiologies apply for biological and psychiatric disease. If stressful situations can evoke the disease, then avoidance can be a controllable, preventive measure.

Whatever the clinical manifestations, certain organs are involved and others are not. The responses are patterned and discreet rather than generalized. What sets the pattern of organ participation? The answer is not clear. The question of organ or psychiatric disease choice remains unanswered. However, they do resemble clearly purposeful responses similar to the response to eating which stimulates blood flow and acid in the stomach. The matter of organ choice becomes a matter of individual makeup. For example, relatively aggressive individuals during tooth extraction experience an increase in saliva, while individuals with a tendency to withdraw from troublesome situations virtually stop secreting saliva.[35]

It has long been known that clinical endocrine disorders are associated with mental disturbances. Hyperthyroid patients may present themselves to the doctor with an initial complaint of nervousness. Hyperinsulinism with lowering of blood sugar provokes acute anxiety. Cushing's syndrome, excessive administration of adrenocorticosteroids, or anterior pituitary lobe hyperfunctioning produce psychiatric disturbances. Pheochromocytoma has features such as headache, nausea, epigastric pain, sweating, pallor, palpitations, and apprehension. Sexual endocrine gland changes, especially in the female, suggest a relationship between the secretion of sex hormones and psychiatric disturbance. The high incidence of mental disturbances during puberty, premenstrual, postpartum, and menopause must be more than coincidence. The endocrine glands have associative mental symptoms, due either to disease, improper functioning, or normal physiological change, and anxiety or depression are the most common.[36]

Biochemical findings can be of interest. Following exercise, patients with anxiety neurosis have a higher blood lactate level than those without the neurosis. Researchers have shown that infusing sodium lactate solution in an anxiety neurotic or in normal individuals precipitates an anxiety attack. The lactate theory of anxiety, as this is now called, is very controversial as many question this cause and effect relationship.[37,38]

Marks and Lader present an excellent review of the physiological changes:

> A number of abnormalities have been reported in patients with anxiety states in response to standard exercise or stress. Stimuli and stresses which produce abnormal responses or unusual responses at lower stimulus levels include pain, cold, muscular effort, carbon dioxide, noise, flash, and anticipation. Abnormal responses to these situations were noted in patient's pulse, minute respiration/volume, ventilatory efficiency, increase in blood lactate concentration, work performance, oxygen consumption, and wincing and withdrawal reactions. On the other hand 24-hour urinary excretion of 17-ketosteroids does not differ from normal. It is not clear whether any of the abnormalities demonstrated so far apply specifically to patients with anxiety neurosis or whether they are the general signs of poor health, chronic illness, or poor state of physical training. . . . Patients with anxiety states have been shown to have increased forearm blood flow at rest. . . . Their skin conductance also shows an increase in spontaneous fluctuations and a decrease in rate of habituation to repeated auditory stimuli.[39] More recent physiological studies do not conclusively confirm the relationship between peripheral physiological testing and anxiety. They do, however, seem to indicate that physiological measurements concerned with direct cerebral function (EEG) correlate better than the peripheral ones do with anxiety.[40,41]

In sum, a relationship between biological and psychological systems has been demonstrated. Although the emphasis was placed on anxiety, the principles outlined are applicable to any emotion. The hope is that this schematic presentation can serve as a prototype of the biological factors which must of necessity be basic in considering any psychiatric condition.

ETIOLOGY

Anxiety neurosis is a common disease. The incidence of this disease in the general population is approximately 5% but many patients with mild forms of anxiety neurosis never consult a physician; therefore, prevalence must be greater.[42] It is claimed that one-third of the adult population suffers from excess anxiety; one-fifth of all patients seen in any day by general practitioners suffers from stress disorders; and 6 to 26% of psychiatric patients are anxiety neurotics.[43]

These figures are rather staggering. Dynamically oriented psychiatrists claim the problem of anxiety is rooted in psychological difficulties. But Lader replies:

> That a third of the populace is affected is no evidence against this argument. However, genetic studies, including twin studies, twins brought up apart, adaptive studies and family surveys show that anxiety states and anxious personalities are strongly determined by hereditary factors. Indeed, in all the flurry of interest in the genetics of schizophrenia and manic-depressive psychosis, it appears that it has been forgotten that the genetic loading in anxiety states is the most pronounced for any functional condition.[44]

Two-thirds of the patients with anxiety are women and the disease mainly affects young adults between the ages of 16 to 40, with an average age of onset in the mid-twenties.[45]

Family studies demonstrate a higher incidence of anxiety neurosis than in the general population, i.e., 15% compared to 5%.[46] One twin study clearly illustrates the role of genetic loading. Monozygotic (MZ) twins showed anxiety symptoms in 65% of the cases studied and dyzygotic twins (DZ) in 13% of the cases studied; while, anxiety neurosis in this study was found in 50% of the MZ twins and in 2½% of the DZ twins. The authors of that study thought that the appearance of anxiety or anxiety neurosis depended upon the interaction of environmental stress and constitution, i.e., the environmental stress factor, when not too severe, elicited adaptive anxiety. But when the stress was severe or hampered by individuals with obsessive compulsive, depressive, or hysterical tendencies, anxiety neurosis (nonadaptive) developed. In that study, the MZ twins showed deviation only along an anxiety axis while the DZ twins showed deviation in other directions.[47] Besides, the dynamic and behaviorist psychiatrists assume that anxiety neurosis is a psychological disease— the result of conflict, faulty development, learning, conditioning, etc. Others propose that anxiety neurosis is a genetic autosomal disease or a pattern relation disease in which the genotype is expressed under stress.

Personality studies on chronic anxiety neurotics are few. Comparing the personalities of patients with chronic anxiety neurosis to those with unipolar and bipolar depression, it was found that the personality of the chronic anxiety neurotic had greater similarity to the unipolar depressive patient than the unipolar to the bipolar or the bipolar to the others. This unexpected finding might have important etiological, diagnostic, and therapeutic implications for all three conditions. In general, the anxiety neurotic was more introverted and less stable, mature, and independent than either depressive group. It was found, however, that the unipolar patient upon recovery was more like the chronic anxiety neurotic than like the recovered bipolar patient. Murray explains:

This is surprising, not so much because of the expected difference between the two classes of depression, but that a recovered or well population should produce scores so much closer to those of an ill one, particularly on factors denoting emotional instability, lack of surgency, timidity and introversion. Certainly the recovered unipolar depressives were significantly less anxiety-prone than the anxiety group, yet they were more so than the recovered bipolar patients. It could be argued that bipolar depressed patients swing into a mildly hypomanic state after recovery from depression and that in this state they assess themselves abnormally. This should have the effect of producing abnormal scores in the opposite direction from the other groups. But, inspection of the scores on those factors where differences were found between the recovered depressed groups showed that the recovered bipolar patients did not score abnormally.[48]

Those similarities between the personalities of chronic anxiety neurotics and unipolar depressives make differential diagnosis very difficult. Further, personality characteristics may be a determining factor in the clinical manifestations, outcome, and type of affective disease that a patient develops.[49]

The patient with an asthenic body type or physical illness is predisposed to anxiety neurosis. Exhaustion, caused by overwork, a debilitating disease, or lack of sleep or rest lowers a patient's ability to cope; hence, anxiety appears. Likewise, the lactate hypothesis stimulated explanations for the cause of anxiety in anxiety neurotics. An acid-base imbalance (alkalosis), hypocalcemia, increase blood lactate and epinephrine level, or a special tissue susceptibility were some of the explanations that were proposed. Are anxiety neurotics susceptible to the effects of lactate?[50] The tacit assumption in the lactate theory of anxiety neurotics, Ackerman claims, is that peripheral physiological alterations are a specific etiological factor for changes in the central mental state (psychic phenomena). And he says:

> One should not be surprised to find it difficult to substantiate a theory in which specific states of peripheral physiologic arousal are proposed as the determining cause of anxiety in anxiety neurotics. First, even a cursory glance at the literature reveals that no study has been able to demonstrate a significant correlation between subjective anxiety states, as measured by validated psychological tests, and specific, consistent alterations in validated autonomic measures.[51]

Ackerman presents data showing that propranolol (Inderal) relieves peripheral autonomic not central, phenomena of anxiety; chlordiazepoxide (Librium) relieves central, not peripheral, manifestations of anxiety; epinephrine infusion in normals could elicit different responses in various individuals; and even lactate infusions when administered by a certain method under specific circumstances could be used as a treatment for patients with long-standing intractable nonsituational anxiety.[52]   Ackerman then goes on to explain that learning, cognition, and conditioning may be critical factors:

> But even though a conditioned phobic response to somatic changes could account for the anxiety precipitated by these stimuli in these patients, it does not account for pathogenesis, psychologically or physiologically, of the primary anxiety neurosis. And it obviously does not fully describe the psychophysiology of anxiety as a mental symptom. Apparently any adequate description of anxiety must be a complex one, accounting for multiple etiologic factors and defining the specific circumstances under which each may be relevant or critical.[53]

The pathophysiology of anxiety and anxiety neurosis remains unexplained.

Psychological viewpoints regarding the nature of anxiety are many. Among others there are: anxiety and the catastrophic reaction (Goldstein); anxiety as a threat to the self-concept (Rogers); unassimilated percepts (McReynolds); related to commitment and awareness (Kierkegaard); a threat to existence as a personality (May).[54,55]   Previously the cognitive theory (appraisal of threat in the absence of an object) was described and listed with the comprehensive theory. Other theories to be briefly outlined are the psychoanalytic or modifications thereof, and the behavioral (learning, conditioning).

Freud's early formulation was that repression created anxiety neurosis. Undischarged sexual energy (libido), he thought, when not satisfied or used appeared as anxiety or symptoms that were anxiety equivalents. He distinguished anxiety neurosis, i.e., the toxic one (the result of undischarged libido) from objective anxiety, i.e., an understandable reaction to anticipated external injury. Objective anxiety is a condition of increased sensory attention or motor tension and could act as a signal leading to proper adaptation or, if adaptation fails, to a repetition of an "old traumatic experience."[56]   This formulation created a mass of contradictions and confusion for Freud and his followers.

To clarify his position Freud divided the mind into superego, ego, and id. Then, he postulated:

> . . . .that the ego is the only seat of anxiety, and that only the ego can produce and feel anxiety. . . .that the three main varieties of anxiety—objective anxiety, neurotic anxiety and moral anxiety—can so easily be related to the three directions in which the ego is dependent, on the external world, on the id and on the super-ego. Our new position, too, has brought to the fore the function of anxiety as a signal indicating the presence of a danger-situation. . . .[57]

Neurotic anxiety, like objective anxiety, became a danger signal; the source of the danger in neurotic anxiety was the patient's sexual and aggressive impulses; hence, Freud reversed his earlier position from repression creating anxiety to anxiety creating repression.[58] Essentially, anxiety neurosis is a complex process. It begins with a partial breakdown of repression of childhood libidinous and aggressive impulses plus concomitant parental prohibitions that were associated with these impulses. The ego responds with anxiety to these perceptions that it interprets as dangerous and an anxiety neurotic process is set in motion. The anxiety is experienced as "free-floating" or "objectless"; thereby, the patient is unconscious of the origin of his suffering. Most modern analysts think that neurosis originates in childhood or even at birth (a developmental concept) but no single developmental stage can be identified as the sole cause of a particular neurosis.[59]

Behaviorism, like psychoanalysis, represents a great number of diverse schools of thought; however, most would agree that all schools are combinations of learning and conditioning theories. Further, behaviorists view anxiety, as well as fear, as a conditioned response to pain; thereby providing a method of associating a mental state with the external stimulus that provoked that response. For example, a person places his finger in a fire and experiences pain (unconditioned response), fear or anxiety (conditioned response). Consequently, upon seeing fire, he feels anxious or more likely frightened (known danger) and thereby avoids placing his finger into the fire. This illustration of the principles of behaviorism is based on the reflex arc. The behaviorist thinks of antecedent conditions (stimulus), response (unconditioned reaction), and associated response (conditioned reaction). A model that Skinner follows when he says:

> Anxiety, as a special case of emotion, should be interpreted with the usual caution. When we speak of the *effects of anxiety*, we imply that the state itself is a cause, but so far as we are concerned here, the term merely classifies behavior. It indicates a set of emotional predispositions attributed to a special kind of circumstance. Any therapeutic attempt to reduce the 'effects of anxiety' must operate upon these circumstances, not upon any intervening state. The middle term is of no functional significance, either in a theoretical analysis or in the practical control of behavior.[60]

Wolpe, although not defining anxiety explicitly, does indicate where it is served:

> Since, almost universally, anxiety is a prominent constituent of neurotic reactions, and since anxiety is served by a primitive (subcortical) level of neural organization, its unlearning can be procured only through processes that involve this primitive level. Neurotic anxiety cannot be overcome purely by intellectual action—logical argument, rational insight—except in the special

case where the unadaptive anxiety depends on a misconception—a conceptual 'wrong equation.'[61]

In sum, behavior theorists use the neurophysiological model and claim that anxiety results from a stimulus response sequence and is an unadaptive habit. Stimuli give rise to anxiety and this anxiety, in turn, begets further anxiety. These conditioned responses perpetuate themselves in a circular manner. This could be viewed as a neurotic biofeedback. Anxiety is "served" at subcortical brain levels; therefore, behaviorists do not feel that neurotic anxiety can be overcome by logical argument or rational insight except where anxiety is caused by intellectual misconceptions.   Learning theorists emphasize environment as the stimulus for anxiety: urbanization, overcrowding, and social insecurity.[62]

Living is stressful.   The stress may be connected with many situations such as frustrations in love and work, marital difficulties, sexual problems, and so on. In addition, the ever-present conflict between duty and desire plus daily routine can lead to tension, which can be cumulative, and ultimately become a factor in producing an anxiety neurosis, or many other medical or psychiatric diseases. Anxiety is a major response to stress.

Stress reaction, like anxiety, is a concept and needs defining. For Selye, a biochemist, stress (stress reaction) " . . . is a biochemical phenomenon, and it is not only independent of anxiety or other mental reactions, but also it doesn't even have to be unpleasant. It's not purely a mental response, and it's not always a response to something bad. A great joy can be just as stressful as a great pain."[63] For students of behavior, Selye's definition of stress is too limited; hence, a broader terminology becomes necessary. Terms such as social stressors, mediating factors, and stress responses are part of the expanded nomenclature. Social stressors refer to life's circumstances (job loss, bereavement, marital difficulties, etc.) that significantly alter the person's social support systems.   These alterations may increase the person's susceptibility to disease; thereby, becoming a precipitating factor. Mediating factors refer to the biopsychological characteristics of the individual that influence his recognition of stressors from any source—social, mental, or physical.   For example, social stressors acting upon an individual with coronary artery disease may be a component in causing a thrombosis, or acting upon a susceptible individual, may precipitate an anxiety attack. Stress responses (which can also be stressors) refer to those responses described as part of the general adaptation syndrome; to specific diseases; and to anxiety, depression, joy, pleasure, guilt, shame, and so forth. Thus this terminology allows an integration of Selye's biochemical level of viewing stress with behavioral scientists' concepts.[64]

What relationship exists between anxiety or anxiety neuroses and the intensity of the stressful situation? One investigator claims a definite progression of components when there is an increase in the intensity of anxiety. He posits the first to appear is the motor component (tension), and in succession, as the intensity of anxiety increases, the following components appear: (1) affective, automatic; (2) secondary symptoms (phobias, obsessions, hypochondriasis, psychosomatic complaints, paranoid delusions, and hallucinations); (3) verbal (increased speech speed). Further, he claims, that as a result of treatment (decreasing the intensity of anxiety) the symptoms disappear in the reverse order of appearance.[65] The implication is that one of the components responsible for the intensity of anxiety and consequent symptomatology is the degree of stressor. Therapy, as it reduces the stressor, is directly related to a reversal of the intensity of anxiety and progression of symptoms.

Kurt Goldstein who worked with brain-injured soldiers noted that they responded with extreme anxiety to even small stressors (and coined the term catastrophic reaction for these stressful situations). He writes:

> Individuals differ as to how much anxiety they can bear. For a patient with a brain injury, the amount is very low; for a child it is greater; and for the creative individual it is still greater. The capacity for bearing anxiety is the manifestation of genuine courage, in which ultimately one is concerned not with the things of the world but with a threat to existence. *In the final analysis courage is nothing but an affirmative answer to the shocks of existence, to the the shocks which it is necessary to bear for the sake of realizing one's own nature.* This form of overcoming anxiety requires the ability to view a single experience within a larger context, i.e., to assume the 'attitude toward the possible,' to maintain freedom of decision regarding different possibilities. This attitude is peculiar to man, and it is because persons with brain injuries have lost it, and have suffered a consequent impairment of freedom, that they are so completely helpless when facing an anxiety situation. They surrender entirely to the anxiety situation, unless they are safeguarded against it through a limitation of their world which reduces their existence to the simplest forms.[66]

DIAGNOSIS

Anxiety neurosis is characterized by a variety of mental states, chemical and physiological manifestations mainly effecting the cardiovascular, respiratory, genitourinary, and central and autonomic nervous systems. The intensity, type, and variability of both psychic and biological manifestations vary from patient to patient, from time to time, and even within the same patient. For example, one patient may be characterized primarily by psychic manifestations, another cardiovascular, another respiratory, another central nervous system, and so forth.

Besides there may be no relationship between the chemical, physiological, and psychological phenomena. Of necessity, then, a number of conditions, usually with recurrent episodes lasting from seconds to days and intermittent periods of remissions are included within this category. These conditions can be divided into acute (panic), subacute (trait), and chronic (state).

Psychological symptoms are described by terms such as nervous, upset, irritable, apprehensive, fearful, or anguish. Physiologically, the patient may complain of shaking, vomiting, fainting, sweating, trembling, dizziness, nausea, grogginess, fatigue, goose pimples, diarrhea, frequent urination, palpitations, increased respiratory rate, shortness of breath, headaches, backaches, muscle spasms, insomnia, fatigue, and vague bodily aches and pains. Practically every bodily system can be affected. Anxiety may be a factor in such diseases as obesity, hypertension, asthma, irritable colon, peptic ulcer, migraine headaches, and eczema anxiety. Chemical changes include increases in glucose, adrenalin, hydrocorticosteroids, red blood cells, and so forth.

Acute anxiety is a terrifying panic in which the autonomic nervous system is overstimulated accompanied by sweating, tremors, fast heartbeat, dyspnea, uncontrolled thought, poor rapid judgments, and impulsive irrational behavior. Duration of an attack can vary from a few moments to an hour. Subacute anxiety (anxiety trait) is expressed and controlled through personality traits such as timidity, apprehensiveness, and overconscientiousness. The tension in this type is not intolerable and may be a lifelong illness for which a physician is never consulted. Chronic anxiety (state) shows some of the personality features of the subacute type—insecurity, apprehensiveness, doubt regarding ability to achieve, excessive self-blame for failures, unnecessary tensions and worries, magnification of difficulties, and anticipation of the worst. Patients also have other characteristics. They are dependent, unstable, immature, and need constant advice and support in their everyday lives. Without direction they are less capable of assuming responsibility, and this results in excessive demands being made upon certain key figures. An example of this is the patient who insists that his wife go to bed at the same time he does. There are bodily complaints for which no organic basis can be found and exaggerated importance is given to visceral functions. Tension shows itself in an increase of muscle tone, hand tremors, strained face, furrowed brow, picking at the fingers, pacing up and down, and repetitious unpleasant movements such as stereotyped tics and grimaces. They cannot fall asleep; suffer from restless sleep, dreams, and nightmares; and arise early in the morning. For some, work is affected: they complain of memory loss, an inability to concentrate, loss of interest, and lack of pleasure. Sexual frigidity is common—amenorrhea or excessive bleeding may develop in the female, and in the male, impotence. The course may vary as one patient may suffer one or two acute attacks or panics in a lifetime while another may suffer innumerable attacks.[67]

Three stages, arbitrarily distinguished in the anxiety neurosis, follow the course of Selye's general adaptation syndrome. The first is alarm reaction or panic in which overresponse to stressors occurs and physiological phenomena predominate. During this stage, hysterical symptoms give relief to the patient; but if these symptoms do not develop and the stresses continue the second stage may appear—the state of resistance or established tension. Here physiological manifestations remain prominent but the patient is tense, irritable, fatigued, and unhappy. Remissions and exacerbations of panic can occur; however, the more determined patient continues to struggle and he maintains his usual life-style. As time passes the clinical features of anxiety become less prominent and the symptoms of fatigue, depression, emotional lability, and weight loss become dominant. Irritability is marked, sleep is disturbed, work productivity diminishes, and relationships are disturbed. The patient cries easily, and is moved to tears by sad stories, sentimental films, and songs. The third stage—exhaustion—cannot be differentiated from states of depression with anxiety. Its manifestations are chronic invalidism or an organ neurosis, that is, the patient shows special concern for such physical symptoms as palpitations, breathlessness, or headaches and becomes convinced that he is suffering from an organic disease. Constant bodily preoccupation, inability to work, or even to stay married can be the advanced manifestations of anxiety neurosis and unfortunately frequently pass unrecognized.[68,69]

DIFFERENTIAL DIAGNOSIS

The unitary theory of disease follows the stages of anxiety neurosis and the entity theory denies the validity of any such progression. Accordingly, one of the most controversial nosological issues revolves around whether anxiety neurosis and depressive neurosis are distinguishable diseases.[70,71] Are they two distinct neurotic affective disorders or are they variations of one disorder? Whatever answer the future provides, the present problem is to develop criteria that differentiate these conditions since therapeutic decisions are predicated on proper diagnosis.

The personality of the anxiety neurotic, as noted above, is less extroverted, stable, mature, and independent than the depressive neurotic. Symptomatology has been analyzed by researchers along two variables—intensity and configuration. Using multivariate statistical techniques, one group of researchers reported that patients in the depressive group were more severely impaired on all factor scale dimensions except the somatization scale (pain in chest, heavy feelings in arms and legs) than the patients in the anxiety group. Interestingly enough patients in the anxiety group did not score higher on the anxiety factor than those in the depressive group, while patients in the depressive group did score higher on the depressive factor than those in the anxiety group.[72]

Symptomatology, upon which the clinician usually bases his diagnosis, places emphasis upon affective, motor, and physiological components. Marks, however, says:

> When anxiety is prominent and other depressive features are slight it can be difficult to know whether a given patient has a depressive illness or an anxiety state. Of a series of patients diagnosed as anxiety states 19 percent were subsequently re-labeled as depressives. The distinction might have some prognostic import. Walker studied 111 outpatients in whom free-floating anxiety was the cardinal symptom and classified them according to outcome. They were treated by reassurance and amyobarbitone only. A group of 24 of these patients with good outcomes were isolated: these patients were thought to be best described as depressives with episodic anxiety. Such patients had no precipitant for their illness and had minor depressive features such as gloomy forebodings, inability to plan, fears of illness and death, and self reproach.[73]

A clue may be found in biographical data in which past episodes of depression, or mania existed in either the patient or his family. Research, using physiological measurements, revealed that forearm blood flow in patients with anxiety neurosis, when placed under conditions of stress, fell with repetition of the stressor; conversely, forearm blood flow rose in depressed patients. There is, however, a suggestion that depressives show a fall in forearm blood flow under stressors, anxiety neurotics show an increase. These paradoxical results, although pointing to flight-freeze patterns of response to stress, further emphasize the need for clear delineation of diagnostic groups.[74] In sum, for the practicing clinician, the diagnosis of anxiety versus depression boils down to his experience and judgment.

Since anxiety phenomena have so much variety, anxiety neurosis must be differentiated from all other psychiatric diseases. Phobias are associated either with specific circumstances or situations in which the patient anticipates contact with phobic objects. Some patients with anxiety neurosis, however, also have increased symptomatology under certain circumstances. On the other hand, some agoraphobics suffer from increased anxiety even when not in the phobic situation. Obsessive compulsive patients have episodic periods of anxiety and depression, and contrary to the general view, hysterical patients can also have pronounced anxiety symptoms. Anxiety symptoms may not only be prodromal to schizophrenia but can also be part of the disease. With most other mental diseases, the overall picture can be apparent enough so that a primary diagnosis is possible.

Anxiety neurosis must be differentiated from many organic diseases. The endocrine system is important in this regard. Hyperthyroidism is characterized by physiological symptoms of anxiety but the symptoms are not as episodic. In advanced cases exophthalmos, widening of palpebral fissure, eyelid lag, enlargement of thyroid and other distinguishing features may be present. Laboratory tests such as T_3, T_4, protein bound iodine, thyroid scan, cholesterol level and basal metabolic rate are abnormal. Acute hyperthyroidism can even be precipitated by an intense emotional experience. Hyperinsulinism, either idiopathic or due to an islet cell tumor of the pancreas, can cause sweats, tremors, weakness, dizziness, and disturbances of consciousness. The same symptoms can occur with any body disturbance which causes hypoglycemia, e.g., starvation. Pheochromocytoma and Addison's disease offer similar diagnostic challenges. Neurological diseases such as temporal lobe and petit mal epilepsy, postconcussion syndrome, Parkinsonism, senility, carotid sinus syndrome, diencephalic lesions, cerebellar and semicircular canal disturbances give rise to symptoms similar to anxiety. Other systemic diseases which must be differentiated from anxiety are gastrointestinal symptoms simulating peptic ulcer, enteritis, or colitis; cardiac symptoms with flushing, pounding pulse, tachycardia, and fainting which are compatible with valvular, muscle, or vascular lesions of the heart. Such drugs as caffeine, alcohol, amphetamine, LSD, mescaline, withdrawal from addictive drugs, and the like can cause reactions similar to and associated with anxiety attacks. The list of conditions which must be considered when differentiating anxiety can be endless but enough has already been said to illustrate the complexity of the differential diagnostic problem.[75-77]

COURSE AND PROGNOSIS

Anxiety neurosis can run the entire gamut from gradually disappearing without serious sequelae in a fairly short span of time (e.g., acute anxiety panic) to a state so severe and intractable that the patient is partially or completely disabled. All gradations exist between these two cases. Although information regarding prognosis is limited and firm evidence is lacking, investigators estimate that from 41 to 59% recover or improve.[78] A five-year follow-up study showed that women have a more favorable outcome than men; men who are under 30 at the time of initial contact with a psychiatrist have a better outcome than older men while women showed no such correlation; the shorter the duration of illness prior to consultation, the better the prognosis; "normal" premorbid personality showed better outcome than "abnormal" personality; and shifts in symptomatology, e.g., gastrointestinal to cardiovascular or vice versa, reflect increased chronicity.[79] However, these criteria provide only an imprecise basis for prediction. An indication of the severity of an anxiety state may be afforded by the somatic manifestations. When marked, the actual disability is likely to be considerable.[80]

TREATMENT

Proper evaluation is the initial step to adequate treatment. Because of the innumerable physical illnesses that may cause anxiety symptoms, evaluation in all cases must include physical and laboratory examinations. In patients suffering from panic, relief from symptoms is an urgent priority. First, the cause of panic must be determined. If the cause is due to situational stress, then the patient must be removed from the disturbing environment. Hospitalization may be necessary, but more often than not, alternate solutions can be found. Second, the patient must be sedated. Propanediols, benzodiazepines, or barbiturates can help during waking hours and hypnotic drugs can facilitate sleep. Early, vigorous treatment is important. Simultaneously, psychotherapy should begin. At first supportive measures should be offered such as suggestion, advice, education, reeducation, explanation, and later, if indicated, intensive forms of psychotherapy. The importance of these initial steps is to prevent recurrent attacks and chronicity.

Subacute forms require a similar program of treatment with less emphasis on drugs and rest and more on psychotherapy and establishing a healthful way of life—a suitable balance of work, family life, exercise, and interpersonal relationships. In subacute anxiety neurosis, resolution of personality and psychological problems is a prime consideration which may necessitate long-term psychotherapy.

Chronic cases have two major considerations: (1) anxiety symptoms and (2) psychological and personality problems. A common sense approach strives towards whatever is practical. Environmental readjustments involve work, family, and a healthy balance in everyday life activities. Adequate sleep, proper diet, and exercise are recommended. Psychotherapy should be an ongoing process from the beginning to the end of treatment. In this manner symptoms of anxiety and intrapsychic and interpersonal problems may be resolved.

Drugs are important in the treatment of anxiety neurosis. Since medication may be used for a prolonged time, the addictive, habituation, and tolerance potential of each drug should be kept in mind. The least possible drug dosage should be used for the shortest period of time. Barbiturates, meprobamates, and benzodiazepines are the drugs used most frequently. The choice of drug and type and time of dosage depends upon the patient's response. A major problem with the antianxiety drugs is drowsiness—the patient must be warned about dangerous occupations or driving a car. If these drugs fail or addiction becomes a concern, the prescription may be changed to a phenothiazine. These are nonaddictive and do not develop increased tolerance. Diphenylmethane antihistamines can also be used as antianxiety agents. A beta adrenergic blocking agent, often used in treating certain heart diseases and hypertension, can also decrease anxiety by blocking the physiological component of anxiety. The tricyclic antidepressants have sedative as well as antidepressive properties. Those with the greatest sedative effects are Tofranil (imipramine), Elavil (amitriptyline), and Sinequan or Adapin (doxepin). In general, any of these classes of drugs may be used alone or in combination. When more than one drug is used, however, the physician should take into consideration synergistic reactions. The dose should maximize relief from symptoms and minimize daytime sedation.[81-85]

Table 4-1 taken from Hollister[86] summarizes the different classes of drugs and their effects. Certain advantages and disadvantages of each class should be apparent and the physician should decide which property is most desired.

TABLE 4-1 Pharmacological Properties of Antianxiety Drugs*

	Pheno-barbital	Mepro-bamate	Benzo-diazepines	Diphenyl-methanes	Pheno-thiazines	Tricyclics
Antianxiety/sedative ratio	+	++	++	±	±	±
Muscle relaxation	±	++	+++	0	–	0
Anticonvulsant action	+++	++	+++	–	–	–
Duration of action	+++	+	+++	+	++	++
Tolerance	++	+++	+	0	0	0
Habituation	±	+++	±	0	0	0
Physical dependence	+	+++	+	0	0	0
Disturbed sleep pattern	++	++	±	++	++	++
Potential suicide use	++	+++	0	++	0	+++

*Signs indicate degree of probability: (– –) opposite effect; (0) none; (±) minimal; (+) slight; (++) moderate; and (+++) great.

Table 4-2 lists the class, generic name, trade name, and usual daily dosage of the various drugs used in the treatment of anxiety.[87,88]

TABLE 4-2 Antianxiety Agents and Daily Adult Dose Range

Drug Class	Generic Name	Trade Name	Daily Adult Dose Range (mg/day)
Barbiturates	Phenobarbital	Eskabarb } Luminal }	30-100
	Butabarbital	Stental } Butisol }	45-120
Benzodiazepines	Chlordiazepoxide	Librium	15-30
	Diazepam	Valium	5-60
	Oxazepam	Serax	30-120

TABLE 4-2 Antianxiety Agents and Daily Adult Dose Range (Con't)

Drug Class	Generic Name	Trade Name	Daily Adult Dose Range (mg/day)
Propanediols	Meprobamate	Equanil ⎱ Miltown ⎰	800-3200
	Tybamate	Solacen	750-3000
Phenothiazines	Trifluoperazine	Stelazine	4-30
	Fluphenazine	Prolixin	3-15
	Perphenazine	Trilafon	4-48
	Prochlorperazine	Compazine	15-75
Betaadrenergic blocking agent	Propranolol	Inderal	10-40
Diphenylmethane antihistaminics	Hydroxyzine	Atarax ⎱ Vistaril ⎰	75-400
	Diphenyldramine	Benadryl	50-200
Tricyclics	Imipramine Amitriptyline	Tofranil ⎱ Elavil ⎰	25-200
	Doxepin	Sinequan ⎱ Adapin ⎰	10-75

Psychotherapy varies depending on the individual case. It may consist of short weekly sessions lasting for several months or as in psychoanalysis—three to five sessions per week for several years. Prolonged treatment is used in cases where personality and psychological factors are major contributors to the neurosis, and some very basic internal changes should, if possible, be made. Other forms of psychotherapy such as family or group sessions may help in some cases, but maximum benefit is usually derived in conjunction with individual therapy.

Behavior therapy using desensitization by reciprocal inhibition or flooding may help. Hypnosis, relaxation, and biofeedback techniques can be tried. If all else fails, however, psychosurgery may be suggested. This is a drastic procedure and, fortunately, is rarely considered.[89,90]

REFERENCES

1. Hine, F.R., Pfeiffer, E., et al., *Behavioral Science: A Selective View.* Boston: Little, Brown, 1972, p. 41.
2. Lazarus, R.S. and Averill, J.R., "Emotion and cognition: With special reference to anxiety," in *Anxiety: Current Trends in Theory and Research,* vol. 2 (edited by Spielberger, C.D.). New York: Academic, 1972, pp. 242-244.
3. Ibid., p. 244.
4. Jaspers, K., *General Psychopathology* (transl. by Hoenig, J. and Hamilton, M.). Chicago: Univ. Chicago Press, 1963, pp. 108-110.
5. Macquarrie, J., *Existentialism.* Baltimore: Penguin, 1972, pp. 118-127.
6. Lazarus, R.S. and Averill, J.R., op. cit., pp. 247-251.
7. Ibid., pp. 260-262.
8. Lesse, S., Psychiatric symptoms in relationship to the intensity of anxiety. *Psychother. Psychosom.* **23**:94-96 (1974).

9. Lazarus, R.S. and Averill, J.R., op. cit., pp. 253–258.
10. Rycroft, C., *Anxiety and Neurosis.* Baltimore: Penguin, 1968, p. 18.
11. Endler, N., "A person–situation interaction model for anxiety," in *Stress and Anxiety,* vol. 1 (edited by Spielberger, C.D., and Sarason, I.G.). New York: Wiley, 1975, pp. 148–151.
12. Spielberger, C.D., "Conceptual and methodological issues in anxiety research," in *Anxiety: Current Trends in Theory and Research,* vol. 2 (edited by Spielberger, C.D.). New York: Academic, 1972, pp. 491–492.
13. Woodruff, Jr., R.A., Goodwin, D.W. and Guze, S.B., *Psychiatric Diagnosis.* New York: Oxford University Press, 1974, p. 45.
14. Macquarrie, J., op. cit., pp. 127–132.
15. Marks, I. and Lader, M., Anxiety states (anxiety neurosis): A review. *J. Nerv. Ment. Dis.* **156**(1):5 (1973).
16. Pitts, F.H., The biochemistry of anxiety. *Scientific American* **220**:69–70 (1969).
17. Bernard, C., *An Introduction to the Study of Experimental Medicine* (transl. by Greene, H.C.). New York: Henry Schuman, 1949.
18. Darwin, C., *The Expression of the Emotions in Man and Animals.* London: J. Murray, 1892.
19. James, W., *The Principles of Psychology,* vol. 2. New York: Holt, 1890, p. 449.
20. Heidbreder, E., *Seven Psychologies.* New York: Appleton-Century-Crofts, 1933, pp. 201–233.
21. Sherrington, C.S., *Integrative Action of the Nervous System.* London: Constable, 1906.
22. Cannon, W.B., *The Wisdom of the Body.* New York: Norton, 1932.
23. Morgan, C.T., *Physiological Psychology.* New York: McGraw-Hill, 1943, p. 356.
24. Prusoff, B. and Klerman, G.L., Differentiating depressed from anxious neurotic outpatients. *Arch. Gen. Psychiatry* **30**:302–309 (1974).
25. Durell, J., "Introduction," in *Biological Psychiatry,* (edited by Mendels, J.). New York: Wiley, 1973, p. 1.
26. Hine, F.R., Pfeiffer, E., et al., op. cit., pp. 11–16.
27. Snyder, S.H., *Madness and the Brain.* New York: McGraw-Hill, 1975, pp. 221–237.
28. Ibid., pp. 255–263.
29. Gellhorn, E., The neurophysiological basis of anxiety: A hypothesis. *Persp. Biol. Med.* **8**:488–515 (1965).
30. Mason, J.W., Organization of psychoendocrine responses. *Psychosom. Med.* **30**:565 (1968).
31. Selye, H., *The Stress of Life.* New York: McGraw-Hill, 1956.
32. Sodeman, W. and Sodeman, Jr., W., *Pathologic Physiology: Mechanisms of Disease.* Philadelphia: Saunders, 1968, pp. 142–143.
33. Ibid., pp. 136–150.
34. Warburton, D.M., Modern biochemical concepts of anxiety: Implications for psychopharmacological treatment. *Int. Pharmacopsychiatry* **9**:189–205 (1974).
35. Wolf, S., "Towards a physiological concept of anxiety," in *Anxiety: The Ubiquitous Symptom* (edited by Hollister, L.E.). New York: Medcom, 1972, pp. 22–25.
36. Beeson, P.B. and McDermott, W., *Cecil-Loeb Textbook of Medicine.* Philadelphia: Saunders, 1971.
37. Pitts, F.H., op. cit., pp. 71–75.
38. Grosz, H.J. and Farmer, B.B., Pitts and McClure's lactate-anxiety study revisited. *Brit. J. Psychiatry* **120**:415–418 (1972).
39. Marks, I. and Lader, M., op. cit., p. 13.

40. Tyrer, P.J. and Lader, M.H., Central and peripheral correlates of anxiety: A comparative study. *J. Nerv. Ment. Dis.* **162**(2):99-104 (1976).
41. Greer, S., Ramsay, I. and Bagley, C., Neurotic and thyrotoxic anxiety: Clinical, psychological and physiological measurements. *Brit. J. Psychiatry* **122**:549-554 (1973).
42. Clancy, J. and Noyes, Jr., R., Anxiety neurosis: A disease for the medical model. *Psychosomatics* **17**(2):90-93 (1976).
43. Lader, M., "The nature of clinical anxiety in modern society," in *Stress and Anxiety*, vol. 1 (edited by Spielberger, C.D. and Sarason, I.G.). New York: Wiley, 1975, pp. 3-26.
44. Ibid., p. 24.
45. Marks, I. and Lader, M., op. cit., pp. 6-7.
46. Woodruff, Jr., R.A., Goodwin, D.W. and Guze, S.B., *Psychiatric Diagnosis.* New York: Oxford University Press, 1974, pp. 52-53.
47. Slater, E. and Cowie, V., *The Genetics of Mental Disorders.* New York: Oxford University Press, 1971, pp. 104-105.
48. Murray, L.G. and Blackburn, I.M., Personality differences in patients with depressive illness and anxiety neurosis. *Acta. Psychiat. Scand.* **50**:189-190 (1974).
49. Ibid., p. 190.
50. Ackerman, S.H. and Sachar, E.J., The lactate theory of anxiety: A review and re-evaluation. *Psychosom. Med.* **36**(1):69-72 (1974).
51. Ibid., p. 74.
52. Ibid., pp. 75-77.
53. Ibid., p. 78.
54. Epstein, S., "The nature of anxiety with emphasis upon its relation to expectancy," in *Anxiety: Current Trends in Theory and Research*, vol. 2 (edited by Spielberger, C.D.). New York: Academic, 1972, pp. 291-337.
55. Beck, A.T., Laude, R. and Bohnert, M., Ideational components of anxiety neurosis. *Arch. Gen. Psychiatry* **31**:319-325 (1974).
56. Freud, S., *New Introductory Lectures on Psycho-Analysis.* New York: Norton, 1933, p. 114.
57. Ibid., pp. 118-119.
58. Ibid., p. 120.
59. Rycroft, C., op. cit., pp. 26-32.
60. Skinner, B.F., *Science and Human Behavior.* New York: Free Press, 1953, pp. 180-181.
61. Wolpe, J., *The Practice of Behavior Therapy*, 2nd ed. New York: Pergamon, 1973, p. 25.
62. Ibid., pp. 1-26.
63. Selye, H., "Stress: Anxiety's breeding ground," in *Anxiety: The Ubiquitous Symptom* (edited by Hollister, L.E.). New York: Medcom, 1972, p. 15.
64. Rabkin, J.G. and Struening, E.L., Life events, stress, and illness. *Science* **194**(4269): 1013-1020 (1976).
65. Lesse, S., op. cit., pp. 97-99.
66. Goldstein, K., *Human Nature in the Light of Psychopathology.* New York: Schocken Books, 1963, pp. 113-114.
67. Marks, I. and Lader, M., op. cit., pp. 10-13.
68. Curran, D., Partridge, M. and Storey, P., *Psychological Medicine: An Introduction to Psychiatry*, 7th ed. Edinburgh: Churchill Livingstone, 1972, pp. 241-243.
69. Cammer, L., Antidepressants as a prophylaxis against depression in the obsessive compulsive person. *Psychosomatics* **14**:201-202 (1973).

70. Derogatis, L.R., Lipman, R.S., Covi, L. and Rickels, K., Factorial invariance of symptom dimensions in anxious and depressive neuroses. *Arch. Gen. Psychiatry* **27**:659–665 (1972).
71. Prusoff, B. and Klerman, G., op. cit., p. 308.
72. Ibid., pp. 307–308.
73. Marks, I. and Lader, M., op. cit., p. 4.
74. Brierley, H. and Jamieson, R., Anomalous stress reactions in patients suffering from depression and anxiety. *J. Neuro. Neurosurg. Psychiatry* **37**:455–462 (1974).
75. Masserman, J., *Psychiatric Syndromes and Modes of Therapy.* New York: Stratton Intercontinental Medical Book Corp., 1974, pp. 37–39.
76. Greden, J.F., Anxiety or caffeinism: A diagnostic dilemma. *Amer. J. Psychiatry* **131**(10):1089–1092 (1974).
77. Winstead, D.K., Coffee consumption among psychiatric inpatients. *Amer. J. Psychiatry* **133**(12):1447–1459 (1976).
78. Greer, S., "The prognosis of anxiety states," in *Studies of Anxiety* (edited by Lader, M.H.). London: Royal Medico-Psychological Association, 1969, pp. 151–157.
79. Noyes, R. and Clancy, J., Anxiety neurosis: a 5-year follow-up. *J. Nerv. Ment. Dis.* **162**(3):200–205 (1976).
80. Curran, D., Partridge, M. and Storey, P., op. cit., p. 247.
81. Hollister, L., Uses of psychotherapeutic drugs. *Ann. Int. Med.* **79**(1):88–98 (1973).
82. Friend, D.G., Practical approach to anxiety. *Drug Therapy* **4**:38–46 (Dec. 1974).
83. Kelly, D., Treatment of anxiety. *Brit. J. Clin. Pract.* **26**(11):505–508 (1972).
84. Blackwell, B., Rational drug use in the management of anxiety. *Rational Drug Therapy* **9**(6):1–7 (1975).
85. Honigfeld, G. and Howard, A., *Psychiatric Drugs.* New York: Academic, 1973, pp. 39–45.
86. Hollister, L., op. cit., p. 90.
87. Ibid., p. 92.
88. Honigfeld, G. and Howard, A., op. cit., pp. 39–45.
89. Kelly, D., op. cit., p. 508.
90. Kelly, D., Progress in anxiety states. *Proc. Roy. Soc. Med.* **66**:252–255 (1973).

5
HYSTERICAL NEUROSIS

The controversy surrounding hysteria begins with its very definition and extends to its etiology, underlying mechanism, course, prognosis, and treatment. Practically every clinical manifestation has been associated with this neurosis. It is one of the most abused, misused, and confused diagnoses in psychiatry. The problem is compounded by loose usage of the term in lay and medical circles, and by the network of pejorative meaning it sometimes assumes in the mind of the practitioner. Because these factors prevent the physician from conducting a comprehensive examination, an urgent need exists to define and to understand hysteria in its proper perspective and to use this knowledge to the patient's advantage.

Unfortunately, psychiatrists contribute to the confusion by eschewing diagnostic criteria for personal preferences,[1] by proposing Briquet's syndrome as a synonym,[2] or by concluding that hysteria is a delusion, a trap, and a nonexistent entity.[3] Hysteria is that entity in which the signs and symptoms are so diverse that they can mimic almost any known disease. However, a diagnosis of hysteria cannot automatically be assumed merely because an organic etiology cannot be discerned. Exclusion alone should not be a basis for diagnosis; there must be positive indications. The dilemma is, what criteria should the psychiatrist follow?

In an attempt to reduce confusion and pejorative connotations regarding hysteria, certain psychiatrists advocate the eponym "Briquet's syndrome" as a synonym. Briquet's syndrome is a polysymptomatic disorder that has specific criteria for diagnosis. Fifty-nine symptoms are divided into ten groups. These groups include symptoms typical of conversion, depression, sexual difficulties, and so forth. For an acceptable diagnosis the patient must have a history of at least 25 medically unexplained symptoms during his or her lifetime and these symptoms must be so distributed that they fit into at least nine groups. Further, these patients must have a complicated or dramatic medical history that began before they reached the age of 35. Only on the basis of these criteria can a patient be diagnosed as having Briquet's syndrome (hysteria).[4] These guidelines eliminate considerations of borderline and transitional states, include symptoms experienced by most people, and exclude those patients with a single acute dissociative or conversion experience as well as those in older age groups.

Briquet's syndrome places emphasis on symptoms, course, and family background. It is a prolonged illness that can last for decades, has a higher incidence in females than males, and is associated with a 25% concordance in first degree female relatives, while male relatives show an increase in sociopathy and alcoholism.[5-8] Using computers, a screening interview has been developed which is purported to help establish the diagnosis of Briquet's syndrome.[9] This is certainly an admirable piece of work and represents a great deal of effort. However, do the symptom cluster and other criteria which are used to diagnose Briquet's syndrome conform to clinical experience? Is Briquet's syndrome really the same disease entity as hysteria? Why use this eponym when many authors both before and since Paul Briquet (1796-1881) have written extensively on hysteria? There are psychiatrists who disregard the work because they consider Briquet's syndrome as a narrowly defined entity which may be a part of hysteria, or because they feel that too much stress is placed on organic-genetic aspects and not enough on psychodynamic factors.[10-14]

The hysterical neurosis is characterized by disorders of sensation, perception, motor function, memory, and consciousness. It is divided into two categories: (1) hysterical neurosis, conversion type, involves the special senses or voluntary nervous system and produces such symptoms as blindness, deafness, anosmia, anesthesias, paralysis, ataxias, akinesias, and dyskinesias; (2) hysterical neurosis, dissociative type, induces an altered state of consciousness or identity, resulting in amnesia, somnambulism, fugue, and multiple personality. Several features are cardinal; to quote Ludwig:

1. Any of the affected functions is potentially capable of being influenced by volitional control.
2. The symptoms of phenomena observed do not reflect known anatomical functions, do not correspond to known neurological pathways or segmental distributions, and do not follow known principles of neurophysiologic response patterns. In this regard, we may make the reasonable inference that the nature of the particular hysterical dysfunction tends to reflect the patient's notion or concept of what such a dysfunction should be.
3. The magnitude or extent of the disability tends not to interfere severely with the preservation of health, to lead to associated physical harm, or to interfere with the maintenance of various survival functions.
4. There is a disturbance of affect, known as *la belle indifférence*, which pertains to a disproportionate lack of concern in relationship to the disabling nature of the symptoms. In many patients, the display of

affect has an almost "organic" quality and resembles that observed in patients with multiple sclerosis or parietal lobe anosognosia. While this affectual state may pervade all patient behavior, it is possible for patients to react with appropriate emotional concern in nonsymptom related areas.

5. Patients with hysteria tend to be highly susceptible to external suggestion. The criterial faculties of the patient seem suspended, and the presentation of an idea, oftentimes absurd, may be accepted automatically and without contradiction.   With appropriate and subtle suggestion, the symptom may be transferred from one area to another, transformed into a different symptom, or eliminated for variable periods of time.

Naturally, like any other psychiatric disorder, it is unlikely that any given hysteria patient will display all of these textbook features. In the formulation of a diagnosis, the clinician will have to make allowances for interindividual variability, the number of these cardinal characteristics present, and the degree to which they are manifested.[15]

Researchers have reported interesting work. Patients with a normal medical background, adequate occupational history, no sexual difficulties, but with symptoms of anxiety, mood disturbance, and conversion symptoms which remitted within one week were investigated. These patients were compared to another group that had sought treatment for organ system symptoms; failed to adjust adequately in sexual, occupational, and interpersonal spheres; suffered from conversion symptoms, anxiety, and depression. Conversion symptoms in this latter group lasted longer than one month in all but one patient.   Both groups were studied by psychiatric interview, psychological testing, and physiological measurements. The significant variable between the groups was the physiological findings. Habituation of heart rate, skin resistance, and electromyelogram to a series of sounds were normal in the first group; but in the group with a history of illness and maladjustments none of the patients was able to habituate to the sound stimulus that was presented 20 times. The authors think that two groups of patients with conversion symptoms should be delineated: (1) acute hysteria for a transient disorder and (2) chronic hysteria that is somewhat similar to but not the same as Briquet's syndrome.[16]

CONSCIOUSNESS AND SELF

Hysteria and depersonalization, perhaps more than other neuroses, raise the issue of self or identity. In these neuroses an integrated self is somehow or other distorted, misinterpreted, or even completely lost; hence, the need to elaborate a concept of self and consciousness. One must have intact perceptual, emotional, ideational, intellectual, and volitional systems in order to be able to experience life as real. A deficit in any one or combination of these systems would lead to disturbances in the patient's ability to conceptualize self or to focus his consciousness.

It is consciousness which provides the means with which the individual defines self and relates that self to the outside world. Yet consciousness is not clearly definable or understood, but responds to internal bodily stimuli and is cognizant of the ambient social world. For conscious activity to exist the body requires an adequate blood supply. The blood must be within certain limits of acid and base balance, and contain quantities of metabolites, sugar, oxygen, and carbon dioxide. Conscious activity and total body status are interdependent. Consciousness is not a "thing" or a static entity but a function or process of the entire body. The brain is the central organ but not the only organ concerned with consciousness.

Dualistic mind-body misconceptions should be discarded. The functional approach recognizes varying *degrees* of sensation, perception, introspection, wakefulness, sleepiness, appreciation of self and the social world, and it does not imply that each of these states exists by itself. What it points to is that these are partial functions of the biopsychosocial processes which lack a total descriptive terminology or adequate conceptual framework.

Biologists regard each and every organism as a self. The self exists in a reciprocal relationship with the environment. It takes matter from the outside, transforms the matter into energy, and uses the energy for its own purposes. The self grows, reproduces, and changes constantly from conception to death.[17]

For psychologists, philosophers, and psychiatrists the self includes everything within the total framework of experience. George Herbert Mead, the social psychologist, considers the self to be different from the physiological organism proper and to arise from social experience and activity. He also stresses that self develops constantly and results from the relationships between each individual organism and its environment.[18] Although biologists emphasize genetics and heredity while psychologists emphasize experience and environment, the bond of agreement between both is that organism and self are inseparable and always in a state of flux or change. In this sense the self, like consciousness, is not a thing or substance but a process, a function in which there is a fluidity and diversity of its constituent parts. The philosopher, John Dewey says:

> There are complex, unstable, opposing attitudes, habits, impulses which gradually come to terms with one another, and assume a certain consistency of configuration, even though only by means of a distribution of inconsistencies which keeps them in water-tight compartments, giving them separate turns or tricks in action.[19]

When that aspect of self which provides a sense of continuity through time, space, and events is faulty, as in hysteria and depersonalization neuroses, the unifying core that brings about meaning and organization is disturbed. The patient's sense of stability is lost and his knowledge of self is gone. There is no "I," "me," "you," or "not I." The self-concept also involves observing oneself as an object and includes judgment of attributes, values, and attitudes. Since the patient loses contact with self, he cannot observe or evaluate himself. Accordingly, he can deny responsibility for his behavior. He claims a lack of control or that this behavior was not "like him." For example, the previously unaggressive individual, now behaving in an aggressive and hostile manner, will deny such behavior to be really his.   The normal person may also dissociate or depersonalize and behave in unaccustomed ways under conditions of fatigue, sensory deprivation, alcoholic intoxication, or hypnagogic states. Afterwards he perceives such behavior as strange.

In depersonalization experiences, as distinguished from dissociation and other mental conditions, the patient's symptoms are consciously disturbing.   One should note, however, that depersonalization and dissociation phenomena can occur in association with other mental diseases and that the diagnosis of hysterical or depersonalization neuroses is reserved for situations in which the condition is not part of some other mental disease. Besides, in depersonalization the patient seems like a puppet to himself: psychic life, thoughts, memories seem "as if" they are not his own. Yet he knows quite well that these are part and parcel of himself or his environment.

Not only is the subjective experience of self disturbed in depersonalization and hysterical phenomena, but the ability to be authentic is also lost. Authenticity is a state of existence in which the individual molds himself into his own image and differentiates his personal conscience from his family, community, or church. He develops a moral sense which may or may not coincide with the social institutions in which he lives. With self and authenticity disturbed, it follows that the individual's ability to make choices is impaired. Without this ability he cannot have personal freedom which requires the capacity to execute feelings, intellect, thoughts, or will. In effect, without a sense of self (identity) and authenticity, the patient has lost the ability to find meaning.[20, 21]

The psychiatrist Pierre Janet recognized that mental activities and events can take place outside of personal awareness. This unaware aspect of self he called subconscious.   Janet further postulated concepts of dissociation, of consciousness, and of self-functioning on a hierarchy of different levels— in which each level can influence thoughts, feelings, and behavior. Janet characterized hysteria as a state with a disintegration of mental synthesis, a reduction in the field of consciousness and capacity for attention, a disorder of memory, and an alteration in sensation, perception, and motor activity.[22] Freud developed the concept of unconscious defense mechanisms and with Joseph Breuer, in 1892, coined the term "conversion" for physical symptoms that have psychic origins.[23] To Jaspers, hysterical phenomena are a break in the labile motility of conscious and unconscious psychic life. In hysteria the psychic life becomes immobile and a portion of it becomes split or dissociated from the main body of the self. This split portion assumes an independent existence, is no longer under conscious control, and contrasts to what happens in normal individuals where experience finds its way into conscious self.[24]

Consensus is lacking regarding the meaning of a changed concept of self and consciousness in the hysterical neurotic. However, dissociation and alienation from reality are recognized symptoms of the disease, and until the patient can "feel" his connection with self and the outside, he cannot achieve health.

HISTORY

Hysteria has stimulated more discussion and articles than perhaps any other psychological illness. It is, however, partially the history of the disease and its etymologic association with women which intensifies its fascination.

Plato, in *Timaeus*, named the disease hysteria. The word means uterus and he thought that the uterus could wander out of the pelvis with hysterical symptoms occurring wherever the womb might lodge.[25] The idea probably came from the ancient Egyptians who recommended that treatment for the disorder be directed at the organ. They made attempts to lure or drive the womb back into its proper place. Since it was assumed to be in another part of the body, they would place sweet smelling substances on the lower part and foul smelling or foul tasting materials on or into the upper part to drive the uterus back into its proper position. The Greeks thought globus hystericus was due to uterine pressure on the throat. Further, they thought the womb resting in the abdominal cavity caused epilepsy; in the heart, anxiety; in the liver, aphonia, gritting of the teeth, an ashen complexion, etc. This theory of uterine starvation or displacement was perpetuated by Hippocrates, Plato, Celsus, Aretaeus, and Soranus. Aretaeus and later Galen of Pergamon observed, moreover, that hysteria could occur in men. Despite their important observation, the sexual—uterine associated—theory of hysteria (by this time about 3000 years old) held sway until the thirteenth century.

At that time, satanism and witchcraft began to dominate medical theory and the logical treatment of hysteria appeared to be exorcism. Subsequently, association of hysteria with the female was strengthened as witches were tortured and murdered through the mid-eighteenth century. The efforts of enlightened physicians, concerned citizens, and a new legal system with a modicum of justice eventually stopped the terror. Thus ended the belief in the supernatural origin, but not the sexual origin, of hysteria.

In the nineteenth century even a physician as famous as Griesinger still considered hysteria a disease of the uterus, although most physicians by then termed it a disease of the mind. In 1853, Robert Carter (1829-1919), an

English physician, thought that the etiology of hysteria was psychological and as-
cribed it to the patient's temperament, to precipitating events and situations, or
to the extent that the patient concealed or repressed the cause. He thought
sexual passion, although not the only etiological factor, was a frequent and important cause. Carter discounted uterine disease as having any relationship to
hysteria and in America, S. Weir Mitchell excluded all sexual etiology. Both Carter
and Mitchell, however, insisted on humane treatment for these patients.

Anton Mesmer explained hysteria as the result of astral influences. He
developed the theory of animal magnetism, now called hypnosis, and used a
special technique, known as mesmerism, to treat patients. Although Mesmer
was expelled from France by a royal commission, because of his treatment
methods, the idea of hypnosis spread. Braid considered hypnosis a psychological
phenomenon; Mary Baker Eddy got the idea for the Christian Science religion
at least in part from her experience with hypnosis; and Charcot thought hypnosis
resulted from organic brain change. In contrast to Charcot, Liébeault and
Bernheim viewed the hypnotic phenomenon as the result of suggestion and for
Coué hypnosis was caused by autosuggestion. There was much controversy
surrounding hysteria and hypnosis.

Let us consider three students of Charcot: the first is Joseph Babinski (1857–
1932), the discoverer of the Babinski sign. He posited that hysterics had a
susceptibility to stimuli that inhibit or dissociate mental processes. The other
two students are Pierre Janet and Sigmund Freud. Janet refuted the sexual
theory of hysteria, but Freud, using at first hypnosis and later different techniques of therapy, "established" repressed sexuality as a basis for hysteria.
He later considered that distortion of inherent infantile sexuality was the etiology
not only of hysteria but of all mental aberrations. The sexual theory of hysteria
had returned in full force.[26-29] Today, in these times of permissiveness, the
theory of repressed sexuality as a cause for hysteria must certainly be rejected,
and the search should continue in different areas.

Freud initially used the term "defense hysteria" and later replaced it with con-
version hysteria. In 1933, the American Medical Association's *Standard Classified
Nomenclature of Diseases* included that term.[30] In 1952 the DSMI used the terms
Dissociative and Conversion reactions subsumed under Psychoneurotic Disorders.
The DSMII subsumes Hysterical neurosis (conversion type) and Hysterical neurosis
(dissociative type) under Neuroses. The latest provisional draft of the DSMIII,
March 30, 1977, makes no reference to the term hysteria. It includes within Axis I
[Clinical Psychiatric Syndrome(s)] the categories: (1) Somatoform Disorders with
subgroups Somatization disorder (Briquet's disorder), Psychalgia, Atypical somatoform disorder, and Conversion disorder; (2) Dissociative Disorders with subgroups
Amnesia, Fugue, Multiple personality, Depersonalization, and Other or unspecified;
(3) Factitious Disorders with subgroups that include Factitious illness with psychological symptoms (Ganser Syndrome, Pseudo-psychosis, or Pseudo-dementia),

Chronic factitious illness with physical symptoms (Munchausen syndrome), Other factitious illness with physical symptoms, Unspecified factitious illness.[31] That draft is not final and until January 1979, when the final version is published, all that can be done, if possible, is to keep up with the latest versions. In any event, it looks as if Briquet's disorder is going to replace hysteria as the official nomenclature.

ETIOLOGY

Genetic studies reveal conflicting evidence on hysteria. Some family studies show familial predispositions to hysteria while other studies which are equally valid show the opposite. Monozygotic and dizygotic twin studies also show conflicting evidence. Ljungberg points out that the incidence of fathers, brothers, and sons of hysterical probands is 1.7, 2.7, and 4.6%, and in mothers, sisters, and daughters 7.3, 6.0, 6.9%, respectively. This is compared with an estimated 0.5% for the general population. The overall male percentage was 2.4% and the overall female percentage was 6.4%. Ljungberg interpreted these findings as supporting evidence for genetic transmission of hysteria.[32] Slater's twin studies showed that in the 12 MZ and 12 DZ partners of the 24 hysterical propositi none were diagnosed as hysterics. However, three of the MZ and two of the DZ partners were diagnosed as neurotic and five MZ and four DZ partners had neurotic symptomatology. These data speak against a specific genetic contribution to the etiology of hysteria. In fact Slater found that the symptomatology had little relationship to prognosis and he questioned whether hysteria was indeed even a syndrome. He found hysterics suffering from focal brain lesions, epilepsy, schizophrenia, depression, and anxiety states. In patients who had signs only of hysteria and nothing else, Slater further conjectured that the diagnosis was in error and he suggested more investigation.[33] In contrast to Slater's findings other investigators found hysteria (Briquet's syndrome) in about 20% of first degree (i.e., parent, sibling, or child) female relatives. They also detected a relationship between hysteria, sociopathy, and alcoholism in close relatives. They suggested that hysteria and sociopathy had a similar etiology and pathogenesis.[34-36] Unfortunately, it is not altogether certain that Ljungberg, Slater, or this latter group were actually discussing the same disease entity.

The type of personality associated with hysterical neurosis varies; passive-aggressive, emotionally unstable, hysterical, schizoid, paranoid are all labels commonly cited.[37] Nevertheless, individuals designated as hysterical personalities are more likely to develop hysterical neurosis than others. Hysterical personalities can be characterized as possessing such traits as immaturity, instability, excitability, suggestibility, superficiality, and egocentricity. These persons respond quickly with enthusiasm, infatuations, laughter, or tears. They see the world only in terms of their own interests. They tend to be possessive, and have a clear grasp of their rights and the duties of others; however, they are in conflict between duty and desire and no outsider can guess which one will be exercised under a given set of circumstances. When frustrated they may resort to self-injury or even suicidal behavior. These persons create passionate scenes with accusations, tears, and protestations that exhaust others. Psychiatrists frequently question whether or not these patients are really depressed since their affect is so labile. They seem to forget quickly and cannot understand how others should be so slow to forgive and forget. Histrionic personalities exaggerate and dramatize. Everything is valued in superlatives—their headaches are terrible, their nerves are shattered, their relatives are the worst or are angels, etc. Their lack of insight plays havoc with social relations or psychiatric therapy. Socially they can follow a downward path like a chain reaction, each stage facilitating descent into the next. They begin as self-deceivers, then liars, and finally swindlers. The pseudologic of these patients, once they become swindlers, is characterized by a capacity to believe their own lies, and to enjoy their artificially created situations. They select occupations that require showmanship—revivalist preachers, actors, actresses, popular lecturers, models, band leaders, and salespersons. However, they are not content for long, whatever the success. No real-life circumstance can meet all their demands. Whatever their attainments they are dissatisfied. Convinced that their achievements do not receive adequate recognition, they blame this on the blindness, stupidity, or ill will of others. Hysterical personalities feel more intelligent and talented than others. From this belief develops a paranoid quality which further disintegrates their social relationships. This longitudinal analysis might help explain why so many different types of personalities are associated with hysterical neurosis. Personality traits however change as the individual ages.[38-40]

In 1937 Kretschmer combined Bleuler's[41] 1924 description with Wittel's[42] 1930 psychoanalytic interpretations and offered a dynamic typology of the hysterical personality which had more than historical interest:

Many symptoms of what is called the "hysterical character" are nothing more than the fixed residua of an early pubertal psyche or unfavourable characterological modifications of the same under the altered demands of later life—namely, the characteristic antithesis between coldness and excess of erotic feelings—that is, an over-lively and over-idealistic psychosexuality with prudish rejection of the physical aspects of sex, enthusiasm for impressive persons, a preference for what is loud and lively, a theatrical pathos, a taste for brilliant roles, heroic fantasies, the playing with the idea of suicide, enthusiastic self-sacrifice, combined with a naive, sulky, childish egotism. An immature psyche of this sort has a greater inclination towards impulsive discharges of affect, and especially towards hypobulic mechanisms. The hypobulic phenomena appear partly as circumscribed hysterical outbreaks (especially in the hysterical attack) and partly as permanent stigmata of the so-called "hysterical character" which, on account of its strongly hypobulic nature, we call capricious, in view of the distinctive contrast between stubbornness and exaggerated suggestibility shown therein.[43]

The neurophysiological theory of the etiology of hysterical neurosis, especially the conversion type, emphasizes an altered state of consciousness as the basic problem. Thus, with dissociation or separation of consciousness, it follows that cognitive performance is impaired in such functions as attention, vigilance, or recent memory, and the capacity to integrate information is disturbed. The neurophysiological theory claims that corticofugal inhibition of afferent stimulation becomes increased, thereby diminishing self-awareness and bodily function. A feedback loop is established (conditioning). Once this mechanism is in operation, the individual responds to biological, psychological, or social threats with the above cognitive disturbances as well as a heightened suggestibility.[44, 45]

This theory agrees with biological explanations comparing hysteria in man to instinctive reactions of animals to danger. There are several instinctive patterns. First, violent motor reactions, where birds released in a room fly about frantically seeking an escape route. This behavior compares to fugue states, convulsions, amnesias, and tremors. Second, the sham-death reflex, where the animal freezes or becomes immobilized. This compares to twilight and dreamy states, paralysis, fits, blindness, deafness, and analgesia. Third, regressive phenomena, occurring in humans as well as animals under stress or danger, may include urinary incontinence, babbling, rocking, and crying. In addition normal humans experience vivid fantasies that may be compared to hysterical psychoses, age-regression phenomena, puerilism, and Ganser syndrome (pseudo-dementia).[46, 47]

Physical factors contribute to hysterical neurosis. Brain damage or severe concussions, especially to the frontal lobes, facilitate the development of the neurosis. Chronic exhausting organic illnesses are not infrequently associated with the symptoms of hysteria. Individuals with low intelligence, whether the result of organic disease or of deprived socioeconomic background, are more prone to hysteria than those of normal intelligence.[48]

Psychological theories of the etiology of hysterical conversion neurosis vary. They differ with each other as well as differing within a single theoretical framework, such as psychoanalysis. Psychoanalytic explanations are concerned with levels of fixation or regression. Psychoanalysts debate whether the problem is at the oedipal or the oral level of infantile sexuality. They do agree that the symptoms are symbolic representations of repressed libido and internal conflict. To the psychoanalyst the symptom expresses both a wish and its denial.[49] Conversely, the behavior therapists are in agreement with neurophysiologists and consider hysteria a disorder of conditioning and learning.[50]

Others think that the symptoms of hysteria and hysterical personality are means of interpersonal communication. The patient assumes a role or plays a game to get what he desires from others. Conversion symptoms, for example, are viewed by the patient and those associated with the patient as socially acceptable; hence, the "sickness" role brings attention.[51] Hysterical personalities by presenting themselves as helpless, weak, or frail are actually controlling, willful, or dominating. They get what they want. By interpreting hysteria as an overt–covert communicative interplay between patient and others and nothing more, these psychiatrists and psychologists make the implicit assumption that the disease and perhaps even life is nothing more than a game of "upmanship."[52] Celani says:

> Hysteria can be viewed as a relatively specific interpersonal style that results from cultural, social, and interpersonal influences. The definition of hysteria has evolved from a symptom-based definition to an interpersonal diagnosis based on specific overt and covert communications that structure the interpersonal environment. The basic communication is one of frailty, weakness, and helplessness and can be used by both sexes, although cultural factors favor its use by females. The interpersonal role used by female hysterics is an overplaying of the feminine role, which tends to structure the interpersonal environment in a manner that ensures male interest and attention while inhibiting male aggression. More importantly, by restricting the range of responses from others, the hysteric ensures that those responses which have been elicited will be confirmatory to and congruent with her own self-attitudes.[53]

Stress is a factor in hysteria. The greater the predisposition to hysteria, the less stress needed to provoke a reaction. Common stresses are engagements, marriages, pregnancies, death, work, and financial responsibilities. Other stresses include emotional strain, accidents, disappointments, and arguments. As a rule when there is an acute episode of hysteria the illness will be preceded by a period of strain associated with either physical illness or psychological stress. Situations in which the physician pays excessive attention to a symptom or illness by prolonged and repeated examinations cast doubt in the patient's mind and can inadvertently provoke hysterical symptoms. The doctor may question a patient regarding a symptom and it will appear; hence suggestion, especially during circumstances of stress, should be avoided.

DIAGNOSIS

Hysterical neurosis is divided into two major categories, conversion and dissociative types. The psychological characteristics of hysterical individuals have already been alluded to. These patients may demonstrate *la belle indifférence*, avoid and evade immediate reality conflicts, are highly self-centered, narcissistic, egocentric, seek sympathy and attention, and are susceptible to suggestion. The physical characteristics of hysterical neurosis, conversion type, are divided according to sensory, motor, visceral, trophic functions, or simulate physical illnesses. The sensory symptoms usually do not follow anatomical nervous pathways. They include anesthesias, paresthesias, and disturbances of special senses (blindness, deafness, anosmia, loss of taste, etc.). The motor symptoms include abnormal movements (tics, choreoform, and oposthotomus). Paralysis may be monoplegic, hemiplegic, or paraplegic. These patients are capable of holding their hands or feet in a flaccid position for so long that contractures or pseudoatrophy result; however, reflexes are retained in the paralyzed area and there are no muscle degenerations. These patients can become mute and aphonic. The simulating characteristics of the hysteric are at times difficult to differentiate from physical illness and a hysterical illness can complicate a physical one. The differential is difficult, and the physician should be especially alert when the patient is seeking financial compensation. Any illness in these patients may be exaggerated or dramatized. Visceral symptoms are anorexia, bulemia (excessive appetite), vomiting, and air swallowing (belching, hiccups, fullness or pain in the abdomen, and flatulence). Characteristic trophic changes are mainly vasomotor disturbances in the paralyzed limb. The extremity can be blue and cold. There can be skin lesions such as blisters or erythemas. These skin manifestations are called dermititis artifacta and can also be produced by hypnosis.[54]

An extreme case of visceral symptoms is anorexia nervosa. There is some doubt whether this entity is part of hysteria since the cardinal feature of self-preservation is apparently lacking. This is a disease of girls in their late teens or early adulthood. The major symptoms are anorexia, amenorrhea, loss of weight, and a distorted attitude towards food and body image. The marked weight loss usually initially results from voluntary dieting, and there may be a family history of dietary problems and obesity. If the weight is not lost in a short time, the patient resorts to additional methods that increase weight loss, i.e., self-induced vomiting, purgatives, or excessive exercise. These patients frequently have a cessation of menstruation which may even precede the weight loss. A vicious progression begins with loss of appetite that is replaced by a repugnance for food so severe that it can lead to emaciation and even death. But an interesting phenomenon in these patients is their endless energy in spite of their emaciation. They can exercise for hours. These patients invariably deny that they are abnormally thin, disregard medical warnings or pleas of close relatives to eat, deny that anything is wrong, and frequently manifest indifference to family, appearance, friends, or work. Difficulties often exist between the patient and her mother. These patients are included in this discussion of hysterical neurosis because dissociation seems to play a large part in these cases.

Although a psychological factor in the genesis of anorexia nervosa cannot be doubted, there may be factors that involve the hypothalamic-pituitary-adrenal-ovarian axis. Some other signs are low basal metabolic rate, hypothermia, hypotension, poor peripheral circulation, and fine, downy (lanugo) hair on their backs. The prognosis is guarded and uncertain because many recover and eventually lead normal lives while others go on to schizophrenia, death from starvation, or suicide.[55-57]

In the hysterical neurosis, dissociative type, the predominant symptom is an altered state of consciousness. The precipitating causes, although similar to those of the conversion type, are usually more dramatic. One form is the double or multiple personality. The patient describes himself, at different times, as being one or another of several different personalities. These different personalities are endowed with different character traits and may or may not be aware of each other's existence. Thus a girl, who turns from Mary to Margaret, may be quiet, studious, and obedient as Mary, and unaware of Margaret's existence. When she is Margaret, however, she may be joyous, headstrong, willful, and refer to Mary in contemptuous terms. There are many novels written on this theme. *Dr. Jekyll and Mr. Hyde, Sybil,* and *Three Faces of Eve* are but a few that are well known.[58]

A fugue is the condition of a person who is found at a distance from his home and claims complete loss of memory of his previous existence. Fugues are nearly always an escape from a disagreeable situation. The patient leaves his residence, arrives in a strange city, remains a period of time, and finally is brought to a doctor in an exhausted, dirty, unkempt state. Nevertheless, even when observed in his dissociated state his behavior appears integrated. If he has money the hysterical patient will eat while the epileptic, schizophrenic, or depressed patient will not. Besides an association with amnesia, fugues also bear a resemblance to somnambulism (sleep walking), a common occurrence in childhood. In these conditions some of the highest cortical centers are active while others, those involved with self-awareness and self-criticism, are isolated.[59]

In hysterical amnesia the patient claims a loss of memory for large sections of his past life, refuses to recognize relatives, and denies knowledge of particular areas such as history or arithmetic. Hysterical pseudo-dementia or pseudo-stupidity is an ill-defined syndrome, typically represented by Ganser syndrome and puerilism, and most frequently seen in jails. The patients give approximate answers (How many legs has a horse? "Three"), and stupid answers (three plus two equals "twenty-two"). Hysterical trances can occur spontaneously or in the hypnotic state. These trances can be highly charged emotional experiences, such as religious conversions, that include visual and auditory hallucinations or "messages" from God. Individuals who get messages within the trance state may divulge highly organized dialogues between themselves and saints or God.[60]

Munchausen syndrome is an eponym for medical and surgical diseases simulated by the patient—a chronic addiction to invalidism. A hospital can provide a stage for drama. The blend of conscious and unconscious motivations in the psychogenesis of all hysterical symptoms is particularly well-illustrated in this phenomenon. Physical signs and symptoms are consciously feigned, but the reasons that impel patients to seek these morbid satisfactions are concealed from them.[61]

Dissociation is a major mechanism in certain other conditions not considered part of hysterical neurosis, dissociative type. These include phenomena such as hypnosis, autohypnosis, and sleep. In hypnosis the change of consciousness is achieved by means of a specific technique, but long automobile rides can also bring it about automatically (highway hypnosis). Sleep, may be partly due to will, perhaps acting autosuggestively, but it can occur simply through tiredness, habit, or other inducements. Other conditions which are dissociative phenomena but not neurosis—some common, some not—may be considered either normal or abnormal. These alterations of consciousness include complex fantasy experiences, nightmares, night terrors, daydreaming, sleepwalking or talking, sleep paralysis (narcolepsy), stupors, delirium, and *déjà vu*.[62]

Although hysteria is an emotional illness that brings personal gain to the patient, it must be realized by the physician that the individual is not a malingerer, i.e., a conscious pretender. Distinctions between conscious and unconscious, reality and fantasy, fact and fiction are apt to be tenuous at best, and both the sick and the healthy can be perfectly comfortable with contradictory feeling, thoughts, and behavior. The psychiatrist must guard against calling a person a malingerer because people are protected by their own human frailties and inherent capacities to see, hear, feel, and believe what they want.

The above should give some impression of the immense variety of hysterical manifestations. In addition to present-day variations of hysteria, the form and content of this disease have varied, as noted, throughout history.

Jasper's chart (following Pierre Janet freely) may help to clarify various hysterical conditions:

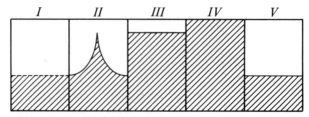

| | I | II | III | IV | V |

(I)   Normal;
(II)   Appearance of a Hysterical Symptom;
(III)   Hypnoid State;
(IV)   Twilight State or Double Personality;
(V)   Chronic Hysterical State without manifest symptoms

Shaded areas indicate the unconscious and unshaded areas the conscious. In column I, normal, the broken line shows the freely mobile state between conscious and unconscious mind. In the other columns a full line is drawn to show the dissociation. Column II shows that conversion hysterical symptoms are manifest. Column III shows the hypnoid state as found in daydreaming. Column IV demonstrates the twilight state or double personality in which consciousness fluctuates from one state to another. Column V illustrates the chronic hysterical state without any manifest symptoms.[63]

DIFFERENTIAL DIAGNOSIS

Diagnosis should be based on both inclusion and exclusion, and the masking physical disease must be excluded or, if present, determined. Psychiatric evaluation seeks indications of an inclination towards hysterical reactions. Although these reactions may seem evident, the basic problem can be anxiety, depression, organic brain damage, psychophysiologic disorders, hypochondria, or chemical or physiological disturbance. The hysterical reaction should be delineated by the symptoms, their value to the patient, and their relationship to his environment. Physical examination and psychiatric assessment are essential for differential diagnosis. Further, Walshe adds:

> An essential feature of the somatic symptoms of hysteria is that they do not correspond to disorders produced by, or capable of being produced by, structural lesions or primary physiological disorder, nor is their behavior compatible with the presence of these. They are, as it were, symptoms that know nothing of anatomy or physiology. They correspond to the patient's notions of his anatomical and physiological arrangements and are clearly influenced in their appearance and disappearance by purely psychological determinants.[64]

Nothing less can satisfy a diagnosis of hysteria.

The difficulty of differentiating hysteria from anxiety neurosis varies. In the presence of *la belle indifférence* there should be no difficulty. However, many hysterical states are associated with anxiety and it is here that the problem arises. In anxiety neurosis the primary symptoms or manifestations are a subjective feeling of anxiety or its equivalent, plus generalized physiological concomitants such as palpitations, tachycardia, sweating, tremors, weight loss, and so on. Where the patient is primarily hysterical, these physiological findings can occur but are not expected; in their absence, the diagnosis of hysteria becomes more likely. When there is objective evidence of anxiety, the problem of how much is hysterical exploitation becomes paramount. This can sometimes be answered by relating the number and degree of physiological symptoms to the amount of distress or the patient's ability to function. With anxiety neurosis the correlation of psychological distress to physiological symptoms and functions will be direct: more symptoms and distress the less ability to function; whereas in hysteria the patient may continue to function in a more or less normal fashion.

Differentiating depression from hysteria is equally difficult. In both conditions patients exhibit diverse symptoms, a degree of normality, distractability, and signs of exploitation of symptoms for particular ends. This becomes especially complicated since the hysteric, capable of simulating depression, can also become depressed. Only careful observation and experience with the patient will allow the physician to determine which is primary: dissociation, dissociation with depression, or depression with dissociation. Helpful clues can be gleaned from the discrepancies among the complaint or complaints, the amount of distress, and the patient's actual level of functioning.

Conversion hysteria must be differentiated from other diseases with bodily complaints: psychophysiologic disorders, postconcussional syndrome, hypochondriasis, and somatization. Psychophysiological disorders consist of a group of diverse diseases—peptic ulcer, ulcerative colitis, essential hypertension, asthma, migraine headaches, skin and mucous membrane diseases, rheumatoid arthritis, thyrotoxicosis—mediated through the autonomic nervous system. Most psychiatrists agree that there is a psychic component in each of these diseases but some psychoanalysts claim that this component has specific psychological meaning. The asthmatic patient, for instance, is described as suffering from a repressed urge to cry for mother and migraine patients from repressed hostility.[65] Other analysts, however, reject this specificity concept of psychophysiological diseases and propose a much more sophisticated hypothesis in which conversion is recognized as only one part of the process. George Engel says:

> . . . it can be seen that the only body parts and functions which are available for the conversion process are those capable of being perceived, consciously or unconsciously, and thereby giving rise to perceptual memory traces which can be used by the ego to symbolize and express hidden wishes. Silent physiological or biochemical processes not accessible to either exteroceptive or enteroceptive perception cannot meet this requirement and hence cannot provide the basis for conversion even though they may be remotely involved in a chain of events initiated by a conversion (e.g., respiratory alkalosis and compensatory excretion of base as remote consequences of the hyperventilation provoked by a conversion sensation of suffocation) . . . . But perceptions of other bodily processes not under voluntary control also can come to represent symbolically the repressed wish, even though these processes originally constituted inborn biological systems, concerned with approach, avoidance, defense, riddance, and adaptation and had no primary symbolic meaning . . . may we conceive of palpitations as a conversion, whether it takes the form of

an overactive heart or merely of a sensation of palpitation without any change in heart action. In the former case the heart action is changed in response to the wish while resulting palpitation symbolizes the wish fulfilled.[66]

In effect psychophysiological diseases, according to Engel, are not only complications of conversion hysteria, i.e., physiological responses associated with the conversion reaction, but are symbolic fulfillment of a conscious or unconscious wish by the autonomic nervous system. Further, since conversion is "an unconscious defense mechanism by which the anxiety that stems from an intrapsychic conflict is converted and expressed in a symbolic somatic symptom,"[67] this would imply that conversion results from an inability of the ego to adequately control anxiety; namely, anxiety is the real problem. Yet Marks writes:

> There is no evidence that patients with anxiety states develop diseases said to be caused by anxiety any more than other people, even though they all have high anxiety. For example, in a 20-year follow-up of 173 patients Wheeler et al. found that they were not predisposed to develop hypertension, heart disease, peptic ulcer, diabetes, asthma, thyrotoxicosis, ulcerative colitis, hysteria, or schizophrenia.[68]

Psychophysiological and conversion hysteria are distinct and different diseases that can, in the last analysis, be differentiated only by clinical manifestations in which the total configuration of both diseases is assessed.

Postconcussional syndrome occurs more often after minor rather than major head injuries and is characterized by headaches, giddiness, fatigue, impaired concentration and memory, depression, and reduced alcohol tolerance. Although most physicians believe it is a mild and transient neurological deficit, some feel it to be either hysterical conversion reaction or malingering. Differentiating these three conditions has practical importance since head injuries which are the result of trauma can lead to discharge from military service, disability on a job, or financial compensation from an insurance company in a personal injury case. There is no clear-cut way to differentiate the three conditions. The only way one can differentiate malingering from the other two conditions is to catch the malingerer performing in a way that contradicts his claimed disability. Conversely, collecting as much information about the patient from him as well as from any other possible source might aid in diagnosing a hysterical conversion; and positive neurologic findings could help diagnosis postconcussion syndrome.[69]

Somatization, a loosely used term, describes patients who complain of generalized weakness, chronic fatigue, lack of energy, inability to feel refreshed after rest, and innumerable aches and pains usually confined to various muscle groups. This condition must be distinguished from neurasthenia, anxiety, hypochondriacal, depressive, or conversion hysterical neuroses. Hypochondriasis is a disease in which the patient is preoccupied with his body, its functionings, and with a conviction of presumed illness in one or more organs. His preoccupation with disease can assume bizarre and grotesque proportions. He may even complain of his stomach "being eaten out" or of bugs crawling on his skin. This condition must be differentiated not only from hysteria but also from all other somatic diseases—psychiatric and physical—and from schizophrenia.[70]

With motor symptoms, hysterical paralysis can usually be distinguished from the organic by the normality of reflexes. The patient withholds strength, so the weakness fluctuates and contractions of the supposedly paralyzed muscles are often visible. Hysterical paralysis of the forearm can be shown by flexing the elbow in supination and allowing the forearm to fall. In both organic paralysis and in normal patients the forearm pronates with the palmar surface of the hand downwards, but in hysterical paralysis the arm falls in the same supine position in which it was held. With leg paralysis the diagnosis can be established by placing the patient in a recumbent position. The patient is asked to sit up using trunk muscles without using hands; in the normal person both legs rise equally; in organic paralysis, the affected leg raises higher than the normal one; the hysteric will keep his paralyzed leg on the floor. A neurologist can help differentiate such organic conditions as tics, tremors, convulsive states, other abnormal movements or extrapyramidal symptoms from hysteria. Similar testing can be devised for gait coordination and sensory disturbance. Hysterical anesthesia can be detected by the fact that symptoms do not follow the nerve distribution (glove and stocking anesthesia). Simulation of disease can be differentiated by its mode of onset, development, and course in the light of the patient's personality and circumstances.[71-73]

Where an original organic disability has become exaggerated or prolonged through hysterical mechanisms, difficulty exists. Only experience and intuition can help here. Organic brain changes provide a fertile ground for physical conversion symptoms of all kinds. However, when any patient over 40 years old shows these symptoms for the first time, other signs of organicity should be determined. The elaborations and exaggerations make it hard to say where organic disability ends and functional disability begins. Commonly involved areas include the head (headaches), chest (breathing difficulties and chest pains), abdomen (indigestion, diarrhea) and the skin (rashes, erythemas, swelling).[74]

Hysterical reactions, may in rare instances, resemble psychoses. Fugues and stupors present the chief differential problems. The personality of the individual, the development of symptoms, and the circumstances must be taken into account. A stupor in a young person is more often schizophrenic than hysterical. In follow-up studies of these conditions misdiagnosis is common, and after a period of time other conditions such as organic brain disease, schizophrenia, epilepsy, manic depressive psychosis, and so on, may become apparent. Hysterical amnesia should be distinguished from amnesia caused by alcohol or epilepsy. Fugues, trances, and twilight states must be distinguished from postepileptic automatism. In postepileptic automatism the behavior is purposeless as compared with the complicated and purposive actions in the other conditions, and the hysteric can adapt rapidly to changing circumstances while the epileptic cannot. Ganser syndrome may simulate organic dementia or schizophrenia and the diagnosis can be difficult if the Ganser syndrome occurs in schizophrenia or organic dementia.[75]

COURSE AND PROGNOSIS

Acute situations may clear up very rapidly and never reappear; however, chronic states may exist for prolonged periods of time, even years. There seems to be a relationship between the length of illness, the degree of secondary gain, the predisposing personality, and environmental stress. Where symptoms vary there is hope and the chief prognostic sign is the level of functioning between attacks. With high performance prognosis is good, and with a low level of function prognosis is bad. Performance is more important then the severity of the attack. The majority of symptoms clear up shortly after an episode, but a certain percentage continue for years. The reasons may be within the patient or his environment. If he gets significant gains from illness it will perpetuate itself. These secondary gains can come from relatives or from compensation payments.[76]

When considering prognosis one should keep in mind that the disease is most common at the two ends of life: early, before the central nervous system has reached maturity; and late, when organic brain changes occur. In youngsters the illness frequently resolves by puberty or late adolescence, but oldsters retain the symptoms which vary only in degree of severity. But motor and sensory types are not now seen as frequently as they were 70 years ago. Other types of hysteria, such as simulation of disease, visceral, and trophic are probably more frequent and more typically represent the fashion of modern-day hysteria. The dissociative reactions are relatively rare in adults but more frequent in children, adolescents, and the elderly.[77]

TREATMENT

Attempting to discuss treatment of this group of patients is similar to a discussion of soup. There are so many varieties and such different qualities that each has to be considered on its own merits. In addition, the effectiveness of any treatment is difficult to evaluate since spontaneous symptomatic recovery occurs in 60 to 80% of patients within one week to a year.[78] Nevertheless, some general principles, methods of symptom removal, and long-term plans for treatment do exist and warrant discussion.

The hysterical patient who appears in the hospital emergency room, especially following a suicidal attempt, should be treated as an acute crisis. Sedatives, narcosynthesis, or hypnosis may be used and a very short period of inpatient care may or may not be advisable. After the crisis abates, either brief supportive psychotherapy or prolonged psychotherapy aimed toward insight and maturity may help.

With the exception of acute emergency situations, treatment should begin only after a thorough examination, and evaluation of the personality, environment, and physical condition of the patient. Various forms of psychotherapy or environmental readjustments may be necessary, including attempts to change relatives' attitudes toward the patient. Generally, it is wise to keep the patient at work and to avoid expensive hospitalization and endless physical or laboratory examinations. Allowing the patient to remain in his home environment may not be advisable. Many show hysterical behavior only in one particular environment—this may be the home. These patients exploit relatives. Yet the physician frequently finds it difficult to get relatives to change their attitudes. He must also deal with his own attitude towards the patient. Because they are demanding, give distorted information, and frequently resist insight into their condition, they frustrate the physician, who may find himself wanting to discharge the patient prematurely. His frustration, though, should not become a reason for discontinuing therapy. The physician must recognize the patient's natural reluctance toward introspection as symptomatic of the illness and constantly guard against his own feelings and attitudes or the treatment may be doomed to failure.[79]

Alleviation of dissociative symptoms makes the patient more amenable to treatment. Patients in trances, fugues, amnesias, twilight states, and so forth can often be brought to full awareness by a powerful stimulus. Among suitable stimuli are noxious substances, such as smelling salts, or a painful electric current administered to any part of the body. Use whatever works: practically anything can and has been used to remove the symptom. Dramatic cures are obtained by faith healers. During mass meetings with "believers" whole groups of people are "cured" at one time (this in contrast to epidemic illness, is epidemic cure). When full awareness returns the treatment should be continued by having the patient undertake some activity—conversing, working, drinking tea, coffee, and so on. Then with continued psychotherapy, areas where the patient has difficulties should be pointed out to him, to help expand his consciousness. Following this, an extensive therapy program should be initiated using whatever methods are appropriate. The hysterical deaf can be persuaded to hear by having them listen to questions through a stethoscope, starting with loud sounds and gradually decreasing the volume until normal tones are reached. It is wise to have others see this result as reinforcement. Aphonia can be overcome by squeezing the patient's chest, suddenly producing an "ah" sound. This proves to the patient that he can produce a sound; then expand from that point. The paralytic can be persuaded to walk and similarly the blind will be made to see. Through various common sense techniques, encouragement, or persuasion most symptoms will disappear.

Supportive psychotherapy, especially suggestion, often gets rid of symptoms but these symptoms may relapse unless a course of prolonged treatment is followed. The longer the symptoms are present, the longer and more exhaustive the course of treatment must be planned. The removal of symptoms is only temporary. They will recur in one form or another unless the underlying difficulty is treated. The success of therapy depends on the degree of environmental stress, the patient's personality, as well as the therapist's ability. With the markedly hysterical patient who is incapable of insight, psychotherapy is the most difficult but it is possible. The most fruitful approach, however, is indirect and environmental. With others psychotherapy may have some success. But with all patients an overly solicitous attitude on the part of the therapist is discouraged, and symptoms should be underplayed within the bounds of reason, kindness, and courtesy.[80, 81]

REFERENCES

1. Lewis, W.C., Hysteria: The consultant's dilemma. Twentieth century demonology, pejorative epithet, or useful diagnosis? *Arch. Gen. Psychiatry* **30**:145–151 (1974).
2. Guze, S.B., The role of follow-up studies: Their contributions to diagnostic classification as applied to hysteria. *Seminars in Psychiatry* **2**:392–402 (1970).
3. Slater, E., Diagnosis of hysteria. *Brit. Med. J.* **1**:395–399 (1965).
4. Guze, S.B., The diagnosis of hysteria: What are we trying to do? *Amer. J. Psychiatry* **124**:491–498 (1967).
5. Woodruff, R., Clayton, P. and Guze, S., Hysteria: Studies of diagnosis, outcome and prevalence. *J. Amer. Med. Assoc.* **215**(3):425–428 (1971).
6. Guze, S.B., Woodruff, R. and Clayton, P., Sex, age, and the diagnosis of hysteria (Briquet's syndrome). *Amer. J. Psychiatry* **129**(6):121–124 (1972).
7. Guze, S.B., The validity and significance of the clinical diagnosis of hysteria (Briquet's syndrome). *Amer. J. Psychiatry* **132**(2):138–141 (1975).
8. Kaminsky, M.J. and Slavney, P.R., Methodology and personality in Briquet's syndrome: A reappraisal. *Amer. J. Psychiatry* **133**(1):85–88 (1976).
9. Woodruff, R., Robins, L., Taibleson, M., Reich, T., Schwin, R. and Frost, N., A computer assisted derivation of a screening interview for hysteria. *Arch. Gen. Psychiatry* **29**:450–454 (1973).
10. Lewis, W.C., op. cit., p. 146.
11. Ludwig, A., Hysteria: A neurobiological theory. *Arch. Gen. Psychiatry* **27**:771 (1972).
12. Margetts, E., Letters to the editor. *Amer. J. Psychiatry* **133**(1):103 (1976).

13. Carter, A.B., A physician's view of hysteria. *Lancet* 2:1241–1243 (1972).
14. Chodoff, P., The diagnosis of hysteria: An overview. *Amer. J. Psychiatry* 131(10): 1073–1078 (1974).
15. Ludwig, A., op. cit., pp. 771–772.
16. Meares, R. and Horvath, T., 'Acute' and 'chronic' hysteria. *Brit. J. Psychiatry* 121:653–657 (1972).
17. Herrick, C.J., *The Evolution of Human Nature.* New York: Harper Torchbooks, 1956, pp. 205–206.
18. Mead, G.H., *Mind, Self, and Society: From the Standpoint of a Social Behaviorist* (edited by Morris, C.) . Chicago: Univ. Chicago Press, 1934, pp. 135–226.
19. Dewey, J., *Human Nature and Conduct: An Introduction to Social Psychology.* New York: Modern Library, 1922, p. 138.
20. Heuscher, J.E., The use of existential-philosophic concepts in psychotherapy. *Amer. J. Psychoanal.* 29:170–175 (1969).
21. Bradlow, P.A., Depersonalization, ego splitting, nonhuman fantasy and shame. *Int. J. Psychoanal.* 54:487–492 (1973).
22. Janet, P., *The Mental State of Hystericals: A Study of Mental Stigmata and Mental Accidents* (transl. by Carson, C.L.). New York: Putnam, 1901.
23. Laughlin, H.P., *The Neuroses.* Washington, D.C.: Butterworth, 1967, p. 649.
24. Jaspers, K., *General Psychopathology* (transl. by Hoenig, J. and Hamilton, M.). Chicago: Univ. Chicago Press, 1963, pp. 381–383.
25. O'Connor, P.J., Hysterical reactions. *Practitioner* 210:58 (1973).
26. Veith, I., *Hysteria: The History of a Disease.* Chicago: Univ. Chicago Press, 1965.
27. Dakin, E.F., *Mrs. Eddy: The Biography of a Virginal Mind.* New York: Scribner, 1929.
28. Twain, M., *Christian Science.* New York: Harper and Brothers, 1907.
29. Wilbur, S., *The Life of Mary Baker Eddy.* Boston: The Christian Science Publishing Society, 1941.
30. Woolsey, R.M., Hysteria 1875 to 1975. *Dis. Nerv. Syst.* 37(7):380 (1976).
31. Provisional classification: Published as a looseleaf manual entitled *DSM-III Draft, 4/15/77.* DRAFT OF AXES I and II of DSM-III CLASSIFICATION as of March 30, 1977.
32. Ljungberg, L., Hysteria: A clinical, prognostic, and genetic study. *Acta. Psychiat. Scand. Suppl.* 112:1957.
33. Slater, E., The thirty-fifth Maudsley lecture: "Hysteria 311." *J. Mental Sci.* 107: 359–381 (1961).
34. Arkonac, O. and Guze, S.B., A family study of hysteria. *New Engl. J. Med.* 268: 239–242 (1963).
35. Guze, S.B., Wolfgram, E.D., McKinney, J.K. and Catwell, D.P., Psychiatric illness in the families of convicted criminals: A study of 519 first degree relatives. *Dis. Nerv. Syst.* 28:641–659 (1967).
36. Woerner, P.I. and Guze, S.B., A family and marital study of hysteria. *Brit. J. Psychiatry* 114:161–168 (1968).
37. Chodoff, P. and Lyons, H., Hysteria, the hysterical personality, and "hysterical" conversion. *Amer. J. Psychiatry* 111:734–740 (1958).
38. Slavney, P.R. and McHugh, P.R., The hysterical personality: A controlled study. *Arch. Gen. Psychiatry* 30:325–329 (1974).
39. Slavney, P.R. and McHugh, P.R., The hysterical personality: An attempt at validation with the MMPI. *Arch. Gen. Psychiatry* 32:186–190 (1975).
40. Celani, D., An interpersonal approach to hysteria. *Amer. J. Psychiatry* 133(12):1414–1418 (1976).
41. Bleuler, E., *Textbook of Psychiatry.* New York: Macmillan, 1924.

42. Wittels, F., The hysterical character. *Medical Rev.* **36**:186–190 (1930).
43. Kretschmer, E., Instinct and hysteria. *Brit. Med. J.* **4002**:578, (September 18, 1937).
44. Ludwig, A., op. cit., pp. 774–777.
45. Bendefeldt, F., Miller, L.L. and Ludwig, A., Cognitive performance in conversion hysteria. *Arch. Gen. Psychiatry* **33**(10):1250–1254, 1976.
46. Ludwig, A., op. cit., pp. 772–773.
47. Kretschmer, E., op. cit., p. 574.
48. Slater, E. and Roth, M., *Clinical Psychiatry,* 3rd ed. London: Balliere, Tindall, and Cassell, 1969, pp. 109–111.
49. Chodoff, P., op. cit., p. 1075.
50. Wolpe, J., "The etiology of human neuroses," in *Contemporary Abnormal Psychology: Selected Readings* (edited by Maher, B.). Baltimore: Penguin, 1973, pp. 293–299.
51. Hollender, M., Conversion hysteria. *Arch. Gen. Psychiatry* **26**:311–314 (1972).
52. Potter, S., *Lifemanship.* New York: Holt, 1951.
53. Celani, D., op. cit., pp. 1417–1418.
54. Malmquist, C.P., Hysteria in childhood. *Postgrad. Med.* **50**:112–117 (1971).
55. Halmi, K., Powers, P. and Cunningham, S., Treatment of anorexia nervosa with behavior modification: Effectiveness of formula feeding and isolation. *Arch. Gen. Psychiatry* **32**:93–96 (1975).
56. Garfinkel, P.E., Brown, G.M., Stancer, H.C. and Moldofsky, H., Hypothalamic-pituitary function in anorexia nervosa. *Arch. Gen. Psychiatry* **32**:739–744 (1975).
57. Lucas, A.R., Duncan, J.W. and Piens, V., The treatment of anorexia nervosa. *Amer. J. Psychiatry* **133**(9):1034–1038 (1976).
58. Batchelor, I.R., *Henderson and Gillespie's Textbook of Psychiatry,* 10th ed. London: Oxford University Press, 1969, pp. 153–154.
59. Ibid., pp. 152–153.
60. Ibid., pp. 152, 154–155.
61. Slater, E. and Roth, M., op. cit., pp. 115–116.
62. Malmquist, C.P., op. cit., pp. 115–116.
63. Jaspers, K., op. cit., p. 403.
64. Walshe, F., *Diseases of the Nervous System,* 9th ed. Baltimore: Williams & Wilkins, 1958, p. 351.
65. Freedman, A.M., Kaplan, H.I. and Sadock, B.J., *Modern Synopsis of Comprehensive Textbook of Psychiatry/II,* 2nd ed. Baltimore: Williams & Wilkins, 1976, p. 797.
66. Engel, G.L., A reconsideration of the role of conversion in somatic disease. *Compr. Psychiatry* **9**:319 (1968).
67. Freedman, A.M., Kaplan, H.I. and Sadock, B.J., op. cit., p. 1292.
68. Marks, I. and Lader, M., Anxiety states (anxiety neurosis): A review. *J. Nerv. Ment. Dis.* **156**(1):15 (1973).
69. O'Connor, P.S., op. cit., pp. 62–63.
70. Coppolillo, H.P., Conversion, hypochondriasis and somatization: A diagnostic problem for internists. *J. Arkansas Med. Soc.* **62**(2):67–71 (1965).
71. Curran, D., Partridge, M. and Storey, P., *Psychological Medicine. An Introduction to Psychiatry,* 7th ed. Edinburgh and London: Churchill Livingstone, 1972, pp. 270–275.
72. Weintraub, M., Hysteria. *Amer. Fam. Phys.* **8**:91–95 (1973).
73. Woolsey, R.M., op. cit., pp. 381–384.
74. Curran, D., et al., op. cit., p. 275.
75. Slater, E. and Roth, M., op. cit., pp. 116–117.
76. O'Connor, P.J., op. cit., pp. 63–64.

77. Curran, D., et al., op. cit., p. 276.

78. Woolsey, R.M., op. cit., p. 385.

79. Moskovitz, R.A., Epithelializing an epithet: Therapies of the hysterical personality disorder. *Dis. Nerv. Syst.* 37:64 (1976).

80. Ibid., pp. 65–67.

81. Curran, D., et. al., op. cit., pp. 276–282.

6
PHOBIC
NEUROSIS

In order to understand phobic neurosis it is necessary to differentiate two independent emotional syndromes—fear and anxiety. Although each emotion has similar components, differentiating them depends upon external circumstances. Anxiety relates more to the individual's appraisal of a threat with no specific apparent object or person discernible and fear relates more to an external identifiable circumstance which may contain a real threat. The differences between anxiety and fear, however, are not that sharp and are often difficult to discern since a real and nonreal threat may be a matter of appraisal. Hence, the controversy exists as to whether or not they are two distinct entities. Some of the evidence will be examined.[1]

Fright is identified in animals such as rats, turkeys, monkeys, etc.; therefore, it has phylogenetic origins. The fright response, however, increases in complexity as the scale ascends to man. It becomes more diverse and even separated from any immediate danger stimulus. The new dimension that is reached with man can be viewed as symbolic fear. Whereas in animals fear can be demonstrated, in man anxiety cannot only be demonstrated but becomes the more predominant emotion. Man still possesses, however, within his genes remnants of his phylogenetic past and reacts with fright not anxiety to certain nondangerous situations. Evolutionary evidence supports the view that fear in man is an instinctive response.[2]

Fear as instinct is opposed by the view of fear as an environmental conditioned response. Fear, according to environmentalists, is the affective component of an emotion learned by association with a painful stimulus. Whereas it is generally recognized that some fears are associated with external circumstances, it is also acknowledged that all fears are not. Hence, a compromise is reached, i.e., fear is a response to a combination of instinct and environment and the response varies in degree depending upon the inherent nature of the individual and the environmental stimuli. Fear is not a homogeneous syndrome but varies with individuals, species, and types of stimuli.[3]

One of the main characteristics of the fright response syndrome is avoidance. Two types of avoidance have been distinguished: active, avoids or escapes the source of the threat; and passive, requires inhibition of a response to avoid punishment. A simple analogy is that some animals rely on flight to escape danger and others freeze and take on a protective coloration to avoid detection. There is evidence that a deficit in active avoidance follows lesions in the lateral portion of the amygdala and a passive avoidance deficit follows lesions in the medial portion of the amygdala. Although these and other similar anatomical findings are controversial, the possibility exists that some component or components of fear are mediated through specific neural mechanisms. If this is so, the separation of anxiety and fear as distinct syndromes is further supported.[4]

The clinician evaluates fear as a relationship between individual and circumstances. Normal people react appropriately to the stimulus, i.e., in dangerous situations fear is a proper response and it varies from mild or moderate to severe. Likewise, the same degrees of response can be considered abnormal when adjudged inappropriate to the circumstance. Normal fear can be adaptive and productive, excessive or abnormal fear can be disruptive and nonadaptive. Excessive fear of a dangerous or even nondangerous situation does not in itself constitute a phobia but involves a response to stimuli that places it in the same class of phenomena as anxiety and depression.

Phobic neurosis, as all emotional experiences, has affective, somatic, visceral, endocrine, and chemical components. The affective state is fear which in most cases persists for as long as the object (animate or inanimate) or situation is within the presence of the individual. Fear-related subjective states are described by a variety of words—fear, alarm, apprehension, dread, dismay, terror, fright, horror, panic, trepidation—which are all closely connected, with each word having its own subtle distinction. Somatic aspects can include crying; paralysis, screaming, running, various facial expressions, tremor, fatigue, tension, restlessness, and excitement. Autonomic or visceral components are pallor, faintness, dizziness, palpitations, nausea, perspiration, changes in blood pressure and respiration, and an increase or decrease of secretions of various exocrine glands. Endocrine secretions and chemical variations include changes in red blood cells, adrenalin, corticosteroids, glucose, thyroid, etc.

Phobias interfere with the individual's way of life. The degree of disability can vary from avoidance of certain animals, which is hardly an inconvenience, to an inability to leave the boundaries of one's home, an extreme restriction. Yet both are considered phobias. To be sure, everyone has a few things he prefers to avoid, and this does not constitute a phobia. If a person has an antipathy for another person and avoids him, this is not a phobia. If he is uncomfortable with most people this may be a phobia; however, if he becomes persistently and inappropriately fearful when confronted with a particular object, animal, or situation that he recognizes as not dangerous, this individual nas a phobic neurosis. In sum, phobias are inappropriate morbid fear emotional responses which are related to diverse internal stimuli, objects, and circumstances, and uncontrolled by rational explanation or thought. Phobias are usually but not necessarily controlled by avoidance.

Danger, from both internal and external stimuli is recognized by certain signs, symptoms, signals, or symbols. Normally, learning proceeds from these indicators and individuals react in a self-preserving, adaptive, and protective manner. As a result, insight and foresight develop. Foresight provides the capacity to avoid or eliminate danger. The individual who possesses foresight, prudence, insight, or understanding usually has a better chance for success than one who lacks these qualities. Innumerable considerations enter into developing insight and foresight, and anxiety and fear stand out as major factors. Consequently, it seems reasonable to assume that those who suffer from an inappropriate amount of anxiety or fear will ultimately be lacking in insight and foresight. This principle applies in other psychiatric conditions in which patients suffer from delusional systems, hysterical dissociations, low intelligence, or organic brain disease. The loss of insight and foresight in these conditions can be considerable. The attempt here is to emphasize the cardinal role that normal anxiety and fear achieve in promoting learning, insight, and foresight and the resulting disability when these affects reach pathologic proportions.[5,6]

Most phobias are not disturbing enough to bring the patient to a physician. This makes it impossible to get accurate figures on the incidence of the disease. However, studies indicate that 77 out of 1000 people in the general population and 2.5% of psychiatric patients suffer from phobias as a major complaint. The degree of disability varies and agoraphobia, the severest and perhaps most disabling of all phobias, has a prevalence in the general population of 6.3 per 1000.[7,8]

HISTORY

Phobia is derived from the Greek word *phobos,* which means flight, panic, or fear. From the fifth century B.C. until the nineteenth century, descriptions of morbid fears may be found. It was not, however, until Aurelius Cornelius Celsus, a first century A.D. Roman encyclopedist, wrote a medical treatise using the term hydrophobia for a symptom of rabies that the term phobia had medical implications. The technical usage of phobia was not formalized until 1871 when Carl Westphal (1833–1890) coined and defined the term agoraphobia, i.e., a fear of assembly or meeting in public places.[9] Prior to this the terms fear and phobia were used very loosely by many writers and it would be foolhardy to attempt even a partial list of such references. Many serious thinkers dealt in some way or other with fear—normal, abnormal, or both. For example, the philosopher, Bertrand Russell referring to one such thinker says:

Spinoza's outlook is intended to liberate men from the tyranny of fear. "A free man thinks of nothing less than of death; and his wisdom is a meditation not of death, but of life." Spinoza lived up to this precept very completely. On the last day of his life he was entirely calm, not exalted, like Socrates in the *Phaedo*, but conversing, as he would on any other day, about matters of interest to his interlocutor.[10]

Others followed Westphal's lead.   In 1877 an Italian psychiatrist, Raggi, coined the term claustrophobia. Kraepelin first subsumed phobias under neurasthenia, later under compulsive insanity.[11]   Aubrey Lewis notes:

Pitres and Régis (1902) recognized two classes of phobia: the diffuse and the special or systematic. The systematic phobia is fixed to a specific object; it may be remittent or intermittent. There are occupational phobias: phobias of places, of natural elements (e.g. storms), of morbidity (e.g. infections), and of living creatures (e.g. snakes, rats). After naming some 70 of these (bedecked with Greek labels) Pitres and Régis emphasized that they belong to a sort of synoptic table, with no pretension to being a nosological classification.

The relation to obsessions was a crux. Pitres and Régis regarded phobias and obsessions not as distinct conditions but as two degrees of the same condition, differing only in the proportion of the two elements—emotional and ideational—which constitute them. Other distinguished psychiatrists have, however, included phobias in the larger class of obsessions . . . .[12]

G. Stanley Hall (1845–1924) was the American who popularized the classification of phobias according to Greek titles.   The lists were endless and of little practical value.[13]

Pierre Janet (1893) applied the term psychasthenia to those conditions which he thought were disorders of will, belief, and sense of reality and included anxiety, phobia, obsessions, compulsions, and certain types of depression. He thought the keystone of these disorders was a personality type that was indecisive, timid, doubtful, hesitant, and lacked reflective tendencies. Janet believed that the obsessive and phobic never completely lost the ability to reflect which distinguished them from hysterics who have an inclination towards obedience and compliance.[14]   Freud (1895) separated phobias from obsessions and divided phobias into two groups: common phobias (those fears everyone has) and contingent phobias (those fears the normal person does not have).[15]   By 1918, he divided phobias into three groups and classified them under anxiety hysteria which he regarded, along with conversion hysteria and obsessional neuroses, as transference neuroses. The first group of phobias concerned objects or situations which were feared by normal people. In this group, the possible danger was obvious and fear was an easily understood reaction.   The second group of phobias involved potentially dangerous situations that were not taken seriously by most people, i.e., traveling in a train or walking on a crowded street (situations where accidents do happen but where the danger is minimal). The third group of phobias was incomprehensible to the normal person and included such fears as a man being afraid to cross the street or a woman becoming fearful when a cat brushed against her dress.[16] Freud says: ". . . that where there is anxiety there must be something of which one is afraid."[17]

Psychiatrists in the recent past have continued to perpetuate the confusion by using imprecise language. Phobia can refer to a symptom, symptom complex, disorder, personality type, disease, etc. Further, the relationship of phobia to anxiety and obsessive compulsive neuroses is still unclear. In the DSMI (1952), phobic reaction was subsumed under Psychoneurotic Disorders; in DSMII (1968), Phobic neurosis was subsumed under Neuroses; in the provisional draft of DSMIII (March 30, 1977), phobic disorders were subsumed under Anxiety Disorders.[18] As with all psychiatric terminology, attempts towards standardized definitions are being developed.

CLASSIFICATION

Several classification systems are in use today. The traditional classifications using Greek or Latin prefixes are still common. Some of the frequently used terms are:

acrophobia—fear of heights
agoraphobia—fear of open places, places of assembly or meeting places
ailurophobia—fear of cats
aquaphobia—fear of water
claustrophobia—fear of closed spaces
cynophobia—fear of dogs
mysophobia—fear of dirt and germs
pyrophobia—fear of fire
xenophobia—fear of strangers
zoophobia—fear of animals

These cumbersome Greek names lead to endless trivia since each object or circumstance must then be named.[19] To avoid this problem, the terms monosymptomatic and diffuse phobias are used. The former designates a specific object or situation to which patients respond with exaggerated fear and the latter refers to patients whose fears are more generalized. The disadvantages of this system are that there are certain phobias which occur in clusters that constitute a definable entity and phobias may be part of another mental or physical illness. Hence, division into monosymptomatic and diffuse phobic states does not allow for sufficiently specific analysis of diverse etiological, prognostic, or treatment considerations.

Categories have been developed to aid in constructing hierarchies for systematic desensitization and other forms of behavior therapy. Questionnaires have been used in which the fears reported by patients are collected and organized into categories. The Fear Survey Schedule III, a 72-item questionnaire, was used by Wolpe and Lang who divided fears into the following categories: animal; social interpersonal; tissue damage, illness, and death; noises; other classical phobias; and a miscellaneous category.[20]   This classification system, although useful for constructing hierarchies for treatment purposes, offers no advantage over monosymptomatic versus diffuse phobias.[21]

Phobias may be divided into two groups based upon whether the stimulus is internal or external. Class I includes those phobias related to external stimuli and is the type most frequently seen by psychiatrists; avoidance of the stimulus is common here. Class I is divided into four groups according to the nature of the stimulus:

$External$.   (1) Animal phobias
(2) Specific situational phobias
(3) Social (interpersonal phobias)
(4) Agoraphobia

Class II includes those phobias related to internal stimuli; therefore, avoidance of the stimulus is impossible. Class II is divided into two groups:

(1) Illness phobias
(2) Obsessive phobias

This classification has disadvantages. How does one classify the patient who has both a phobia of spiders and of heights? This combination as well as other mixed combinations do occur and the above system has no specific category for them. Also the distinction between stimuli source is arbitrary. The patient's reactions in many cases cannot, in reality, be separated on the basis of whether the source of the stimulus is internal or external. For example, is the student with an obsessive urge to undress, who so avoids going to school, responding to an internal stimulus (obsession) or to the external stimulus (going to school)? Is he avoiding school because of the obsession or because he fears the classroom situation? Even in view of the contradictions, this method of classification does offer a practical clinical approach to the study of conditions in which phobias are the main complaint and not part of another illness.[22]

A major advantage of this system is that certain useful correlations have been found between Class I phobias (i.e., those phobias associated with external stimuli) and the age of onset, clinical features, physiological measurements, treatment, and possibly prognosis. Although these correlates need more substantiation than is presently available, they are a beginning, and could help in the future to isolate and define the various types of phobias into distinct disease entities. Of course, to the average clinician physiological measurements are not available, hence, they are of little practical value. Further, the meaning of physiological findings is not clear. Yet, this classification does break down the phobias into manageable proportions, allows more precise definitions and correlations, and offers the hope for better case management. It will, therefore, be used in this book.

ETIOLOGY

There have been few systematic studies of phobias. One difficulty with these studies is the wide diversity of clinical manifestations. Can a fear of spiders rightfully be compared to a fear of leaving one's home or to a fear of illness? Another difficulty is that investigators use different criteria. Also, some psychiatrists consider phobias and anxiety as synonymous and others consider phobias as part of obsessive compulsive neurosis. Simply stated, patients with fear as a primary emotional component (e.g., patients who suffer from animal phobias) must be carefully compared and investigated with patients who have similar fears as well as with patients who have apparently dissimilar fears (e.g., patients who suffer from a fear of illness). Sufficient systematic studies of this type have not been done.

Although the phylogenetic origin of phobias has been established, the genetic basis is not clear. Twin studies show that in cases where one twin is phobic the other member is not.[23] Personality evaluations do not correlate with any one type even though phobics are described as being timid, shy, dependent, immature, and as having high introversion scores on the Eysenck Personality Inventory.[24] More studies need to be done on psychiatric as well as nonpsychiatric groups before any conclusions can be drawn regarding the role of heredity in phobias.

The relationship between mood changes and phobias has been investigated. Animal and situational phobias were found to be relatively unaffected by anxiety or depressive affective illness while social phobias and agoraphobia could be markedly increased. Withdrawal is easily understandable with depression and socialization in the depressed group was easier with strangers than with friends. With anxiety states on the other hand, social phobias and agoraphobia showed more of an increase in the presence of strangers than with relatives or friends. Patients with anxiety states have more phobias before and during the illness than those with depression. Also, the most significant increase of agoraphobia was associated with patients who had anxiety states; hence, anxiety seems to be more primary to social phobia and agoraphobia than depression.[25] These findings have additional relevance since physical illness can precipitate an affective illness; therefore, curing a physical illness may help remove phobias.

Psychoanalysts view phobias as involving more than sensory perceptual associations. To them phobias represent a failure of repression and a symbolic displacement of the conflict to an object, situation, or idea. The phobic symptoms unconsciously include both the forbidden wish and the fear of the wish.[26] Salzman thinks that the hard-core problem of the phobias is the obsessive compulsive character structure and the individual's fear of losing control over his impulses. He does not emphasize, as Freud does, the sexual and aggressive impulses but any impulse that threatens the integrity of the individual. Further, he says that phobias:

> . . . may develop around tender impulses, power drives, or the need to maintain pride and self-esteem. Loss of control and concern about humiliating and threatening consequences which might result are factors that produce a phobia . . . . The phobia, by an absolute injunction, prevents an individual from confronting any situation, place, or person potentially capable of producing anxiety and that may temporarily put the individual out of control. It is a ritualized avoidance reaction which, like all rituals, attempts to exert some control over nature through the agency of magic. The phobia is a ritual of "no doing" or inaction.[27]

For analysts, the phobic object or situation is secondary; symbolism, fear of losing control, and the obsessive compulsive personality are primary.

Behaviorists explain phobias on the basis of conditioning, modeling, sensory association, and learning. A neutral stimulus, by contiguous association with a traumatic or painful stimulus, evokes the same response as the traumatic stimulus. The effects of such an association provides the basis for classical conditioning. Phobias can be acquired by direct learning or imitation (modeling), e.g., a mother who exhibits fear towards an object will provide a model for the child. Phobias by sensory association tend to generalize, get progressively broader, and reappear in other situations. Finally, phobias can be learned on the basis of cognition in which the patient is aware of the consequences to which his behavior will lead; hence, he avoids certain situations. This formulation of learning involves symbolic and cognitive processes; hence, behaviorists who explain phobias using learning theory are, like psychoanalysts, using symbols but interpreting them differently. In addition, behaviorist explanations are becoming more complex and not entirely physiological.[28,29]

Culturally, the family and society can influence the kind of circumstances to which individuals will react fearfully.[30] Many phobias start without any apparent change in the patient's life situation, some begin with a trivial incident, and a substantial number start with a major change, i.e., divorce, serious illness, death of a close person, marriage, pregnancy, childbirth, etc. With such a wide degree of stressors the relationship of the person's psychological state at a specific time and circumstance is the biggest consideration.

DIAGNOSIS

The clinical syndromes of phobic neuroses vary. Class I phobias, as previously noted, are correlated with the source of stimulus, age of onset, physiological measurements, prognosis, and preferred type or types of treatment. Those phobias related to external stimuli (Class I) are as follows.

(1) Animal phobias

Young infants fear loud noises and sudden movements, older children fear strangers, but fear of animals usually does not begin before the age of eight. This contrasts with all other phobias, which usually start between adolescence and middle age. Before puberty the distribution of animal phobias is equal in both sexes, after that time they predominate in women. The phobias are usually limited to a single type of animal, e.g., birds, dogs, mice, cats, insects, etc. It is questionable whether such a universal fear of snakes or sinister animals should be included under this category.

Psychophysiological measurements reveal that patients with animal phobias acquire eyeblink conditioning more rapidly and extinguish the response more slowly than the normal; show normal habituation and spontaneous fluctuation on the galvanic skin resistance test to successive auditory stimuli; and demonstrate normal forearm blood flow. These measurements confirm the absence of diffuse anxiety. Adults rarely seek treatment for this condition alone and respond to desensitization, flooding (implosion) or psychotherapy.[31]

(2) Specific situational phobias (miscellaneous specific phobias)

These phobias are monosymptomatic, do not include animate objects, have an equal incidence in either sex, can start at anytime from childhood through old age, and persist fairly consistently. They are related to isolated situations—heights, wind, dark, closed spaces, thunder, running water, etc.—and remain limited to a specific situation.

Physiological measurements are not available but are probably similar to those found in animal phobias since these patients do not show signs of generalized anxiety. Likewise, treatment similar to that used with patients who have animal phobias is effective and response to treatment is good.[32]

(3) Social phobias

These phobias usually start after puberty, have their highest incidence in late adolescence, have equal sex distribution, and may begin anywhere through the late thirties. A distinguishing characteristic is that social phobias occur in the presence of another individual, not in groups or crowds. In a one to one situation a patient with a social phobia may be unable to eat, speak, or write and besides being fearful they may shake, blush, vomit, get dizzy, tremble, etc. These symptoms, when severe enough, can lead to avoidance of friendships with consequent loss of social relationships and even work. In extreme cases complete social isolation can occur with the one exception that they usually maintain their family contacts.

Physiological measurements reveal increased spontaneous fluctuations and decreased habituation on the galvanic skin resistance test, increased resting forearm blood flow, and more rapidly acquired eyeblink conditioned response than normals. These data indicate a high level of generalized anxiety.

Comparing social phobia, animal phobia, and agoraphobia reveals that animal phobia has the fewest and agoraphobia the greatest number of psychiatric symptoms associated with it. Social phobia seems to stand somewhere in between the other two. It occurs, as does agoraphobia, at an older age than animal phobias. In addition, social phobia occurs less frequently in women than either animal phobia or agoraphobia and its anxiety level is closer to agoraphobia than to that of animal phobia. The response to treatment in social phobia is somewhere in between animal phobia which shows the best response to treatment and agoraphobia which shows the worst response to treatment.

Some questions center on whether social phobias are a coherent group or merely a stage of agoraphobia. Both are symptomatologically alike and relate to the presence of people. At times both types show up in the same patient. The differences are that agoraphobia has a high incidence in women, more symptoms, more generalized anxiety, depression, unreality symptoms, and a poorer prognosis than social phobias.[33]

(4) Agoraphobia

The term agoraphobia is sometimes defined as a fear of open spaces but this is incorrect both clinically and etymologically. A medical journal editorial says:

> The Hellenistic agora was a meeting of the people, and by derivation the word came to be used for the place where the meeting was held. It is only because of the fine weather of Greece that the agora was in the open, and if the term agoraphobia were derived from Anglo-Saxon it would no doubt also carry the meaning of fear of enclosed spaces .... The Greek term agora also came to mean the gift of public speaking, and it is interesting that among agoraphobic patients the act of speaking in public is the most terrifying ordeal of all.[34]

The central, but not sole, feature of agoraphobia is fear of going into various kinds of public places. It is actually a cluster of features that includes many phobias occurring in various combinations that can be associated with anxiety, panic, depression, obsessions, and depersonalization. Hence, confusion in diagnosis occurs and agoraphobia is often called anxiety hysteria, locomotor anxiety, street fear, phobic-anxiety-depersonalization syndrome, anxiety syndrome or phobic-anxious states, anxiety states, anxiety neurosis, severe mixed psychoneurosis, pseudoneurotic schizophrenia, borderline states, and nonspecific insecurity fears. Although agoraphobia may have symptoms similar to any of the above conditions, it is distinct and different. It is a concept that includes various components found in all phobias. The fear of going into open meeting places is the central or hard-core component and the other components may or may not be present, in varying degrees, in a specific case.[35]

This is the most common and most distressing phobia seen by psychiatrists. In a survey of agoraphobics in Britain it was found that 19% had relatives with similar phobias.[36] Studies indicate that agoraphobics come from stable close-knit families with overprotective mothers; conversely, psychopaths come from broken homes. Premorbid personality has been described as shy, passive, dependent, and anxious, however, a minority of agoraphobics were outgoing, active persons prior to becoming ill.[37]

Agoraphobia occurs mainly in women and usually starts between the ages of 18 and 35. These patients have a higher incidence of childhood phobias than control groups. Frigidity is not an uncommon precursor and concomitant of the illness. These patients are disabled to varying degrees such as a partial disability in which the patient is unable to enter an airplane or supermarket to a severe disability in which the patient cannot leave his home.[38]

Agoraphobia can begin abruptly after severe stress, for no apparent reason, or slowly in association with moderate anxiety. Dependence on others is conspicuous and symptoms may appear when the relationship with a significant individual is threatened. This individual is closely bound with the patient's sense of security. These patients go to extreme lengths to have someone home with them at all times or constantly visit with their mother or another close relative. When this dependence is related to the husband, he may have to change his shift to avoid night work, not travel long distances from home, or be forced to do all the shopping. In severe cases, the patient becomes housebound and may need a constant companion. When this dependence on a significant person is threatened other phobias may appear and some patients begin to manifest symptoms characteristic of anxiety, depersonalization, depression, obsessions, compulsions, etc.

Agoraphobia is most intense in enclosed spaces as stores, airplanes, vehicles, restaurants, theaters, buses, churches, and in situations where the patient finds himself surrounded by crowds. He then gets flushed, flustered, tremulous, pale, and panic-stricken. Waiting in a crowd may lead a patient to leave in flight, fear, embarrassment, and humiliation. The patient fears fainting, helplessness, and uncontrollable behavior. Once he faints, phobias become intensified and the patient can become wholly incapacitated to the point where he may refuse to go shopping, walk outdoors, or even leave the home. Hyperventilation can cause tetany and fainting. In extreme cases, sleep is broken and restless, and dreams are terrifying. The patient may become anorexic, lose weight, and become exhausted until he appears pallid, haggard, and drawn. These symptoms

can fluctuate depending upon internal and external stressors, and partial remissions and episodic exacerbations occur. The patient is in a constant state of
flux but there are phases in which he is relatively comfortable. In cases
that last longer than one year partial rather than complete recovery is the
usual outcome.[39]

Physiological measurements suggest a high anxiety level in agoraphobic
patients. Slow habituation and a large number of spontaneous fluctuations
on the galvanic skin resistance test and a slight increase in forearm blood flow
confirm the high anxiety level. The eyeblink conditioning response, however,
is acquired and extinguished at normal rates. Findings of high anxiety levels
and/or association with multiple panic attacks or obsessions are associated with
a poor prognosis.[40, 41]

The following is a description of Class II phobias or phobias in which the
patient suffers from an internal stimulus which cannot be avoided:

(1) Illness phobias

Patients of both sexes suffer equally from the fear of a specific illness such
as cancer, heart disease, venereal disease, stroke, etc. There is endless rumination
about these diseases and the amount of pain and suffering that they will bring.
The phobic illness differs from the obsessive in that the phobia does not have
subjective resistance, and differs from hypochondria in that the phobic's concern
usually involves a specific illness whereas the hypochondriac's concern is more
generalized.[42]

(2) Obsessive phobias

These are repetitive fears that the patient knows are foolish, inappropriate,
and not typical of him. Examples are a fear of hurting others, stabbing one's
baby, swearing, contamination, undressing in public, forcing intercourse on
someone, etc. These phobias are generally found in association with neuroses
such as anxiety, depressive, or obsessive compulsive, and are usually included
under one of these categories for diagnostic purposes, with the phobic symptoms
as ancillary diagnostic criteria. Even though these phobias are usually considered
with the other diagnostic categories, Marks says:

> These obsessions could strictly be called phobias; they are disproportionate
> to demands of the situation, cannot be explained away and are beyond
> voluntary control.[43]

The proper diagnostic category for obsessive phobias has not been satisfactorily
determined.

All phobias, irrespective of stimulus source, must be viewed from a holistic
viewpoint. School phobia, also called school refusal, is an excellent example
of this principle. School phobias, most prevalent in boys between the ages of
7 and 16 with a peak age of onset between 11 and 12, is characterized by

outright refusal to go to school and acute fear and anxiety emotional responses that may include inability to sleep or eat, abdominal pain, nausea, vomiting, headaches, diarrhea, sore throat, leg pains, etc. Etiological factors are multiple: personality defects, fear of leaving mother or separation anxiety, fear that something dreadful will happen to either parent while at school, or an actual situation in school that threatens the child with either failure, loss of self-esteem, or physical harm. A school phobic must be differentiated from a truant, who is absent from school without permission and often even knowledge of the parents, and from a school withdrawal who is kept home by the parents for whatever reason. Treatment for the school phobic varies, i.e., individual or family psychotherapy (dynamic or behavioral), and environmental readjustment (either within that school or change to a different school). School phobia, like all other phobias, is not a simple phenomenon but a complex biopsychosocial entity that conforms to the comprehensive model of disease.[44-46]

DIFFERENTIAL DIAGNOSIS

Most people have some irrational fears. These are not serious nor can they be considered neurosis. Specific animal or situation phobias usually require very little effort to diagnose. Multiple phobias, social, and agoraphobias, however, require careful differential diagnostic evaluation.

Both anxiety neurosis and phobic neurosis must be distinguished from fear. In normal fear a real danger must exist. The distinction between anxiety neurosis and phobic neurosis (animal, specific, or social situation) is that irrational fear in the latter exists related to a specific object, situation, or a social circumstance. Irrational fear is cardinal for the phobia and anxiety or "nervousness" for anxiety neurosis. Anxiety neurosis is a more generalized and diffuse disease. In agoraphobic neurosis, the dependence on others and the inability to visit public places are the outstanding differentiating characteristics. Both anxiety and phobia can be symptoms of almost every type of mental condition, and for diagnosis the totality of the situation must be considered. To decide what is the primary and what is the secondary condition is often difficult.

Phobic states in which anxiety and depersonalization predominate should be distinguished from temporal lobe epilepsy and diseases of the temporal lobe. When the attacks of phobia have a very sharp onset and last no more than seconds, it is usually wise to suspect an organic origin. Self injury and incontinence of urine and feces are more common in epileptics. Further, the orderliness of events in epileptic attacks contrasts with phobia in which there is a variability in symptom progression.[47]

The distinction between illness phobia and obsessive compulsive neurosis is not so clear-cut. In some cases, the patient's compulsive thinking and behavior is secondary to a phobia as when he must wash all the food he eats because he fears the food is unclean; in another case the patient's thinking and behavior may stem from obsessive rumination (as when he keeps thinking he is covered with germs and thus constantly scrubs his hands); and in still other cases, the patient claims he has no idea why he is engaging in such behavior except that it makes him feel better. Some psychiatrists believe the symptoms may appear sequentially. In a sequence where obsessions are primary, the patient may begin by obsessionally thinking about germs, then he directs his thinking by phobically avoiding contact with objects he considers covered with germs, and finally he no longer considers avoidance sufficient and washes his hands compulsively. Transition from obsessive thinking to phobic avoidance and compulsive behavior, and finally to delusional thinking takes place at the point where the patient considers himself "contaminated." He then appreciates less the absurdity and irrationality of his fears, and is schizophrenic.[48]

The stage at which the patient is able to keep the symptoms in check is the important differentiating feature. In phobias related to external stimuli, the patient can be made comfortable by avoiding the object or situation which causes him distress. The obsessive patient is unlikely to find avoidance effective. Furthermore, phobic symptoms emerge and disappear more readily than the obsessive, and the phobic can accurately describe when the symptom first appeared and when he is symptom-free. This is less true of the obsessive patient. Although the onset of symptoms in the obsessive may be dated, it is more likely to be a slow progression or an exaggeration of a preexisting meticulousness and rigid personality. In addition, obsessive symptoms usually remit less frequently and completely, and more slowly than in phobics. Generally, in the obsessive patient, community relationships decline first, next family relationships become estranged, and finally, ability to work declines or is lost. In phobics, especially agoraphobics, the sequence may differ. Work may suffer first due to fear of traveling, entering elevators, or other similar difficulties, then community relations and finally family relationships are affected. The longer the illness lasts, the less the family can tolerate the demands of the phobic.[49]

At times phobics become depressed and even suicidal, or suffer from depersonalization. During depersonalization the patient believes that he has lost his identity. He may feel like an automaton or outside himself, or that the world is unfamiliar or strange. Phobics may experience other states such as conversion hysteria or fugues but these states are not very common.

COURSE AND PROGNOSIS

Controlled follow-up studies are few, therefore, not much is known about the natural history of the various types of phobias. Case descriptions and personal experiences that include course and prognosis are the major source of information.[50] This method has disadvantages, i.e., it lacks critical definitions, criteria, reliability, etc. One five-year follow-up study of untreated phobics showed that many improved without treatment; childhood phobias (100% improved or recovered within five years) did not last as long as adult phobias; and the rate of improvement for untreated cases approximated the rate of treated cases (about 43%). Further findings indicate that prognosis depends upon degree of generalization of the phobia and the degree of fear—more generalization and greater fear result in poorer prognosis.[51] Yet another study showed a significant correlation (35%) between childhood symptoms or traits and the same symptoms or traits present in adulthood, e.g., fear of thunder, animals, and injections.[52] No attempt was made in the latter study to evaluate improvement or recovery rates; hence, the two studies cannot be compared. It does, however, demonstrate the lack of consistent research methods.

Generally, in phobias due to external stimuli, animal and situational phobias have a better prognosis then social phobia with agoraphobia having the worst prognosis. Prognosis of phobias due to internal stimuli (illness and obsessive types) is not known but clinical observations mitigate against a good prognosis. Acute phobias usually remit, but once they persist over one year complete remission without treatment is not likely. Agoraphobics can improve with treatment to the point where they may lead useful lives, but rarely do they improve to the point where there is a complete removal of the symptoms.[53]

TREATMENT

The best treatment is prevention. Besides inheriting the right genes, prevention involves creating an environment from infancy onward in which the behavioral patterns are such that the individual faces and solves difficulties immediately in the here and now. Consistent with this belief is the notion that following a traumatic circumstance, the person should reenter the situation as soon as possible which may stop excessive fantasizing regarding the trauma and hopefully prevent a reinforcement of the phobic situation. Even in the face of the above attitudes, phobias do become established. Once established, treatment becomes more difficult.[54]

Many treatment modalities exist. Each is consistent with the general orientation of the psychiatrist. For animal, situational, and uncomplicated social phobias, variations of individual, family, and group psychotherapy, and relaxation techniques are used. The following are some of the more common methods: (1) systematic desensitization—gradually exposing the patient to the feared situation or object both in imagination and in reality; (2) flooding—sudden exposure to the phobic stimuli; (3) supportive or insight psychotherapy; (4) vigorous muscular activity (running) prior to increasing exposure to a phobic situation; (5) desensitization with muscle relaxation techniques with or without concomitant psychotherapy, hypnosis, or drugs.[55-59]

The management of the agoraphobic is difficult. These patients should be under the care of a psychiatrist and not the general practitioner. It is unfortunate that in many cases the patient has been housebound 10 to 20 years before seeing a psychiatrist and by then intractable avoidance may be superimposed on the original illness. An acute agoraphobic attack needs immediate treatment. Hospitalization may be necessary. Adequate dosages of antianxiety drugs should be administered, i.e., enough to relieve the panic. Psychotherapy should be initiated. Some time after the acute episode subsides and a doctor-patient relationship is established, groups with patients who have similar symptoms may be recommended. For the chronic state of agoraphobia, tranquilizers are of little help since tolerance develops; however, drugs should be used on occasions when the fear can be reduced enough to allow the patient to function outside the home—attending a wedding, going to church, entering a store, and so on. Where there is evidence of depression tricyclics are indicated. Various types of behavior therapy may be tried such as desensitization, flooding (implosion), or operant conditioning. These should be supplemented by psychotherapy. At times, when weight loss is a prominent feature, insulin may be necessary. As a last resort, in patients considered incurable, leucotomy may be performed.[60–63]

REFERENCES

1. Sarason, I.G., "Test anxiety, attention, and the general problem of anxiety," in *Stress and Anxiety*, vol. 1 (edited by Spielberger, C.D., and Sarason, I.G.). New York: Wiley, 1975, p. 179.
2. Lazarus, R.S. and Averill, J.R., "Emotion and cognition: With special reference to anxiety," in *Anxiety: Current Trends in Theory and Research*, vol. 2 (edited by Spielberger, C.D.). New York: Academic, 1972, p. 255.
3. Ibid., pp. 256–257.
4. Ibid., pp. 257–258.
5. James, W., *The Varieties of Religious Experience: A Study in Human Nature* (edition authorized by Longmans, Green and Co.). New York: Modern Library, 1902, p. 96.
6. Macquarrie, J., *Existentialism*. Baltimore: Penguin, 1972, pp. 120–134.
7. Agras, S., Sylvester, D. and Oliveau, D., The epidemiology of common fears and phobia. *Compr. Psychiatry* 10:151–156 (1969).
8. Terhune, W., The phobic syndrome: A study of eighty-six patients with phobic reactions. *Arch. Neurol. Psychiatry* 62:162–172 (1949).
9. Errera, P., Some historical aspects of the concept of phobia. *Psychiatric Quart.* 36:325–336 (1962).
10. Russell, B., *A History of Western Philosophy*. New York: Simon and Schuster, 1945, p. 574.
11. Laughlin, H.P., *The Neuroses*. Washington, D.C.: Butterworth, 1967, p. 550.
12. Lewis, A., A note on classifying phobia. *Psychol. Med.* 6:21 (1976).
13. Hall, G.S., A study of fear. *Amer. J. Psychol.* 8:147 (1897).
14. Janet, P., *Psychological Healing: A Historical and Clinical Study*, vol. 1 (transl. by Paul, E.S.). London: George Allen & Unwin, 1925, pp. 272–273.

15. Freud, S., "Obsessions and phobias; their psychical mechanisms and their aetiology (1895)," in *Collected Papers,* vol. 1, 6th impression (edited by Jones, E. and transl. by Riviere, J.). London: Hogarth, 1950, pp. 128–137.

16. Freud, S., *A General Introduction to Psychoanalysis* (transl. by Riviere, J.). New York: Garden City Publishing Company, 1943, pp. 345–348.

17. Ibid., p. 348.

18. Provisional classification: Published as a looseleaf manual entitled *DSM-III Draft, 4/15/77.* DRAFT OF AXES I and II of DSM-III CLASSIFICATION as of March 30, 1977.

19. Laughlin, H.P., op. cit., pp. 553–555.

20. Wolpe, J. and Lang, P.J., A fear survey schedule for use in behavior therapy. *Behav. Res. Ther.* 2:27–30 (1964).

21. Wolpe, J., *The Practice of Behavior Therapy,* 2nd ed. New York: Pergamon, 1973, pp. 108–115.

22. Marks, I.M., *Fears and Phobias.* New York: Academic, 1969, pp. 105–106.

23. Ibid., p. 79

24. Ibid., p. 80

25. Schapira, K., Kerr, T.A. and Roth, M., Phobias and affective illness. *Brit. J. Psychiatry* 117:25–32 (1970).

26. Freud, S., "Analysis of a phobia in a five-year old boy (1909)," in *Collected Papers,* vol. 3, 7th impression (edited by Jones, E. and transl. by Strachey, A. and Strachey, J.). London: Hogarth, 1950, pp. 49–289.

27. Salzman, L., *The Obsessive Personality: Origins, Dynamics and Therapy.* New York: Science House, 1968, p. 129.

28. Marks, I.M., op. cit., pp. 85–94.

29. Mischel, W., *Introduction to Personality,* 2nd ed. New York: Holt, Rinehart and Winston, 1976, pp. 79–82.

30. Marks, I.M., op. cit., pp. 80–81.

31. Marks, I.M., The classification of phobic disorders. *Brit. J. Psychiatry* 116:379–380 (1970).

32. Ibid., p. 384.

33. Ibid., p. 383.

34. Editorial, *Brit. Med. J.* 5938:177 (1974).

35. Marks, I.M., Agoraphobic syndrome (phobic anxiety state). *Arch. Gen. Psychiatry* 23:538–539 (1970).

36. Marks, I.M. and Herst, E.R., A survey of 1,200 agoraphobics in Britain. *Social Psychiatry* 5(1):18 (1970).

37. Marks, I.M., Agoraphobic syndrome (phobic anxiety state). op. cit., pp. 540–541.

38. Ibid., pp. 539–542.

39. Ibid., pp. 542–552.

40. Agras, W.S., Chapin, H.N. and Oliveau, D.C., The natural history of phobia. *Arch. Gen. Psychiatry* 26:315–317 (1972).

41. Marks, I.M., The classification of phobic disorders. op. cit., p. 381.

42. Ibid., p. 384.

43. Ibid., p. 384.

44. Marks, I.M., *Fears and Phobias,* op. cit., pp. 173–177.

45. Lassers, E., Nordan, R. and Bladholm, S., Steps in the return to school of children with school phobia. *Amer. J. Psychiatry* 130(3):265–268 (1973).

46. Waldron, Jr., S., Shrier, D., Stone, B. and Tobin, F., School phobia and other childhood neuroses: A systematic study of the children and their families. *Amer. J. Psychiatry* 132(8):802–808 (1975).

47. Slater, E. and Roth, M., *Clinical Psychiatry,* 3rd ed.   Baltimore: Williams & Wilkins, 1970, pp. 460–462.
48. Laughlin, H.P., op. cit., pp. 558–562.
49. Detre, T.P. and Jarecki, H.G., *Modern Psychiatric Treatment.*   Philadelphia: Lippincott, 1971, pp. 228–229.
50. Ambrosino, S.V., Phobic anxiety-depersonalization syndrome. *N.Y. State J. Med.* 73:419–422 (1973).
51. Agras, W.S., Chapin, H.N. and Oliveau, D.C., The natural history of phobia, op. cit., pp. 315–317.
52. Abe, K., Phobias and nervous symptoms in childhood and maturity: Persistence and associations. *Brit. J. Psychiatry* 120:275–283 (1972).
53. Marks, I.M., *Fears and Phobias,* op. cit., pp. 265–267.
54. Ibid., pp. 180–182.
55. Van Egeren, L.F., Feather, B.W. and Hein, P.L., Desensitization of phobias: Some psychological propositions. *Psychophysiol.* 8(2):213–228 (1971).
56. Gillan, P. and Rachman, S., An experimental investigation of desensitization in phobic patients. *Brit. J. Psychiatry* 124:392–401 (1974).
57. Orwin, A., Treatment of a situational phobia—a case for running. *Brit. J. Psychiatry.* 125:95–98 (1974).
58. Razani, J., Treatment of phobias by systematic desensitization: Comparison of standard vs. methohexital-aided desensitization. *Arch. Gen. Psychiatry* 30:291–293 (1974).
59. Frankel, F.H. and Orne, M.T., Hypnotizability and phobic behavior. *Arch. Gen. Psychiatry* 33:1259–1261 (1976).
60. Hussain, M.Z., Desensitization and flooding (implosion) in treatment of phobias. *Amer. J. Psychiatry* 127(11):1509–1514 (1971).
61. Marks, I.M., *Fears and Phobias,* op. cit., pp. 267–270.
62. Carey, M.S., Hawkinson, R., Kornhaber, A. and Wellish, C.S., The use of clomipramine in phobic patients: Preliminary research report. *Cur. Ther. Res.* 17(1):107–110 (1975).
63. Silverstone, J.T., Lorazepam in phobic disorders: A pilot study. *Cur. Med. Res. Opinion* 1(5):272–275 (1973).

7
OBSESSIVE COMPULSIVE NEUROSIS

Obsession denotes unwanted repetitive thoughts, images, fears, or impulses. Compulsion denotes unwanted repetitive acts or complex behavioral patterns. Obsessive compulsive neurosis is an independent psychiatric disorder. It consists of the following components: (1) patient experiences obsessions alone, obsessions with compulsions, or compulsions alone; (2) patient realizes the nonsensical nature of his mental processes and behavior; (3) patient has conscious resistance to those unwanted repetitive phenomena; (4) patient usually feels distress, embarrassment, anxiety or fear emotional responses when he cannot complete obsessive or compulsive phenomena; (5) patient's will power and ability to control his mentation and/or behavior decreases in the areas involving the obsession or compulsion. In effect, the obsessive compulsive neurosis meets the criteria of a disease entity.[1]

Anancastic or anancasm are all-inclusive terms. They cover obsession, compulsion, obsessive compulsive neurosis, and obsessional personality. For example, anancastic personality is synonymous with obsessional or rigid personality. Alternatively, anancastic or compulsive symptoms include both obsessions and compulsions. Synonyms for obsessive compulsive neurosis include obsessional state, constitutional syndrome, or neurosis; obsessional-ruminative state; phobic-ruminative state; compulsion neurosis; and psychasthenia. Terminology varies among psychiatrists as well as in different countries.[2-4]

Further definitions are necessary. Akhtar posits the following forms of obsessions and compulsions:

(A) Obsessions: Six forms of obsessions were identified:
1. Obsessive doubt: An inclination not to believe that a completed task has been accomplished satisfactorily. (Each time he left his room a 28-year-old student began asking himself 'Did I lock the door? Am I sure?' in spite of a clear and accurate remembrance of having done so.)

2. Obsessive thinking: A seemingly endless thought chain, usually one pertaining to future events. (A 24-year-old pregnant Hindu girl tormented herself by thinking 'if my baby is a boy he might aspire to an academic career that would necessitate his going far away from me, but he might want to return to me and what would I do then, because if I . . . ,' and so on.)

3. Obsessive impulse: A powerful urge to carry out actions which may be trivial or socially disruptive or even assaultive. (A 41-year-old lawyer was obsessed by what he understood to be the 'nonsensical notion' of drinking from his inkpot, but also by the serious urge to strangle an apparently beloved only son.)

4. Obsessive fear: A fear of losing self-control and thus inadvertently commiting a socially embarrassing act. Unlike the obsessive impulse, there is no actual urge involved here. Marks* (1969) holds that these are 'fears about one's own feelings.' (A 32-year-old teacher was afraid that in the classroom he would refer to his unsatisfactory sexual relations with his wife, although he had no wish to do so.)

5. Obsessive image: The persistence before the mind's eye of something seen, usually recently. (A 47-year-old housewife kept 'seeing a car's licence plate that had come to her attention. Another patient 'saw' her baby being flushed away in the toilet whenever she entered the bathroom.)

6. Miscellaneous forms: Phenomena obsessional in nature but unclassifiable in the above five categories. (A 23-year-old student could not rid her consciousness of a currently popular tune.)

(B) Compulsions: Two distinct categories were identified:

1. Yielding compulsion: A compulsive act that gives expression to the underlying obsessive urge. (A 29-year-old clerk had an obsessive doubt that he had an important document in one of his pockets. He knew that this was not true, but found himself compelled to check his pockets again and again.)

2. Controlling compulsion: A compulsive act that tends to divert the underlying obsession without giving expression to it. (A 16-year-old boy with incestuous impulses controlled the anxiety these aroused by repeatedly and loudly counting to ten.)[5]

Obsessional doubting is more common than any other form of obsession, and a patient may fluctuate between several forms. For instance, a patient may wonder, after leaving her home whether she closed the door (obsessive doubt); then, may have the urge to kill her child and reject the urge as ridiculous (obsessive impulse); then, fear undressing in public (obsessive fear); and finally, either check the door several times to make sure it is closed (yielding compulsion);

*Marks, I.M., *Fears and Phobias*. New York: Academic Press, 1969, pp. 163–165.

or count to ten in order to divert herself from the obsessive fear, thought, or urge (controlling compulsion). Although these forms differ from one another, content can be the same irrespective of form.[6] The most common content of anancasm involves preoccupation with:

(1) Health maintenance (diet, exercise, sleep, or weight); disease (cancer, heart, insanity, venereal); dirt, germs, contamination, and death.
(2) Sexual deviations (exhibitionism, homosexuality, pedophilia, incest, etc.); and dysfunctions (frigidity, impotence, premature ejaculation, dyspareunia, etc.).
(3) Aggression towards self (suicide, injuries), others (homocide, accidents), larger community (wars, natural calamities).
(4) Family welfare (health, finances, and relationships).
(5) Religious matters (contemplation of God's existence, performance of rituals, church attendance, questions of faith, etc.).
(6) Work and its rewards (position, security, acceptance, etc.).
(7) Impersonal abstractions (numbers, mathematics, geometric designs, etc.).
(8) Orderliness and cleanliness (books on the shelf, shirts in the dresser, extreme precision in arrangement of life's daily routines, hand washing, house cleaning, etc.).

Content is extremely variable not only with individuals but also with different cultures. The frequency of specific content may vary with culture.[7, 8]

Certain normal activities are distinguished from obsessive compulsive phenomena. Children's play is often repetitive. They hop a certain number of times on one leg and then switch to the other, or take a stick and tap it in a prescribed manner. Adults experience haunting melodies or recurring memories. Daily routines are for the most part repetitive and normal—morning ablutions, dress, transportation to and from work, a "procedure" at work, and so on. It is, however, necessary to distinguish these from other forms of rituals. Repetitive behavior can become connected with fantasies of good and evil. Children, for example, can imagine that cracks in the sidewalk represent deep gulfs in the earth and should they not walk or hop in a certain manner, they will fall into the gulf or be stricken. In time, they cannot stop this ritual even though they realize it is nonsensical. At this point it is pathological. Adults have superstitions. Acts such as throwing a pinch of salt or spitting three times in a certain manner can take the meaning of good or evil. Although irrationality is admitted, only when a certain degree of discomfort accompanies the superstition is neurosis present. Primitive people have many superstitions and they obey certain rituals (rain making, dance ceremonials, etc.) which they believe influence their daily lives. If they think that an outside force, not an inner thought or impulse, is governing and directing their actions, they are psychotic. The progression from normal repetitive behavior to uncontrollable obsessions to psychosis must be evaluated in terms of the individual in a specific circumstance and society. Religious observance, ceremonials, and traditions share with other rituals the potential of being performed for normal or abnormal purposes.[9]

Brain-damaged patients tend toward a rigidity and orderliness that resembles compulsive behavior. Repetition is found in association with encephalitis, traumatic injuries to the brain, senility, space-occupying lesions within the brain, substances toxic to nerve tissue, and so on. There is also an increase in repetitive behavior during fatigue and hypnagogic states. These are not compulsions. Furthermore, patients suffering from schizophrenia and manic-depressive psychosis demonstrate stereotyped mannerisms. This phenomenon, when strictly defined, does not meet the criteria of compulsions but rather is part of the phenomenology of these illnesses. Conversely, cases of organic brain disease and schizophrenia may have true obsessions and compulsions.

In sum, obsessive compulsive neurosis must be defined rigidly, or else it becomes meaningless. Essentials are an uncontrollable repetitive urge, thought, image, fear, or act that the patient resists. Content varies with individuals and cultures. Finally, obsessive compulsive neurosis should be distinguished from normal repetitive behavior, superstitions, ceremonials, and rituals as well as stereotyped behavior associated with other diseases—mental or physical.

HISTORY

French psychiatrists were the first to describe and evolve a concept of obsessive compulsive states. In 1838, Jean Étienne Esquirol described the first case of obsessive doubting and grouped it with monomanias. Jean-Pierre Falret later named it "the illness of the doubt." In 1861, A. Benedict Morel coined the term "obsession" and insisted that it was an emotional illness. In 1867, Richard von Krafft-Ebing introduced the term into German psychiatry and observed that obsessions were influenced by depression. In 1870, Wilhelm Griesinger used the term to describe recurring thoughts that occurred in the form of questions and were beyond the control and against the better judgment of the patient. In 1878, Carl F. Westphal integrated the thinking of his predecessors and proposed that obsessional ideas were independent of any affective state, existed in consciousness in spite of and against the patient's will, and were recognized by the patient as abnormal and strange. Westphal emphasized cognition and negated the dependence of obsessions on affects. This idea contrasted with Krafft-Ebing who associated obsessions with depression and French psychiatrists who insisted on the affective basis for obsessions. Controversy existed, although both German and French schools agreed that the obsessional process was involuntary, automatic, and resisted by the patient. The Germans separated intellectual from emotional disease. Thought and action were voluntarily controlled, they reasoned, whereas sensations and affects were involuntary. Therefore, German psychiatrists defined obsession as a disease of intellect and believed, in contrast to the French, that the occurrence of anxiety or depression was secondary and without causal significance.[10-12]

In 1903, Pierre Janet introduced the term and concept of psychasthenia which included obsessions, phobias, and other neurotic syndromes, but excluded hysteria. In attempting a psychology of conduct he tried to avoid the division of mind into compartments and pondered over the total individual in an environment. Psychasthenic patients have lowered energy and tension levels, split consciousness, general weariness and inadequacy, lack of perseverance, and a tendency to depersonalize. Obsessive ideas, Janet thought, encountered resistance such as doubts, hesitations, or uneasiness, caused by a weakness in the patient's power of reflection and decision-making. Yet the patient's ability to reflect is never completely lost, so obsessive ideas never have a totally free reign. Lowered energy levels lead to a decrease in higher mental ability; especially will and attention. Consequently, the patient cannot control his thoughts, images, fears, impulses, or actions; nor can he perceive self and environment realistically, or behave appropriately. Janet defined a clinical entity and offered an explanation.[13, 14]

Sigmund Freud, like Janet, was concerned with the meaning of obsessional neurosis. In 1895, he considered obsessions and phobias as symbolic rituals which replaced repressed sexual feelings that emerged into consciousness.[15] In 1908, Freud traced the origin of obsessive compulsive neurosis and personality to the anal-sadistic stage of development. He claimed that due to conflict between parents and child over bowel training, the child becomes fixated at the anal level and is predisposed to anal personality traits (orderliness, parsimony, and obstinacy), or later in life, when repression fails, regresses to the fixated anal level of development and develops symptoms of the neurosis.[16] Freud held this formulation of obsessional neurosis throughout his life.[17] Psychic mechanisms such as symbolization, displacement, reaction-formation, undoing, and isolation result from failure of repression and regression.

In 1925, Kurt Schneider defined obsessions as contents of consciousness accompanied by subjective compulsions that cannot be shed even though recognized as senseless. In 1936, Lewis posited that recognizing the obsession as senseless is not the essential character since obsessions are not always senseless or absurd and he criticized Schneider's failure to mention that obsessive ideas were contrary to and in spite of the patient's will. According to Lewis (1957) the essential feature was resistance or struggle against the obsession or compulsion. Rituals and ceremonials, when accompanied by obsessions, ward off the overwhelming painful obsession and are secondary. The more a repetitive act is enjoyed the less likelihood of its being obsessional. Freedom of will separates the obsessional from the schizophrenic and resistance is experienced as a loss of free will.[18-20] The current definition relies heavily on the concepts of Westphal, Schneider, and Lewis. The intention here is not to negate the value of Janet, Freud, and others toward furthering our understanding, but rather to emphasize the struggle and the years that it took to distinguish obsessional states.

CLASSIFICATION

The problem of classifying obsessive compulsive neurosis relates to the need to: (1) establish increased reliability by clearly defined criteria for the disease and its components; (2) separate a distinct disease entity; (3) distinguish symptoms, traits, and disease; (4) search for ways to increase validity. The first part of this chapter attempts to carefully define obsessional neurosis and its component parts within a holistic framework; hence, no further elaboration on this point is necessary.

Obsessional states have been described, defined, or classified as follows: Esquirol (1838)–*"folie de doute,"* grouped with monomanias; Morel (1861)– manifestation of *"delire émotif"*; Krafft-Ebing (1867)–abnormal influence on thoughts and will in depressive states (*"Zwangsvorstellungen"*); Griesinger (1868)–compulsion to question (*"Zwangsvorstellungen"*); Westphal (1877)– classical description subsumed under thought abnormality; Freud (1895)– separates obsessions and phobias as separate entities; Janet (1903)–holistic concept and separates psychasthenia from neurasthenia; Dornblüth (1911)– subsumes the following under psychasthenia: true obsessive phenomena, true compulsive phenomena, tics, instinctive acts without compulsion such as craving for food, drink, etc., and sexual anomalies (perversions); and Lewis (1936)– defined distinct disease entity.[21] Yet, it was not until 1952 in the DSMI that obsessive compulsive reactions (subsumed under Psychoneurotic Disorders) were officially separated from phobic reactions, and it was not until 1968 in the DSMII that obsessive compulsive neurosis (subsumed under Neuroses) came into existence. The DSMIII (draft of March 30, 1977) subsumed obsessive compulsive disorder under Anxiety Disorders.[22]

Curran in the 1972 seventh edition of his book writes regarding personality problems:

We use this term to cover broadly a whole range of neurotic states and abnormal personalities. Since they present to the practitioner as personality problems, we feel this approach to be more practical than the traditional one of considering neurotic states as if each were an illness in its own right. Traditionally, these states are listed as follows: anxiety neurosis, neurotic depression, . . . , hysteria, and obsessional neurosis. Of these, obsessional neurosis seems to us the only one which has the qualities of a real illness, and which cannot be satisfactorily conceived of purely in terms of personality reaction; we have, therefore separated it from our considerations of anxiety, hysteria and reactive depression, ...[23]

Similarly in developing a hierarchical system of classification Foulds subsumes compulsive and ruminative symptoms under neurotic symptoms while subsuming states of anxiety under Dysthymic States. He considers Dysthymic States (class I) the most normal of the categories with Neurotic Symptoms (class II) following. He defines four classes with the most disturbed patients in class IV (Delusions of Disintegration).[24] In addition, obsessive compulsive neurosis meets the criteria for a disease as defined in this book (see Chapter 3).

Traits and symptoms should be separated. Traits are sharply defined enduring characteristics that may be interpreted as normal or abnormal. The individual who is excessively orderly, precise, disciplined, penurious, clean, neat, rigid, overconscientious, and so forth can either be a normal or an abnormal personality. When the preceding traits are integrated appropriately within the personality, they promote adequate socialization and competent work. In order for this to be true, these traits must be present without the person feeling a subjective sense of obsession or compulsion and there should be no desire to resist these traits. On the other hand, the same traits can be ego-alien, counterproductive to socialization and work, and felt as an obsession or compulsion which is unwanted and resisted. Then the person is an obsessive compulsive personality. The obsessional personality is an extreme case in which a great deal of time and energy is lost with minutiae, performance is decreased, and efficiency is lost. Traits are universal, ego-syntonic, and enduring; symptoms are ego-alien and distressful to the patient or to others who are closely associated with him.[25, 26]

The obsessional personality cannot delegate responsibility to others and this trait causes work difficulties and/or family problems. He insists that things be done his way. Extreme persistence at a task is another trait which can cause problems. Obstacles do not stop him irrespective of reality because he is reluctant to change. Once moving in a direction, he continues until the task is completed and, in this sense, has mental inertia. Although a high moral and ethical value can be set on many of these characteristics—dependability, reliability, punctuality, precision, and scrupulousness—the obsessional personality may harm himself or others for a principle. He simply cannot let go. Traits, in this context, are symptoms of an abnormal personality.

Merely defining phenomena, although important, is not enough. Classification systems need valid correlations. Fortunately psychiatrists are now beginning to make these correlations. For instance, Akhtar divided obsessive compulsive according to form and content. He found that patients with obsessions alone not only had the best prognosis but also had a greater strength of personality (ego-strength) than patients with compulsions. Further, he found that patients with controlling compulsions had greater ego-strength than those with yielding compulsion and that the ego-strength of patients with both types of compulsions was somewhere between those having only one type. To clarify, in order of decreasing ego-strength, the hierarchy descends from obsession alone to controlling compulsion, combination of controlling and yielding compulsion, and finally to yielding compulsion alone.[27]

Although no classification system of obsessional neurosis is generally accepted, the following is proposed.

(1) Acute obsessional neurosis: Symptoms appear for short periods of time and completely disappear within two to six months. They may reoccur at infrequent intervals.

(2) Subacute obsessional neurosis: Symptoms are lifelong enduring personality traits that are ego-alien, distressing, and disturbing to the patient or to others.

(3) Chronic obsessional neurosis: Symptoms that last longer than six months, usually vary in intensity but never completely disappear, and may or may not be associated with obsessional personality traits.

ETIOLOGY

Due to the rarity of the disease—0.05%-1.0% in the general population and 1-2% in psychiatric practice—and lack of controlled studies, very little systematic knowledge is available. It is, however, reasonable to assume that the disease is equally distributed between the sexes and the incidence of other mental illnesses in first degree relatives of obsessive neurotics is significantly higher when compared with families suffering from other types of neuroses. Evidence indicates that patients with this least common neurotic entity are often of above average intelligence, frequently exceptionally talented, and prone to abstract thinking. Finally, the age of onset, on average, is in the early twenties and these patients are frequently first born or only children.[28]

Many other conditions have been correlated with obsessive compulsive phenomenology. About 31%, approximately one third of the patients with the neurosis, have premorbid obsessive compulsive personality traits. Interestingly enough, many individuals with this premorbid personality never develop this neurosis, while those without any evidence of an obsessive personality do develop this neurosis. Obsessional neurosis and personality are associated with depression, anxiety, depersonalization, hypochondria, phobia, schizophrenia, organic brain disease, anorexia nervosa, migraine headaches, and duodenal ulcerations. Evidently the personality-illness relationship is not specific and the personality can only be considered as one factor associated with the illness. In fact, the symptoms in children with obsessive compulsive neurosis seem to be exaggerations of personality traits found in their parents. These parents are described as motorically underactive but verbally overactive, placing high value on social correctness, living within a form of social isolation, emphasizing cleanliness, adhering to high moral standards, and depreciating the value of maleness.[29-31]

There are hypotheses which. evaluate mood as the basic disturbance in obsessive compulsive neurosis. Some claim that obsessive compulsive phenomena occur when patients suffer from a high level anxiety and that the neurosis reduces the anxiety to a tolerable level.[32] Others stress depression as primary, because clinically, obsessive compulsive neurosis is often associated with depression. As depression lifts, frequently the obsessional behavior disappears. Since obsessional patients do not passively avoid situations that provoke ritualistic behavior, some psychiatrists believe that anger (perhaps self-anger) is the fundamental mood disturbance. Others, based on clinical findings with patients in whom doubt and indecision are persistent, speculate that this leads to fear as the predominant affect. They conjecture that fear of consequences or an inability to predict leads to doubting, indecision, rumination, and ultimately rituals, which further increase the patient's insecurity and weaken his will. The point emphasized by these groups is that altered affects—depression, anger, or fear—are the most important determinants of obsessive compulsive neurosis, not anxiety. These affects or moods even take precedence over events in the environment that the patient may claim provoke his ritualistic behavior.[33]

Controversy exists as to whether depressed patients who suffer from aggressive obsessions are more prone to suicide than those without the obsessions. Obsessional patients with depression are usually less severely depressed than nonobsessional depressives and the latter are more often associated with psychosis. Suicidal obsessions however, are common with depression. Although many psychiatrists support the viewpoint that suicidal and homocidal obsessions in depressed patients were protective against suicidal attempts, Videbech in an extensive review of the literature and research did not find any significant difference in the incidence of suicidal thoughts, attempts, or actual suicide between the groups.[34] Therefore, psychiatrists who treat these patients cannot relax suicidal precautions.

Other issues exist regarding depression with anancasm. First, in depressed patients the transition from obsessions to delusions, or vice versa occurs in about 10% of the cases. This raises the controversial question of whether obsessions are a stage in the development of schizophrenia.[35, 36] Second, what is the function of obsessive personality as it relates to obsessions in depressions? Videbech claims a positive correlation between anxiety, hypochondriacal attitude, agitation, and the strength of obsessive personality in anancastic depressed patients; while nonanancastic depressed patients demonstrate a positive correlation only between agitation and the strength of the obsessional personality.[37] In contrast, Vaughn claims that obsessive compulsive personality reduces anxiety in the presence of obsessions in depressions; whereas, obsessions in depressions, without the obsessive personality, are associated with an increased incidence of anxiety, agitation, overactivity, rapid mood change, and a decrease in incidence of motor retardation.[38] The role of personality, therefore, becomes a crucial and controversial issue regarding clinical manifestations of obsessions in depression. Previously, it was mentioned that obsessive compulsive neurosis without depression reduces anxiety.

Other models are proposed in addition to those that emphasize the role of mood and personality to explain obsessional neurosis. Some of the proposed models are that obsessional neurosis: (1) is an avoidance response that was acquired following an initial traumatic experience; (2) is the result of positive reinforcement; (3) is caused by the patient's judgment that an unfavorable outcome or consequence will occur (a fallacious appraisal of threat); (4) is a means of avoiding decisions, conflicts, and ambiguity; (5) is a relative inability to organize and integrate experience, a tendency to be overspecific and less abstract; and so forth.[39, 40] Another model that attempts to explain the thought processes of obsessional neurotics is personal construct theory. Construct theory utilizes a repertory grid methodology in which a subject identifies elements. These elements are organized into constructs or categories. Construct theory seeks to elucidate the subject's own categories, i.e., to find out the way he constructs his own experiences. Personal construct theory attempts to discover how the subject arranges his own dimensions in contrast to trait typology which arranges the subject into categories according to the psychiatrist's or psychologist's preconceived theory.[41]

Makhlouf-Norris using construct theory methodology studied patients with obsessional neuroses. The patient's constructs were grouped into clusters. In primary clusters *all* component constructs significantly relate to one another within the cluster. Primary clusters are relatively independent and the relationship of the remaining constructs to these were divided into:

> . . . (a) a construct significantly correlated with one or more constructs (but not all) in a cluster was considered a related off-shoot or a 'secondary' construct; (b) a construct significantly correlated with one or more constructs in two or more clusters was considered a joint off-shoot or a 'linkage' construct; (c) a construct not significantly correlated with any other construct was considered an 'isolate.'[42]

Further, three topographical organizations appeared: monolithic, segmented, and articulated. Monolithic and segmented are nonarticulated typologies and are found in obsessional neurotics. Articulated typology is found in normal control subjects.

The monolithic typology is illustrated in Fig. 7-1. It consists of one primary, one secondary, and two isolate clusters. The monolithic structure is interpreted

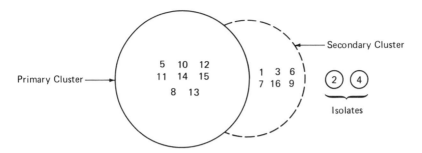

Fig. 7-1.   A monolithic structure of constructs consisting of one primary, one secondary, and two isolates (redrawn from Makhlouf-Norris, Jones and Norris). Numbers inside clusters represent constructs.[43]

as very restricting and the person cannot make independent judgments that have opposing implications. The person is rigid and not capable of altering his opinion even when confronted with experience or fact that invalidates his opinion.

The other typology found in obsessionals is the segmented system which is illustrated in Fig. 7-2. In this organization there are several primary clusters and two isolates that are nonarticulated; therefore, independent judgments are made without reference to other positions of the self. These persons have no means by which one part of self can influence another. They lack an over-all cohesive identity and avoid making decisions which require prediction. These patients need to know and to control events; hence, the obsessional behavior could be a symbolic means of control, knowing, and a device to reduce uncertainty. It also may imply a divided will in which one part acts in opposition to the other.[44, 45]

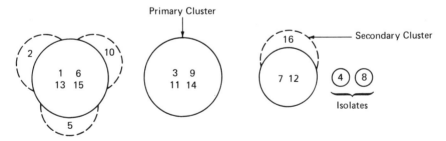

Fig. 7-2.   A segmented structure of constructs consisting of three primary, four secondary clusters, and two isolates (redrawn from Makhlouf-Norris, Jones and Norris). Numbers inside clusters represent constructs.[46]

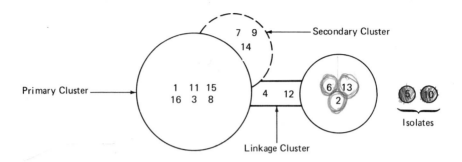

Fig. 7-3 An articulated structure of constructs consisting of three primary, one secondary cluster, and one linkage cluster (redrawn from Makhlouf-Norris, Jones and Norris). Numbers inside clusters represent constructs. [48]

Normal topographical organization, illustrated in Fig. 7-3, consists of several primary clusters, a single secondary cluster, and two isolates. It is an articulated system that allows the individual to have separate but related constructs. These constructs within a cluster have connection with and implications for those within other clusters. The linkage cluster enables the person to cope with congruent as well as incongruent implications. A free, labile, and integrated mental system exists. [47]

In monolithic and segmented systems the person's identity is not integrated but rather consists of specific parts that are nonrelated. The self is fragmented. With the monolithic structure, judgments with opposing implications cannot be made. With either the monolithic or segmented structure, change does not readily occur since the systems are isolated from each other. Makhlouf-Norris says:

> Construing the self as non-ideal could well serve to reduce uncertainty concerning the self. To construe the actual-self as a failure or unhappy is to some extent self-validating. If a person predicts that he will fail in some situation or be unhappy, he is unlikely to mobilize his resources and direct himself so as to achieve success or happiness. Thus his prediction will be validated by doing nothing. To construe the self as successful or happy risks invalidation, because an attempt to achieve success or happiness may fail. *The need for self-certainty may be such as to lead to construing the self in a way which predicts undesirable outcomes which are certain to be validated, rather than predict desirable outcomes which are open to test and to the risk of invalidation.* [49]

Self-identity and will in obsessive compulsive patients is disturbed. Personal construct theory demonstrates that obsessional behavior serves a dual function.

By guaranteeing failure, it assures certainty. The obsession and compulsion are undesirable but can always be validated; therefore, the self's need for certainty is satisfied.

Psychoanalytic theory differentiates obsessive compulsive neurosis from other neuroses according to ego defenses, nature of repressed impulses, or a combination of these two items. For example, the hysterical patient mainly employs repression, projection, and reversal, whereas the obsessive patient uses principally the mechanisms of isolation, rationalization, reaction-formation, and undoing. The obsessive also projects and displaces affects but these are not as consistent or as specific as the other defenses. Isolation separates the affect from the content of an idea or image. Thus, the obsessive patient does not have an absolute amnesia, like the hysteric, but he mentions facts detached from emotional experience. Using rationalization, he explains his actions in a reasonable manner. In this way, the obsessive can explain away impulses or thoughts that are unacceptable to his conscious ego. Reaction-formations are deeply embedded in the obsessive neurotic. These reaction-formations usually take place by undoing, i.e., a constant preoccupation with balancing two opposites with each other. A good day must be followed by a bad day. Unconscious hostilities make this patient appear gentle and kind. Undoing can take the appearance of superstition and magical thinking.

Psychoanalysts trace the origin of this neurosis to the toilet training period of the child. Obsessives are referred to as anal personalities since their development has become fixed at this stage. Both sexual or libidinal and aggressive instincts regress to this level of development. Regression then becomes primary and the other described defense mechanisms follow in its path. This, the analysts say, not only explains the little value that these patients place on the emotional aspects of sex but also why they are obstinate, orderly, and frugal. Frugality continues the anal habit of retention, orderliness derives from control over excretion, and obstinancy carries on the rebellion against a demanding environment.   Furthermore, obsessive compulsive neurosis represents a dynamic equilibrium between ego-alien images or fantasies (incestuous, coprophilic, and sadistic) and rituals that are exaggerations of morality. This results both from an ego ideal in which expectations are too high and from a tyrannical superego. These patients place a high value on such traits as cleanliness, punctuality, and consideration for others. A balance of asocial impulses and thoughts with moralistic attitudes characterizes the obsessive. The struggle to maintain this balance explains why these patients suffer from doubts, indecisiveness, and ambivalence. Hand washing is a response to coprophilia, touching to hurting, kindness to anal-sadistic impulses, and so on.[50] Salzman says:

> While the factors suggested by many theorists can be identified in the obsessive-compulsive mechanism, the overriding purpose of the behavior

is to attempt to achieve some security and certainty for the person who feels threatened and insecure in an uncertain world. The possibility of controlling oneself and the forces outside oneself by assuming omniscience and omnipotence can give one a false illusion of certainty. Therefore, the main ingredient is one of control . . . . In my view, the obsessive-compulsive dynamism is a device for preventing any feeling or thought that might produce shame, loss of pride or status, or a feeling of weakness or deficiency—whether such feelings are hostile, sexual, or otherwise. I see the obsessional maneuver as an adaptive technique to protect the person from the exposure of any thought or feeling that will endanger his physical or psychological existence . . . .[51]

Classical behaviorists and learning theorists base their explanation of obsessive compulsive neurosis on the repetitive nature of stimuli as well as responses, anxiety reduction conditioning, and the establishment of a reverberating circuitry in the brain. An aberration in the arousal and central inhibition of the nervous system, they feel, is basic to the development of this type of psychopathology. This unstable arousal system leads to abnormal neural connections, which in turn leads to the formation of habits and the establishment of pathological reflexes and cognition. Accordingly, impulses, thoughts, and acts become fixed into a learned pattern of behavior.[52]

However, psychological or physiological stress may be an etiological factor. The kinds of stress which are thought to be precipitants vary from author to author and include such stresses as those that provoke anxiety, demand an environmental alteration or a change of an established habit, necessitate an increase in responsibility or require a flexible attitude, difficulties in marriage, or sex. Other stresses include pregnancy, delivery, illness, death of a near relative, frustration, and overwork. These stresses may be acute or cumulative.[53]

DIAGNOSIS

Diagnosis is easy. Precisely defining and classifying the disease assures that confusion can be avoided. With resistance as the essential characteristic and unwanted repetitive ideas, images, impulses, or acts as the accompanying phenomena, clarification is explicit. Further, if the patient identifies with the obsession or compulsion and lacks resistance, he is delusional. Overevaluated emotional ideations, images, or impulses, however, fall somewhere between obsessions and delusions since the patient accepts them without struggle but has intermittent doubts.[54] Form and content, as well as classification into acute, subacute, and chronic also aid in clarifying terminology.

Obsessional neurosis is a mismatch between patient and environment. The patient has the thought that his hands are dirty; he washes; the thought reoccurs and he washes again. As the number of washings increases, the patient becomes caught in a circle of irrational thought and behavior. He decides that only three washings are allowable. This breaks down. A fear develops that there was a miscount or a doubt arises as to whether the towel was clean. Gradually, matters may go from bad to worse. Compulsive *slowness* in which a patient can take hours to dress, undress, bathe, leave the home or office, cross a road, cripples the lives of the patient and his family. The family reacts; at first, they may ridicule or criticize, then express concern or distress, and finally—sometimes after years—either passively accept the patient's condition or else reject him. Divorce or removal of the patient from the home may occur depending on family tolerance, relationship, and severity of symptoms. The patient usually seeks psychiatric treatment about seven years after the illness begins.[55, 56]

Other terms are used besides the ones referred to earlier in this text. Obsessions occur in which the patient broods over the meaning of life, the existence of God, and the destiny of man. He ponders over such everyday occurrences as what tie to wear, what to feed the dog, or whether he has locked the door. Prolonged inconclusive repetitive thinking that occurs to the exclusion of other interests is called obsessive *rumination*.[57] It can extend to the point where the patient feels compelled to scrutinize the advantages and disadvantages of every aspect of a situation or problem so that he does not have to arrive at a decision. He may also end up by questioning whether the original facts or premises were correct. Mixed feelings or ambivalence result when the patient simultaneously has opposing attitudes toward the same person, object, or situation. Ambivalence is characteristic of obsessional *convictions*. These are convictions based on the false premise that word, thought, and deed are the same, e.g., to think or say something evil about someone is equivalent to causing some misfortune to him. Another example of obsessional conviction is called morbid pathological or obsessive—delusional jealousy. The patient is preoccupied with the conviction that his spouse is sexually unfaithful. He constantly harrasses the spouse, keeps meticulous observations of her behavior, and searches for signs that he can interpret as infidelity. Besides this there is a cyclic pattern—rage, guilt, remorse, and depression—during which either homocide, severe beatings, or suicide become distinct possibilities. In effect obsessional convictions represent illogical, magical, superstitious, and even delusional thought. The difference between delusional and obsessional conviction is that in the latter, the patient is ambivalent and resists the belief. A progression of obsessional thinking, doubting, or rumination can lead to indecision, ambivalence, and conviction. The patient may become fixed at any point along this spectrum.[58–60]

Coexisting with obsessive mental activities are compulsive acts. Some common compulsions involve checking and rechecking of doors and locks to make sure they are closed, testing and retesting electrical and gas appliances to make certain they are off, and most typically, repeated hand washing to remove germs and disease from the body, clothing, or anything touched. When these patients have to "check out" in such a way that the act has to be repeated a set number of times, in a certain prescribed manner, an obsessional *ritual* is present. There are rituals for bedtime, daytime, bathroom, work, sex, and so on. These patients persist in this activity against their better judgment and even to the exclusion of useful activity. Hours can be lost in nonproductive activity or rituals. These patients maintain consistency by performing repetitive acts. They feel that with order less is apt to go wrong even though the performance can increase rather than decrease their tension or anxiety. They straighten curtains, tablecloths, furniture, towels, and so on. Such acts when based on superstition compel the patient to repeat each act a certain number of times thereby insuring that all will go well. In severe cases these activities may be completely disabling. Where there are compulsive rituals there can be obsessional doubting which may take the form of endless rechecking.[61]

Obsessions and compulsions have more than a surface meaning. They are an outward manifestation of inner disturbances and are usually symbolic. The symbolism may be a complicated series in that each symbol in its turn cancels out the meaning of its predecessor in an attempt to keep the basic conflicts hidden from consciousness. The clinical cluster of overt symptoms can, therefore, be constantly changing but the underlying common denominator is that they are always obsessional.

DIFFERENTIAL DIAGNOSIS

When obsessional symptoms appear the doctor decides whether they are due primarily to an obsessional neurosis or secondary to another disease. Of course, repetitive behavior—tics, mannerisms, doodling, and rituals—is found in other neurotics, psychotics, patients with organic brain disease, and in normals. These conditions should be differentiated from obsessional behavior. Without resistance the behavior cannot be considered obsessional. Once it is determined that the behavior is obsessional, the physician must then decide what is primary, e.g., is the patient obsessive compulsive with a secondary depression, or depressive neurotic with secondary obsessions? At times the determination can be difficult, but for the most part the evidence for one disease or another will be clear enough. Where clinical judgment indicates that no one entity is primary, two or more diagnoses may be posited, e.g., schizophrenia (paranoid type), obsessive compulsive neurosis, and hysterical personality type.

Previously obsessive compulsive personality trait and symptoms, and obsessive compulsive, phobic and hypochondriacal neuroses were distinguished from one another. Phobic responses due to external stimuli are characterized by avoidance of the object or situation, whereas, illness phobias are not as easily distinguished since the stimulus source is internal. Where fear of illness (nosophobia) exists more or less independently from other obsessive features and is localized around a single symptom, organ, or disease, phobic neurosis may be the diagnosis. The hypochondriac, in contrast, does not usually center around one symptom, organ, or disease. Marks says:

> It is not at all clear how nosophobias relate to more general forms of hypochondriasis, and whether they aren't simply a special form of it . . . the definitive status of illness phobias awaits further clinical and psychophysiological study. It is undoubtedly true that numerous patients present with a single fear of disease which is part of a depressive illness, and that these fears wax and wane with the depression and should be regarded simply as a depressive concomitant. Yet others may be part of an abnormal personality, obsessive neurosis or other psychiatric disorder. It is not known how small the residue is of patients who have illness phobias as the main complaint without other complicating factors . . . .[62]

Bodily complaints require extensive differentiation from innumerable physical illnesses as well as those mental illnesses that have bodily complaints as part of their clinical picture.

Depression, schizophrenia, and chronic organic brain disease are associated with obsessive compulsive neurosis. Depression is the most common complication of obsessional neurosis, and with endogenous depression obsessional symptoms can be so prominent that they mask the depression. Thus, it can be very difficult to determine which disease is primary and which is secondary. This situation is complicated because some patients acquire and some lose obsessional symptoms during a depression and both obsessive compulsive neurosis and endogenous depression can have a recurrent or cyclic course. Only by careful evaluation of the total situation—the symptomatology, personality, precipitating stresses, and so on—can the determination between primary obsessive compulsive neurosis and affective disease be made.[63]

Schizophrenic patients frequently have obsessive compulsive symptoms, and some say that obsessive compulsive neurosis is a bridge between schizophrenia and the other neuroses. Yet others maintain that obsessive compulsives rarely become schizophrenic. Mistaken diagnoses between these two conditions occur during the early stages. There can be difficulty in delineating obsession from delusion but it is usually possible; and schizophrenia differs from obsessional neurosis by being a formal thought disorder with associational, affective, perceptual, behavioral, and verbal disturbances. Obsessionals are verbally coherent and have resistances to their alien ideas or actions. These manifestations are the principal considerations by which the two conditions are distinguished.

Patients with organic brain disease sometimes develop repetitive thoughts and behavior. This finding led some to postulate that brain pathology is an etiological factor in obsessive compulsive neurosis. Most would agree however, that the evidence for this is quite slim.[64] Besides, organic brain-damaged patients do not seem to have true obsessive compulsive symptoms.   Although their symptoms are repetitive and are recognized by the patient as alien to himself, the symptoms do not have the compulsive quality nor the strong sense of resistance as found with the neurosis.   Major characteristics of organic brain disease are impairment in memory, orientation, judgment, and intellectual functions; a labile and shallow affect; personality change; and neurological findings may or may not be present.

COURSE AND PROGNOSIS

Although the onset of the disease usually occurs around the age of 25, frequently there are precursory symptoms in childhood.   These initial manifestations include symptoms other than obsessional, such as headaches, pain in the chest and abdomen, hypochondriasis, fatigue, anxiety, and depression.   Clearly, however, these same symptoms occur in children who subsequently have no difficulties in later life as well as those who develop other types of mental illness.

The mode of onset varies. Most develop insidiously, and some acutely. The course can progressively worsen or remain static; can fluctuate but never be symptom free; or be phasic with complete remissions.   The prognosis varies. The factors that tend to lead to a favorable prognosis are a normal premorbid personality, a phasic course, satisfactory resolution of precipitating disturbance, and those cases in which anxiety or depression are prominent features. Factors that indicate a poor prognosis are an obsessional premorbid personality, early age of onset, and a clinical picture showing severe symptoms. Factors unrelated to prognosis are positive family history, childhood symptoms, sex, intelligence, unmarried status, acute versus insidious onset, and previous attacks.[65]

Note that prognosis is dependent on accurate diagnosis. In instances where obsessive symptoms are secondary to other illnesses, the prognosis is dependent on these others. Where true obsessional neurosis exists whether acute, subacute, or chronic, the above factors have relevance. Remissions, exacerbations, and fluctuations in severity of symptoms may occur in relation to stressors. Finally, although many consider the prognosis for subacute and chronic obsessive compulsive neurosis to be the poorest of all neurotic conditions, this may be unduly pessimistic.   Many have spontaneous remissions and treatments are available that can help.[66]

TREATMENT

Obsessive compulsive neurosis can be difficult to treat. This should be enough reason for physicians to make proper evaluation of the patient. Whether obsessive compulsive neurosis is the primary illness or secondary to another condition, treatment should be directed towards the primary diagnosis and must include methods that are as broad and diversified as possible. No one method is satisfactory and the psychiatrist should be willing and able to try whatever modes are available. A rigid treatment approach is discouraged. Where obsessive compulsive phenomena are secondary, as with anxiety or phobic neuroses, psychotherapy (supportive and dynamic), environmental readjustment, behavior therapy and drugs can be helpful. In schizophrenia phenothiazines, insulin, and psychotherapy are indicated. In depression tricyclics, electroconvulsive and psychotherapy are the best treatments. In organic brain disease, treatment, if at all possible, is directed towards amelioration of the underlying pathology. The hope with all these illnesses is that by treating the primary condition remission of the obsessive compulsive condition will occur.

Obsessive compulsive neurosis may require the entire psychiatric treatment armamentarium. It may be individual, using supportive behavioral and dynamic techniques; or family, group, and community methods. It is preferable to use either individual alone or in combination with one or two of the other methods.[67, 68] In situations where severe stress exists, such as at work or at home, it may be possible to alleviate the symptoms by changing the environment. Drugs can be important. Tricyclics are used as a prophylaxis against depression and as a means of bringing relief from obsessional symptoms when no depression exists.[69–71] Claims are made that two new drugs are helpful in obsessive compulsive neurosis: a benzodiazepine (bromazepam),[72] and a tricyclic (chlorimipramine, Anafranil).[73–75] Relaxation methods such as exercise, autogenic or progressive relaxation techniques may help. Behavioral methods such as deconditioning, desensitization, reciprocal inhibition, and reinforcement are used but results are for the most part disappointing. However, behavioral therapists are claiming some success with response prevention. In this method the patient is allowed to come into contact with situations in which a compulsive ritual is performed but prevented from carrying out the act. For example, patients with a hand washing compulsion are placed in a hospital room with a sink in which the taps are turned off.[76–78] Claims are made for success with electroconvulsive therapy[79] and psychosurgery.[80] In summary, all of the above are used in the treatment of obsessive compulsive neurosis. None of the treatments is known to be very satisfactory but it is hoped that they might be of some help. The use of dynamic psychotherapy in the treatment of this illness is currently in disrepute in some circles. Although the results have not been good, psychotherapy has relieved discomfort, helped patients with interpersonal relationships, increased their sense of self-awareness, and added insights into themselves and their social environment. This is an essential ingredient in the treatment of this neurosis. Psychotherapy can add an additional dimension to any of the other treatments and thereby contribute something toward successful therapy. It should not be neglected.

REFERENCES

1. Slater, E. and Roth, M., *Clinical Psychiatry*. Baltimore: Williams & Wilkins, 1970, p. 126.
2. Ibid., p. 127.
3. Anderson, E.W. and Trethowan, W.H., *Psychiatry*. Baltimore: Williams & Wilkins, 1973, p. 224.
4. Woodruff, R.A., Goodwin, D.W. and Guze, S.B., *Psychiatric Diagnosis*. New York: Oxford University Press, 1974.
5. Akhtar, S., Wig., N.N., Varma, V.K., Pershad, D. and Verma, S.K., A phenomenological analysis of symptoms in obsessive-compulsive neurosis. *Brit. J. Psychiatry* 127:343–344 (1975).
6. Ibid., p. 346.
7. Ibid., pp. 346–347.
8. Videbech, T., The psychopathology of anancastic endogenous depressions. *Acta. Psychiat. Scand.* 52:349–357 (1975).
9. Walker, V.J., Explanation in obsessional neurosis. *Brit. J. Psychiatry* 123:675–680 (1973).
10. Laughlin, H.P., *The Neuroses*. Washington, D.C.: Butterworths, 1967, pp. 312–313.
11. Meyer, A., *The Commonsense Psychiatry of Dr. Adolf Meyer* (edited by Lief, A.). New York: McGraw-Hill, 1948, pp. 130–132.
12. Carr, A.T., Compulsive neurosis: A review of the literature. *Psychol. Bull.* 81(5):311 (1974).
13. Janet, P., *Les Obsessions et la Psychasthénie*. Paris: Felix Alcan, 1903.
14. Bailey, P., The psychology of human conduct: A review. *Amer. J. Psychiatry* 8:209–234 (1928).
15. Freud, S., "Obsessions and phobias; their psychical mechanisms and their aetiology (1895)," in *Collected Papers*, vol. 1, 6th impression (edited by Jones, E. and transl. by Riviere, J.). London: Hogarth Press, 1950, pp. 128–137.
16. Freud, S., "Character and anal erotism (1908)," in *Collected Papers*, vol. 2, 7th impression (edited by Jones, E. and transl. by Riviere, J.). London: Hogarth Press, 1950, pp. 45–50.
17. Freud, S., *New Introductory Lectures on Psycho-Analysis* (transl. by Sprott, W.J.H.). New York: Norton, 1933, p. 137.
18. Black, A., "The natural history of obsessional neurosis," in *Obsessional States* (edited by Beech, H.R.). London: Methuen, 1974, p. 20.
19. Lewis, A.J., Problems of obsessional illness. *Proc. Roy. Soc. Med.* 29:325–336 (1936).
20. Lewis, A.J., Obsessional illness. *Acta. Neuropsiquiat. Argent.* 3:323–335 (1957).
21. Johnson, A., "Obsessive-compulsive-ruminative-tension states," in *Psychobiology and Psychiatry* (authored by Muncie, W.). St. Louis: Mosby, 1939, pp. 586–609.
22. Provisional classification: Published as a looseleaf manual entitled *DSM-III Draft*, 4/15/77. DRAFT OF AXES I and II of DSM-III CLASSIFICATION as of March 30, 1977.
23. Curran, D., Partridge, M. and Storey, P., *Psychological Medicine: An Introduction to Psychiatry*, 7th ed. Edinburgh and London: Churchill Livingstone, 1972, p. 234.
24. Foulds, G.A. and Bedford, A., Hierarchy of classes of personal illness. *Psychol. Med.* 5:181–192 (1975).
25. Travis, T.A., Noyes, Jr., R. and Clancy, J., The obsessive personality: One of a series. *Postgrad. Med.* 54(6):73–77 (1973).

26. Slade, P.D., "Psychometric study of obsessional illness and obsessional personality," in *Obsessional States* (edited by Beech, H.R.). London: Methuen, 1974, pp. 95-109.
27. Akhtar, N.W., et al., op. cit., p. 347.
28. Templer, D.I., The obsessive-compulsive neurosis: Review of research findings. *Compr. Psychiatry* 13(4):375-383 (1972).
29. Black, A., op. cit., pp. 32-36.
30. Templer, D.I., op. cit., pp. 376-380.
31. Adams, P.L., Family characteristics of obsessive children. *Amer. J. Psychiatry* 128(11):1414-1417 (1972).
32. Carr, A.T., op. cit., p. 312.
33. Mellett, P.G., "The clinical problem," in *Obsessional States* (edited by Beech, H.R.). London: Methuen, 1974, pp. 55-94.
34. Videbech, T., op. cit., pp. 344-345, 357-359.
35. Ibid., pp. 343-344, 363-371.
36. Templer, D.I., op. cit., pp. 379-380.
37. Videbech, T., op. cit., p. 369.
38. Vaughan, M., The relationship between obsessional personality, obsessions in depression, and symptoms of depression. *Brit. J. Psychiatry* 129:36-39 (1976).
39. Carr, A.T., op. cit., pp. 313-317.
40. Fransella, F., "Thinking and the obsessional," in *Obsessional States* (edited by Beech, H.R.). London: Methuen, 1974, pp. 177-184.
41. Mischel, W., *Introduction to Personality,* 2nd ed. New York: Holt, Rinehart and Winston, 1976, p. 109.
42. Makhlouf-Norris, F., Jones, H.G. and Norris, H., Articulation of the conceptual structure in obsessional neurosis. *Brit. J. Soc. Clin. Psychol.* 9:265 (1970).
43. Ibid., p. 268.
44. Ibid., p. 273.
45. Makhlouf-Norris, F. and Norris, H., The obsessive compulsive syndrome as a neurotic device for the reduction of self-uncertainty. *Brit. J. Psychiatry* 121:277-288 (1972).
46. Makhlouf-Norris, F., Jones, H.G. and Norris, H., op. cit., p. 270.
47. Ibid., p. 273.
48. Ibid., p. 270.
49. Makhlouf-Norris, F. and Norris, H., op. cit., p. 285.
50. Fenichel, O., *The Psychoanalytic Theory of Neurosis.* New York: Norton, 1945, pp. 268-310.
51. Salzman, L., *The Obsessive Personality: Origins, Dynamics and Therapy.* New York: Science House, 1968, pp. 13-14.
52. Beech, H.R. and Perigault, F., "Toward a theory of obsessional disorder," in *Obsessional States* (edited by Beech, H.R.). London: Methuen, 1974, pp. 113-141.
53. Black, A., op. cit., pp. 38-39.
54. Slater, E. and Roth, M., op. cit., p. 126.
55. Kringlen, E., Obsessional neurotics: A long-term follow-up. *Brit. J. Psychiatry* 11:709-722 (1965).
56. Goodwin, D.W., Guze, S.B. and Robins, E., Follow-up studies in obsessional neurosis. *Arch. Gen. Psychiatry* 20:182-187 (1969).
57. Woodruff, R.A., Goodwin, D.W. and Guze, S.B., op. cit., p. 79.
58. Ibid., pp. 78-79.
59. Docherty, J.P. and Ellis, J., A new concept and finding in morbid jealousy. *Amer. J. Psychiatry* 133(6):679-683 (1976).

60. Herceg, N., Successful use of thiothixene in two cases of pathological jealousy. *Med. J. Aust.* 1(16):569–570 (1976).

61. Woodruff, R.A., Goodwin, D.W. and Guze, S.B., op. cit., pp. 79–80.

62. Marks, I.M., *Fears and Phobias.* New York: Academic, 1969, p. 160.

63. Templer, D.I., op. cit., p. 379.

64. Ibid., p. 380.

65. Black, A., op. cit., pp. 36–46.

66. Curran, D., Partridge, M. and Storey, P., op. cit., pp. 298–299.

67. Suess, J., Short-term psychotherapy with the compulsive personality and the obsessive-compulsive neurotic. *Amer. J. Psychiatry* 129(3):270–275 (1972).

68. Fine, S., Family therapy and a behavioral approach to childhood obsessive-compulsive neurosis. *Arch. Gen. Psychiatry* 28:695–697 (1973).

69. Cammer, L., Antidepressants as a prophylaxis against depression in the obsessive compulsive person. *Psychosom.* 14:201–206 (1973).

70. Freed, A., Kerr, T.A. and Roth, M., The treatment of obsessive neurosis. *Brit. J. Psychiatry* 120:590–591 (1972).

71. Ananth, J., Solyom, L., Solyom, C. and Sookman, D., Doxepin in the treatment of obsessive compulsive neurosis. *Psychosom.* 16(4):185–187 (1975).

72. Burrell, R.H., Culpan, R.H., Newton, K.J., Ogg, G.J. and Short, J.H.W., Use of bromazepam in obsessional, phobic, and related states. *Cur. Med. Res. Opinion* 2(7):430–436 (1974).

73. Yaryura-Tobias, J.A. and Neziroglu, F., The action of chlorimipramine in obsessive-compulsive neurosis: A pilot study. *Cur. Ther. Res.* 17(1):111–116 (1975).

74. Capstick, N., Clomipramine in the treatment of the true obsessional state. *Psychosom.* 16(1):21–25 (1975).

75. Wyndowe, J., Solyom, L. and Ananth, J., Anafranil in obsessive compulsive neurosis. *Cur. Ther. Res.* 18(5):611–617 (1975).

76. Mills, H.L., Agras, W.S., Barlow, D.H. and Mills, J.R., Compulsive rituals treated by response prevention. *Arch. Gen. Psychiatry* 28:524–529 (1973).

77. Fine, S., op. cit., pp. 695–697.

78. Marks, I.M., Hodgson, R. and Rachman, S., Treatment of chronic obsessive-compulsive neurosis by *in-vivo* exposure: A two-year follow-up and issues in treatment. *Brit. J. Psychiatry* 127:349–364 (1975).

79. Gruber, R.P., ECT for obsessive-compulsive symptoms (possible mechanisms of action). *Dis. Nerv. Syst.* 32:180–182 (1971).

80. Bridges, P.K., Goktepe, E.O., Maratos, J., Browne, A. and Young, L., A comparative review of patients with obsessional neurosis and with depression treated by psychosurgery. *Brit. J. Psychiatry* 123:663–674 (1973).

8
DEPRESSIVE NEUROSIS

Defining depression is not a simple matter. Affects such as sadness, unhappiness, dysphoria, sorrow, loneliness, or an inability to enjoy are not the only criteria. In fact many patients who are called depressed do not complain of, nor do they feel, any of these affects. Instead, they have other complaints. These include self-accusation, self-reproach, loss of incentive, low self-esteem, guilt, and worthlessness. The facial expressions of depressed patients—dull, saddened, emotionless, flattened, stern, and with wrinkled brow—often but not always mirror their verbalized moods. Depressed patients may lack energy, speak slowly and briefly, or have difficulty in thinking, concentrating, and performing. Their judgment may be impaired and they may complain of generalized aches and pains as well as headaches, chest pains, backaches, gastrointestinal or cardiovascular problems. There can be disturbances of sleep, eating, sexual drive, personal relationships, and work. Any one or combination of the above manifestations may indicate the existence of depression. There are absolutely no clear-cut symptomatological criteria for a precise definition.[1, 2]

In summary, the depressed patient can manifest varying degrees of sadness, distortion of self-concept, psychomotor retardation, somatic and visceral complaints, and interpersonal difficulties. Depressed patients are extremely challenging to the psychiatrist because they appear in various "guises or disguises"—complaining or not, smiling or not, pained or not. They seem to share no single symptom or cluster of symptoms which clearly points to a consensual definition that says "depression." In the last analysis, depression is not yet defined. Psychiatrists, recognizing this difficulty, therefore, define depression in accordance with the predominant symptomatic modes of behavior.

A holistic definition of depression not only considers the emotional and cognitive nature of the disease but also recognizes the relationship between the individual and the social structure of his life-style. Structure consists of the patient's daily life in all its various aspects—some more important than others—and all are interrelated. Due to the interrelatedness of all the parts, a

171

breakdown or loss in one aspect will effect other aspects and so the whole. Thus, a man who loses his job and becomes depressed may also respond by losing his incentive to work, losing interest in his wife and children, withdrawing from lifelong friendships, decreasing his food intake, sleeping less, becoming constipated, etc. Depression is a disease that can and often does effect every aspect of the individual—biological, psychological, and social.[3]

The true or essential nature of depression is unknown and controversy exists. For instance, are the dysphoric feelings that are part of daily mood fluctuations which all people experience, similar to the variations in feeling experienced during depressed states? This question is often asked. To even raise this question may implicitly suggest that depression is an emotional or affective disorder and that it subscribes to the faculty theory of mind, places depressive affect as the primary emotional disturbance, and views all other faculties as either unessential or secondary. If this presumption is accepted, however, the question has immense importance. Besides defining depression as an affective disorder it opens the way to regarding depressed states in accordance with either the unitary or entity theory of disease. The unitary position maintains that normal blends into abnormal by gradual degrees and the difference between the two states is quantitative. In contrast, the entity theory maintains that normal and abnormal are qualitatively different states. Each state possesses specific characteristics and the phenomena are viewed either as a symptom, syndrome or symptom-complex, disease, illness, or a combination of these. Between these two positions, a third position exists which claims that up to a point the unitary theory is correct but at a quantitative point, a new quality arises and then the category or entity viewpoint becomes true. This last group takes a compromise position. Each viewpoint has its adherents and opponents and there is a great deal of debate revolving around these considerations.[4]

Aaron Beck views depression as an intriguing disorder, paradoxical, and mysterious. He says:

> The puzzling features of depression have pointed to new concepts of this disorder that promise to lead to new understandings and new therapies. No other condition of humankind seems to defy what are generally considered the basic principles of human nature. The suicidal wishes run counter to the instinct of self-preservation; the not infrequent reports of infanticide by depressed mothers make a mockery of the maternal instinct. Basic biologic drives—such as hunger, sexual urge and sleep—are disrupted and the 'social instincts' are extinguished, as indicated by the depressed patient's seclusiveness, loss of interest in other people and reduction in his or her capacity for love. The pleasure principle—the goal of maximizing satisfactions and minimizing pain—is reversed: not only is the depressed person's capacity for enjoyment stifled, but he or she appears to behave in ways that increase personal suffering.[5]

This description reads well but it does not define depression. If there ever was an "as if" disease, this is it. Psychiatrists, psychologists, and lay people refer to depression "as if" they know what it is.

HISTORY

The term depression has assumed most of the diagnostic burden which was once carried by melancholia. With the exception of involutional melancholia, no current references exist to this term in our diagnostic nomenclature. The clinical manifestations of melancholic persons have not changed despite the virtual disappearance of the term. Why, then, has the term fallen into disuse? Perhaps a historical survey will answer this question as well as enhance the understanding of current concepts and practices regarding depression.

Hippocratic writings in the fourth century B.C. coined and described the term melancholia, although descriptions of it are found in ancient Egyptian, earlier Greek, and Hebrew writings.[6, 7] Hippocrates attributed the condition to an imbalance of black bile and phlegm. Melancholia was an entity that included mental and physical symptoms. Galen in the second century A.D. developed a physiological psychology in which he attributed melancholia to either an excess of normal black bile in the very substance of the brain or to an abnormal, thick and black bile in the blood derived from burning (adjustion) and exhaled to the brain. This humour was thought to affect body build and personality. The melancholic individual was lean, swarthy, miserable, downcast, and slow moving; he suffered from visceral, somatic, and rhythmic disturbances (recurrent melancholic attacks, sleep disturbances, and so on).[8, 9]

The humoural theory dominated medical thinking throughout the Renaissance, however, in the seventeenth century other explanations for melancholy began to appear. Thomas Willis (1621-1675), the father of cerebral physiology, regarded "animal spirits" that flowed out of the blood and into the brain as the cause of melancholia.[10] Felix Platter considered melancholia a form of mental alienation in which imagination and judgment were perverted in such a way that the patient became sad and fearful. He regarded the brain as the organ of mental disturbance.[11] Robert Burton (1577-1640), a clergyman, wrote the most extensive exposition of melancholia when in 1621, he published *Anatomy of Melancholy*. He thought of melancholy in Galenical humoural theoretical terms that were still prevalent and he based some of his writings on those of Timothy Bright (1551-1615). The causes of melancholy, Burton thought, were God, the devil, witches, the stars, old age, bad diet and air, inheritance from parents, retention and evacuation, immoderate exercise, loneliness, idleness, excessive or inadequate sleep, fear, shame, disgrace, envy, malice, immoderate pleasures such as love of play, wine, and women, self-love, too much study, poverty, loss of friends and money, etc. For him melancholia included everything from normal grief and sorrow to what today is called neurotic and psychotic depression. He placed special emphasis on love melancholy. Treatment was for the body and soul hence, spiritual guidance, drugs, surgery, productive occupations and activities, travel, and so forth were advised.[12, 13]   In an article written in 1961, a modern author compared Burton's thoughts with a recent study of depression and concluded that little has been learned about the etiology or symptomatology of depression in the past 340 years![14]

In the eighteenth century, G.E. Stahl thought that mental disorders were due to an abnormal relationship between body and soul. The soul, he thought, could be inhibited by a strange motive or idea which arose from the senses, bodily function, or mood. This concept pointed out the effect of psychic life on organic processes and vice versa. Thus, melancholia could be caused by psychic or somatic phenomena in which sadness is the predominant idea or mood. While Stahl's concern was mainly metaphysical, numerous others were developing nosological systems.[15, 16] Regarding one such classification Lewis says:

> Dreyssig's classification (1770-1809) shows well the changes of meaning that the term 'melancholia' was undergoing. He collects all mental disorders into three forms—mania, melancholia, imbecility; melancholia is a partial insanity, or a partial failure of judgment and reasoning capacity, limited to one or a few subjects; it may be true or false; true melancholia is bound up with a lasting sad mood, false melancholia with indifference or cheerfulness; raging melancholy as the highest form approaches mania. This is clearly a very important distinction between 'true' and 'false' melancholia. The proximate cause of melancholia he took to be a disturbed balance between the power of judgment and the power of imagination. It is distinguished from hypochondria and hysteria on the ground that in the latter, irritability is especially increased in the abdominal viscera. As to the relationship between mania and melancholia just alluded to, the famous aphorisms of Herman Boerhaave contain a similar opinion. Boerhaave regarded mania as a higher form of melancholia . . . .[17]

George Cheyne, in 1733, accepting Burton's description of melancholy, referred to these various disorders as the "English malady." He felt that English men were particularly prone to this disease because of climate, fertile soil, richness and heaviness of food, wealth and abundance, inactivity and sedentary occupations, and preference for urban living. In effect, they called melancholia that included hypochondriacal melancholy and other mental disorders the "English malady" because it showed British superiority over other nationalities. It was a form of snobbery.[18] Throughout this century a great deal of psychological work was done and it became apparent that mental life had laws which were in need of closer correlation with the new findings in physics and chemistry.

Philippe Pinel in the latter part of the eighteenth century characterized the melancholic temperament as dejected, gloomy, disheartened, and preoccupied. Melancholia, at times, becomes incompatible with social functioning and thus includes exalted (chiefly paranoid) and depressive states. He regarded depression and mania as mood disorders. However, Immanuel Kant thought that melancholia was not quite a disorder of mood but could lead to it; like hypochondria it could be a delusion of misery.[19]

Early in the nineteenth century melancholia was broadly defined and attributed to disturbances of bile or phlegm; an abnormality of the soul; a dysfunction of the brain; a mental, mood, or thought disorder; and so on. Esquirol followed Pinel's classification of four types of mental disorders, i.e., mania, monomania or fixed delusion, dementia, and idiocy. When Esquirol came on the scene the term melancholia had lost significant meaning because it included too many symptoms. He attempted to restrict definition within a reasonable framework. He coined the term lypemania as a substitute for depressive states. He equated lypemania to melancholia with delirium, i.e., a chronic afebrile brain disease manifested by sad, debilitating, or oppressive emotion. Further he felt that lypemania sometimes led to mania. Thus Pinel and Esquirol set the stage for their followers Falret and Baillarger who for the first time proposed the concept of manic-depressive illness.[20]

Jelliffe says:

> German psychiatry is all too prone to push Kahlbaum (1863) into the foreground as the leader in the separation of syndromes and disease entities, particularly as bearing upon the manic-depressive entity. But the writings of J.P. Falret are unequivocal and frequent upon this theme.[21]

In 1851, Jean Pierre Falret described periodic melancholia and, in 1854, Baillarger described *"folie à double forme"* which Falret later called *"folie circulaire."* Falret pointed out the remissions and exacerbations that occurred during the course of this disease: the sudden onset, the increase in duration of each attack with advancing age, and the mistaken belief that *"folie circulaire"* always resulted in continuous insanity. He believed that the attacks, intermittent not periodic, were able to be delayed, aborted, or even cured, although the disease was essentially incurable. He characterized the attacks as either mania or melancholia with intervening lucid intervals of varying duration, capable of complete suspension of intellectual and affective faculties. Further, he thought the disease was hereditary, more common in women than men, and followed a definite course.[22]

Kahlbaum coined the term "cyclothymia" and insisted upon the disease entity concept. He considered all forms of melancholia as different stages of one disease assuming different forms during its course. Thus in stable melancholia, which he called dysthymia, all psychic manifestations came from a morbid affect. In contrast melancholia, not stable melancholia, was, to him, the initial or transitory stage of melancholy. Other types of melancholia were named– melancholia simplex, melancholia with delusions, melancholia attonitas and so forth–but the splitting of all forms of melancholia from dementia praecox by Hecker and Kahlbaum clearly opened the path for Kraepelin's synthesis.[23]

Kraepelin in the earlier editions of this book attempted to separate disease entities. In the third edition in 1889 mania, melancholia, periodic and circular psychoses were separate entities. However, in the sixth edition in 1899, melancholia was included with anxious depressions of the involutional (menopausal) period and belonged with senile deteriorations. Depressions of earlier years belonged to the dementia praecox or manic-depressive group. In this edition the term manic-depressive appeared for the first time. In 1904, in the seventh edition, Kraepelin still limited melancholia to anxious depressions of later years and excluded it from other psychoses. However, he widened manic-depressive insanity to include periodic, circular, most simple manias, and manic-depressive insanity, mixed forms. In the eighth edition in 1913, melancholia covered the presenile and earlier period. He included within manic-depressive insanity: periodic, circular, simple mania, the greater part of melancholia, and amentia. Kraepelin was now more convinced that all of the above were part of a single morbid process, had prognostic importance, and passed from one form to the next. Although he died before the ninth edition was published in 1928, the synthesis was essentially complete in the eighth edition.[24] Jelliffe writes:

> In the 1913 formulation, the favorable prognosis of the attacks, the tendency to repetition, the great significance of constitutional (hereditary history) are emphasized. We find the manic phase, the depressed phase, the circular phases, the mixed states and the allied forms all carefully described.[25]

The manic-depressive psychosis included almost all abnormalities of mood, i.e., chronic depressions, episodic illness, manias, and other types of depressives. However, other twentieth century psychiatrists began to doubt the all-inclusiveness of depression under one such heading.

Adolf Meyer, at first using the Kraepelinian system gradually discarded it in favor of his own. He introduced the term depression into American psychiatry; thereby discarding the term melancholia. By 1908, his genetic-dynamic interpretation of reaction types was developed. He distinguished depression in each case according to etiology, symptom-complex, course, and prognosis within the framework of total man in an environment (psychobiology).[26] Depression may occur in different forms: (1) pure forms subsumed under holergasias or thymergasias (psychoses); (2) static constitutional types (personality disorders); (3) as an accompanying reaction to other developments such as organic psychosis, toxic reactions, content-determined reactions, and merergasias (neuroses).[27]

These distinctions, he thought, would result in more careful individual case studies since they included symptoms, biological status, personality, external circumstances, and so on. Meyer thought that depressive reactions protected the individual where adaptation had failed.

There were others. Kretschmer by 1928 proposed the term pluridimensional diagnosis. He considered physical type (pyknic), biographical data, environment, experience, and personality (cycloid) before making a value judgment regarding a symptom or group of symptoms. Ewald, Thalbitzer, and Hart used the terms endogenous, exogenous, qualitative, and quantitative to describe states of depression. Stransky in 1911 proposed the theory of endocrine pathogenesis and Kleist adhered to a genetic basis for manic-depressive insanity. Many others also proposed various theories of diseases of organs or abnormal physiological states to explain melancholia.[28]

Psychoanalytic formulations of depression begin with Karl Abraham (1877–1925). In 1911 he stressed that aggressive (sadistic) impulses toward the loved object are repressed and directed towards the ambivalent introject. He formulated the dynamics that began with feeling hatred for the environment (projection). This evoked guilt and anxiety, whereupon the aggression was turned inward towards the introject and led to self-reproach and depression.[29] In 1917 Freud hypothesized that depression was similar to the process of mourning, and that both conditions were a response to the loss of a love object. Grief, in contrast to melancholia, involved the withdrawal of love into the patient's self and abandonment of the object cathexis. Thus there was an ambivalent identification of self with the lost object and a narcissistic regression. This desire to incorporate the love object was fixed at the oral stage. The ambivalence which represented unresolved hostile feelings was turned inward and resulted in despair, worthlessness, at times suicide, and other depressive symptoms.[30] To Abraham in 1924, the depressed patient simultaneously regressed to the anal-sadistic level where hostile and sadistic impulses were prevalent and to the oral level where ambivalence predominated. The etiological factors which Abraham considered important were a constitutional predisposition to oral eroticism, a special fixation at the oral level, a severe narcissistic injury, a disappointment in love before resolving the oedipal complex, and a repetition of this disappointment in later life. Further the hostility was directed against the original lost love object although the recent love object precipitated the attack. With time the introjected love object was "worked through" and the depression lifted.[31] Rickman and later Rado restated these views in terms of ego psychology. In their formulations the self-accusation and depreciation of the depressed patient were due to an unconscious attempt to placate an overly harsh superego. Thus, in melancholia, the hostility or anger was directed towards the ego, and in mania it was directed towards the external environment. In effect in melancholia there was a pathological separation of ego and superego, and in mania there was a fusion.[32-34]

The search for an understanding into the nature of depression in the past 50 years has amassed a great deal of information but has not solved the problem. Joseph Zubin in 1952 outlined the following five basic problems of depression: (1) the need to rigorously define the concept; (2) the techniques necessary to detect an incipient depression; (3) the need to quantify the degree of depression; (4) the type of personalities susceptible to depression; (5) the development of a method to study depression in the pure state.[35] Almost 20 years later, he says:

Today in 1970, despite the facts that investigations of depressions have increased quantitatively, if not qualitatively, that antidepressant drug therapy has bloomed, and that epidemiological investigations have flourished, the five basic problems of 1952 remain unsolved and continue to defy our most energetic attempts at resolution. The reason for this slow progress is not a lack of methods and techniques but rather that the basic feature of depression is an inner feeling of sadness and dejection; the rest is epiphenomena. As we have been unable to determine the cause of this inner sadness, if we could induce it experimentally, we might eventually be able to determine its cause, elimination, and prevention. For the present, however, we are left with a subjective, intuitive feeling which manifests itself directly, if at all, by verbal report and indirectly by such different types of behavior as fearfulness, diminished appetite, psychomotor retardation, and a host of others.[36]

Besides those basic problems, practical considerations exist such as treatment, prevention, and prognosis. Earlier treatments included rest, chess, bibliotherapy, travel, exercise, emetics, purgatives, music therapy, bloodletting, and so on. From 1925 till 1950 the major treatments included psychotherapy, insulin coma, fever therapy, psychosurgery, prolonged narcosis, hypoxemia, electronarcosis, and electroconvulsive therapy. Packs, tubs, seclusion rooms, physical restraints, and barbiturates were used. The very diversity of treatments for depression is depressing. In the last 25 years a series of new drugs has augmented the treatment armamentarium and these drugs may have some preventative capacity. However, at present, definitive treatment or prevention is not available. Then, there is prognosis. Not much can be said about the psychiatrist's ability to predict accurately the outcome of a specific attack of depression. All areas are basically unsolved.

The road from "melancholia" to "depression" has been long and tortuous. The trials and tribulations of melancholia reflect and exemplify the vicissitudes of psychiatry's history. Even a study as abbreviated as this evidences the astounding difficulty of objectively defining depression. Without a satisfactory definition how can cause or proper classification be determined? Are there qualitative and quantitative differences among the various types of depression? How can the psychiatrist select proper treatment for a patient? Many unanswered questions remain, but unquestionably history teaches us to view depression with caution and respect, and to resist any dogmatic formulation regarding this most painful illness.   There is hope—psychiatrists must constantly reassure themselves—that someday the riddle of depression will be solved.

CLASSIFICATION

The twentieth century has witnessed various classifications of depression. Kraepelin placed reactive depression under congenital neurasthenia, a subdivision of constitutional psychopathic states.   Psychogenic or reactive depression was reserved for patients who responded to external situations with depressive symptoms and improved as the situation improved.   Manic-depressive psychosis, he thought, was not primarily due to external stress and, once started, continued independent of precipitating cause and ran a definite course.   Reactive and neurotic depressions were not considered synonymous.[37]   Beck says:

> The most definite precursor of the concept neurotic-depressive reaction was that of reactive depression.   In 1926, Lange listed psychogenic and reactive depression separately in his classification of depression.   He differentiated psychogenic depression from the endogenous variety on the basis of greater aggressiveness, egocentricity, stubbornness, and overt hostility.   In addition, he stated that there were no discernible variations in mood in the psychogenic depressions.   Changes in the milieu influenced this condition, and it became better when the personality conflict was solved . . . .[38]

Many authorities became involved in the controversy between a separate or a fused status for reactive and neurotic depression; however, by 1934, these two conditions were merged.   The American Psychiatric Association in 1934 classified reactive depression under psychoneuroses.   However, this designation lacked general acceptance by many psychiatrists and the concept neurotic-depression was still closely allied to the manic-depressive disorder and not classified under psychoneuroses.[39]

In 1945, the War Department classification adopted the term neurotic-depressive reaction.   Incorporated in this designation were psychobiological and psychoanalytical concepts.   They considered depression as the attempt to allay anxiety through introjection and repressed aggression and as a nonpsychotic response precipitated by a recent event that was associated with a loss.[40]   The Veterans Administration later adopted this classification and introduced the term psychotic-depressive reaction.   In 1952 the Diagnostic and Statistical Manual of the American Psychiatric Association (DSMI) maintained the separation of psychoneurotic and psychotic-depressive reaction.   The DSMI considered psychoneurotic-depressive reaction as synonymous with reactive depression and differentiated it from psychotic-depressive reaction. The psychoneurotic reaction had a discernible precipitating cause and allayed anxiety. The psychotic reaction (endogenous) was related to the patient's life history (mood swings), personality structure (cyclothymic), precipitating event, and the presence of malignant symptoms.   Further, psychotic depression was a separate entity from manic-depressive psychosis, depressed type.[41]

The DSMII (1968) had the term depression scattered throughout the diagnostic categories.   These categories were listed: neurotic and psychotic depression; manic-depressive psychosis—manic, circular, and depressive types; involutional melancholia; depressions in old age, schizophrenia (schizoaffective), and organic brain disease; depressive reactions to physical illness or drug ingestion; and depression in association with other mental or physical illnesses.   Differences between psychotic and neurotic depression depended on whether reality testing or functional adequacy were impaired enough to be considered psychotic and both diseases were related to a precipitating event. They were also differentiated from manic-depressive illnesses and involutional melancholia.   The latter two conditions did not have an observable precipitating stressor.   Involutional melancholia was distinguished by absence of previous depressive episodes and its occurrence during a particular period of life. Schizoaffective disorder, a subtype of schizophrenia, is a mixture of schizophrenic symptoms with pronounced elation or depression.   Although these distinctions are arbitrary, and have etiological implications which may be misleading and wrong, it does help to limit and define the various disorders. The DSMIII (March 30, 1977 proposal) subsumes under Affective Disorders three major categories: episodic, intermittent and atypical affective disorders.   Episodic affective disorders are further subdivided into manic disorder (single episode or recurrent), depressive disorder (single episode or recurrent), and bipolar affective disorder (manic, depressed, or mixed).   Intermittent affective disorders are divided into the following types: depressive (depressive character), hypomanic (hypomanic personality), bipolar (cyclothymic personality). Atypical affective disorders are divided into depressive, manic and bipolar.   Terms such as neurotic, psychotic, endogenous, and reactive are eliminated.   The DSMIII will publish its final draft in January 1979.[42]

Besides symptomatology as a criteria for classification other methods attempt to distinguish the various types of depression.   They use statistical, genetic, biochemical, and physiological criteria. The literature on these methods is voluminous and at this time only a synopsis of their conclusions can be presented.

Statistics as used in studies on psychiatric classification are usually based on psychometric test scores and multivariate analysis.   The multivariate analytic techniques—also called analysis of variance or anovar—most frequently applied are factor (including principal component analysis), discriminant function and cluster analysis.   To attempt an explanation of this difficult topic is beyond the scope of this book. Those who wish to read an excellent synopsis of statistical methods written for readers of medical journals are referred to Wulff, and those who wish to read a critical and lucid account of multivariate analysis as it applies to psychiatric classification should read Kendell.[43,44]

Statistical methods attempt to determine whether depression is a single entity with a variety of symptoms or two or more distinct entities. Macfayden in an excellent review of research articles concluded:

> . . . from the overview of the studies that employ factor analysis to validate depressive constructs that only a few patients exhibit predominantly un-contaminated endogenous features as identified in each research paper, and at least one other factor is necessary to account for the variability . . . .[45]

Factor analysis, she finds, is only suggestive of two or more types of depressive illness. Discriminant function and cluster analysis similarly do not answer the question. Further she adds:

> While an 'endogenous' depressive group was identified consistently in most of the research papers, and several well-controlled investigations indicated the existence of two or more depressive entities, it was concluded that the lack of control of and comparability between diagnoses, symptoms, statistical methods, and experimental designs mitigate against a meaningful comparison of research results.[46]

Perhaps genetic, physiological, or biochemical studies will shed light on the problem of classification.

Macfayden reviewing recent articles on genetic findings in depressed patients concluded:

> . . . studies suggest that the number of episodes, sex, family history, age of onset, and presence of mania are all important factors that differentiate depressive subgroups. However, the number of episodes and sex differences have been considered important mainly in the Winokur studies; family history has been found to be similar in unipolar and bipolar groups and to differ in others, even within a unipolar or bipolar sample; age of onset has been considered important in most of the research with a critical cut-off at 40 years, but discriminates in samples of unipolar, bipolar, and combined samples; both unipolar and bipolar patients conform to a polygenetic model, which forces the conclusion that the presence of mania does not differentiate consistently a subgroup on some variables.[47]

With regard to biochemical, physiological, and drug response Macfayden concluded that those studies similarly did not strongly support any subtype classification of depression.[48] Psychiatrists and psychologists must, therefore, rely on clinical manifestations until research offers a better method of classification.

Terminology needs clarification.   Primary affective disorders include only persons with no previous psychiatric illness other than possibly previous episodes of depression or mania.   Secondary affective disorders occur in patients with other preexisting psychiatric or physical illnesses.[49]   Unipolar affective disease with one or many attacks (multiphasic) involves depression alone.   Bipolar disease involves at least one episode of hypomania or mania and at least one episode of depression.[50] The above terminology eliminates the neurotic/psychotic and endogenous/reactive dichotomies and replaces them with a new dichotomy (unipolar/bipolar).   Although the new label does not define homogeneous sub-types any more clearly than the older ones, it seems to be gaining acceptance among psychiatrists and as noted will probably be used in the DSMIII.   What-ever the name, it does not change the clinical manifestations that patients present nor the problem of subtypes of classification for depression.

Utilizing available information clinicians must have a consistent classification system.   The clinician, therefore, is forced into categories.   Depression, then, cannot in one instance be considered a dimension of personality and in another instance a disease entity.   The relevant problem is to delineate practical and useful categories and to clarify the relationship among them.   Neurotic and psychotic are useful categories.   Foulds clarifies the categories by positing that:

> . . . the relationship between neurotic and psychotic depression may well be an inclusive one, such that all those with psychotic depressive symptoms have 'neurotic depressive' symptoms, but not all those with 'neurotic depressive' symptoms have 'psychotic depressive symptoms.'[51]

Although psychotic and neurotic depressions overlap, they do have meaning as defined in the DSMII.   The terms postpartum, involutional, or senile link depression with certain periods in the life cycle; retarded and agitated are re-lated to motor activity and link depression to certain clinical features; manic-depressive (cyclic depressions cannot be differentiated on the first attack) and schizoaffective disorders are distinguished; and so forth.   Until a better method is devised that correlates symptomatology with etiology, course, prognosis, and treatment, the present classification will suffice.   It does lend itself to multiaxial diagnosis, multifactorial etiological considerations, and multiple forms of therapy.

ETIOLOGY

Etiological considerations are difficult to establish because the definition and classification of neurotic depression is not distinctly separated from all other types of depression.   This imprecision forces a general discussion of all affective disorders, distinguishing the various entities whenever possible.   The underlying assumption is that at the present time not enough is known to attribute particular etiological factors to each entity and that some of the same factors are operant with all types of depression. The hope is that, until definitive relationships are established between etiology and diagnosis, this approach will be helpful in attaining that objective.

Physiological changes concomitant with depression offer excellent examples of the common bond between body functions and an affect. The mechanism by which this is accomplished, however, is not so clear. Hypothalamic function may be altered in depressed states. The hypothalamus is concerned with homeostasis, regulation of certain biological rhythms, metabolism, and autonomic nervous system functioning. In depressed states the following may occur: a diminution in the secretion of gastric juice, saliva; a decrease in intestinal peristalsis and basal metabolic rate; delayed water secretion; lag in the glucose tolerance curve; and a disturbance of sodium, potassium, and cholesterol metabolism. Further hypothalamic functional disturbances are: sleep rhythm irregularities; slowed heart rate; lower body temperature; loss of appetite, weight; metabolic, menstrual, and sexual changes; and so on. Besides these functions, the hypothalamus is concerned with the mediation of emotion. Since the hypothalamus is concerned with homeostatic and emotional functioning, it must have importance for psychosocial adjustment. This becomes more apparent in view of the relationship among the hypothalamus, pituitary, and other endocrine glands.[52]

The similar physiological changes that occur in both manic-depression. depressed type, and in hibernation in lower animals are interesting and numerous. Both conditions are characterized by lower metabolic rates, weight loss, hypothermia, bradycardia, hypotension, and diminished body activity. During hibernation, these changes are attributed to altered hypothalamic function and it has been suggested that in manic-depressive illness a similar alteration occurs in humans.[53]

Studies of depression indicate a lowered threshold of central nervous system arousal, a disruption of rapid eye movement (REM) during sleep, and disappearance of the deepest stage of nonrapid eye movement sleep (delta rhythm). Investigators speculate that lowering the central arousal state could in part result from sodium accumulation in the neurons. They find increased intraneuronal sodium in depressed, and especially in manic, states. Moreover, they think replacing sodium with lithium carbonate in the intraneuronal membrane may correct the physiological abnormality. Hence, these investigators explain manic and depressed states as a genetically determined electrolyte disturbance.[54]

The biogenic amine hypothesis of depression was stimulated by two findings: first, tubercular patients became euphoric when treated with iproniazid; second, hypertensive patients treated with rauwolfia alkaloids (reserpine) became depressed. Iproniazid, a monoamine oxidase inhibitor (MAOI), elevates catecholamines and indolealkylamine in brain and other tissues. Rauwolfia alkaloid depletes these amines. A relationship among affective states, catecholamines, and indolealkylamines seems warranted.

The catecholamines [norephinephrine (NE), epinephrine (E), and dopamine (DA)] and indolealkylamines [tryptamine, serotonin (5HT)] are neurotransmitters. They are chemicals that diffuse across the synapse and either excite or inhibit the succeeding neuron. Synapses are found in the central nervous system (CNS), autonomic nervous system ganglia, and neuromuscular junction. Many other substances are neurotransmitters but the individual synapses where these compounds function and how they function are not known. But the evidence indicates that these transmitters have a relationship to hunger, sleep, and pleasure as well as to emotional states of dysphoria and mania. The emphasis in this section will be on the action of NE, DA, and 5HT in the CNS, since they seem to be the most important transmitters involved in the affective states.[55]

NE, DA, and 5HT do not readily pass the plasma-brain barrier. Synthesized, stored, released, and inactivated within the neuron, they are concentrated in the phylogenetically older parts of the brain. NE and 5HT have high concentrations in the hypothalamus; DA is highest in the corpus striatum (caudate and putamen); and 5HT has its highest concentration in the pineal gland and enterochromaffin cells of the gastrointestinal tract. The cell bodies for DA, NE, and serotonin are almost exclusively localized in the pons, medulla oblongata, and tegmentum of the midbrain. There are catecholamine cell groups located in the hypothalamus, but the dopaminergic nerve terminals are from cells primarily in the substantia nigra. The amines found in the limbic system, cerebellum, and spinal cord arise from long axons whose cell bodies are found in the lower brain stem. Cell bodies from one area of the brain can, then, innervate areas that are anatomically distinct from each other such as the hypothalamus, cerebellum, spinal cord, amygdaloid nucleus, and so on.[56]

The neurotransmitters originate from amino acids. Catecholamine synthesis starts with L-tyrosine (L-TYR) hydroxylation to 3,4-dihydroxyphenylalanine (DOPA). This reaction takes place in the brain, adrenal medulla, and tissues receiving sympathetic innervation. DOPA is decarboxylated to 3,4 dihydroxyphenylethylamine (dopamine) granules of vesicles which can be catalyzed by enzymatic action to NE. NE is released from the intraneuronal granules into the synaptic cleft. The NE interacts with receptors on the postsynaptic membrane and is either returned (reuptake) to the presynaptic terminal or inactivated by further enzymatic action. The enzymes involved in the inactivation reaction are catechol-3-0-methyltransferase (COMT) and monoamine oxidase (MAO). The end products are 3-methoxy-4-hydroxymendelic acid (VMA) and 3-methoxy-4-hydroxyphenylglycol (MHPG). The intermediate products of NE metabolism are normetanephrine (NM), E, and metanephrine (M). Serotonin synthesis starts with tryptophan uptake into the brain where it is hydroxylated to 5-hydroxytryptophan (5HTP) and then catalyzed to 5HT. 5HT is stored in nerve granules. When released into the synaptic cleft it can either be metabolized by MAO to 5-hydroxyindole acetic acid (5HIAA) and by tryptophan pyrrolase (TP) to kynurenine and related metabolites, or in a similar fashion to NE; a reuptake process occurs. The metabolites VMA, MHPG, NMN, MN, kynurenine and 5HIAA are all excreted in the urine.[57, 58]

The biogenic amine theory is based upon the assumption that these amines are decreased during depression and increased during mania. If the depletion theory of depression is valid, then a biochemical method for diagnosis of depression is available. Since the metabolites of biogenic amines are excreted in urine, determining the amount excreted and correlating it with the symptomatology should verify whether the hypothesis is right or wrong. The assumption is that the metabolites reflect the level of biogenic amine in the brain. Low metabolites would indicate decreased brain amines, hence depression; and high metabolites would correspond to mania. However, it is probable that only a small fraction of these compounds in the urine come from the brain and the urinary metabolites reflect more the activity of the adrenal medulla, and the peripheral autonomic nervous system. It is uncertain which fraction of the metabolite found in the urine originates in the NE or 5HT in the brain. This led to spinal fluid studies based on the assumption that the metabolites in the fluid would better reflect brain activity. Studies indicate that M, NM, and VMA do not correlate with clinical depression and that 5HIAA gives mixed results depending on the investigator. Only MHPG seems to reflect CNS norepinephrine metabolism and correlates with the clinical picture of an affective disorder. However, these results do not allow for definite conclusions.[59,60] Mendels, in reviewing studies using drugs to deplete NE and 5HT in laboratory animals, subhuman primates, and humans says:

> While they do produce significant depletion of the target amine, and cause a variety of behavioral symptoms, it is clear that the depletion of either brain NE, dopamine, or serotonin is in *itself* not sufficient to account for the development of clinical depression. Such depletion, even if severe and accompanied by a major reduction in amine turnover produces few *persistent* behavioral changes compatible with clinical depression. In fact, when one considers how much amine reduction is necessary to produce behavioral deficits in animals, it seems unlikely that such a severe depletion could occur in depressed patients and not be more readily detectable, unless it were sharply localized in one area of the CNS. While these results do not rule out the possibility that amines play an important role in affect regulation, they do emphasize the need to consider other systems which may interact with changes in amine function.[61]

The conclusion seems to be that the biogenic amine theory is far from proven and new chemical hypotheses are constantly being proposed.[62-64]

Depressive illness is frequently associated with several different personality types. Cycloid or cyclothymic personality traits consist of alternating states of euphoria and dysphoria that have no apparent relationship to external situations. These individuals appear unstable, labile, and constantly fluctuate in mood. Obsessive compulsive personalities are stubborn, overconscientious, meticulous, overserious, somber, studious, narrow in their interests, have difficulty in adjusting to change, bound by high moral codes, and so forth. A variation of this personality type may manifest itself by overcompliance, politeness, obsequiousness, and subservience. Although these may be the most common personality types associated with depression, other traits such as hostility and oversuspiciousness to the extreme of being paranoid are also observed.[65, 66]

Family background and twin studies are important in discerning a genetic factor in depression. First-degree relatives of depressed patients have a higher incidence of depression than those in the general population. Twin studies indicate a higher concordance rate for MZ than DZ twins especially with bipolar illness (manic-depressive)–bipolar MZ concordance (72%), unipolar MZ concordance (40%). Although the evidence is not conclusive, it does indicate that a genetic factor is present in depression and supports separating categories. The data are in accordance with current biochemical and physiological hypotheses of depression since each enzyme and hormone is thought to be transmitted by a specific gene hence a deficiency in one gene causes one type of depression. That should not, however, minimize the role of the interaction between stressful environment and genes nor the possibility of depression being a polygenic, autosomal, or even an X-linked chromosomal disease.[67, 68]

Age and sex may have relevance in the etiology of depression. Children can become profoundly depressed by trivialities but they are almost immune to prolonged changes of mood. The capacity for prolonged mood changes begins around puberty and by adolescence reaches a degree severe enough to lead to suicide. From adolescence to the late twenties the incidence of neurotic depression rises sharply and women are more vulnerable than men by a three or four to one ratio. The incidence of neurotic depression peaks in the female around 25 and in the male around 40. In middle life the tendency is for longer durations and more frequent attacks; however, the incidence in women consistently drops from 30 to 75 and in men there is a small dip from 25 to 30 and then a slow increase until about 40 at which point the incidence again begins to drop slowly until age 75. At 40 women have a two to one ratio to men. By 60 there is a three to two ratio, and by 70 it is a four to three ratio. Around the age of 75 both sexes have the same incidence of neurotic-depressive illness. This correlation of age and sex with neurotic depression seems especially important when compared to psychotic depression. In the latter the incidence rises more slowly in both females and males with a female–male ratio of two to one from adolescence to 50. At 50 the incidence peaks in the female, remains about the same until 70, and rapidly declines by 75. In the male, the incidence of psychotic depression peaks at 60 and slowly declines until 75. The female to male ratio at 60 is about eight to five and remains the same until 75. This difference in age and sex with neurotic and psychotic depression may have some important etiological and diagnostic (categorical type) consequences; however, to date they are not proven.[69] A study which analyzed neurotic illness into the age distribution of its categories supports the hypothesis that increasing age produces somatization of neurotic illness which could lead to misdiagnosis of the neuroses, failure of the patient to be referred to a psychiatrist, and a distortion of the age distribution curve towards an earlier peak and decline.[70]

Other data correlate with depression. Certain substances such as rauwolfia alkaloids, sulfonamides, steroids, L-dopa, and mandelamine may cause depression. Physical illnesses commonly associated with depression are viral diseases (mononucleosis, hepatitis), chronic heart and kidney conditions, anemias, malignancies, avitaminosis, multiple sclerosis, rheumatoid arthritis, endocrine disorders, and so on. Any type of surgery, including organ transplants, can be followed by depression. Postpartum depression or "baby blues" is well known. Novelists can get depressed after "delivery," i.e., publication of their book. Herman Melville went into a 20 year depression after publication of *Moby Dick*. Both Thomas Hagen, author of *Mr. Roberts*, and Lockridge, author of *Raintree County,* committed suicide after their work was successful. Last, depression can be associated with any psychiatric condition, for instance, anxiety neurosis, neurasthenia, hypochondriasis, organic brain syndromes, schizophrenia, and so on.[71]

Psychodynamic models of depression with their earlier concepts of hostility turned inward toward an ambivalently loved person have been revised. These modified concepts still maintain, however, that the most immediate cause of a depression is a loss, a minor or major disappointment, a single frustrating event, a series of unpleasant experiences, etc. Rooted in ego psychology, these concepts stress helplessness, hopelessness, low self-esteem, narcissistic injury, and an inability to reach ego ideal goals. They stress the depressed individual's negative view of self in the here, the now, and the past as well as the futility of the future. Each concept places emphasis on one or another aspect of ego functioning as the prime cause of depression.[72]

Separation or loss studies are extensive and have stimulated a great deal of investigation. Separation is viewed as either a precipitant of depression or, when the loss occurs in childhood, as a predisposition to adult depression. Controversy exists as to whether or not a precipitating event that involves separation predates the appearance of a depressive illness. Many individuals with separation loss do not develop depressions. Depression may develop without separation, and separation may develop as a result of depression.[73]

The concept that a loss in early life predisposes a person to adult depression was expressed, as previously noted, by Abraham and Freud. René Spitz found that infants between 6 months and 1 year of age, separated from their mothers and placed in foundling homes, had a higher incidence of mental disturbance, physical illness, and even death than those living with their mothers or those over 1 year of age. He called this type of depression anaclitic.[74] John Bowlby's earlier studies concluded that the primary bond was between mother and infant and that there was a high degree of correlation between emotional problems in childhood and lack of a mother-infant relationship which permitted clinging and following patterns. When the bond was broken anxiety and depressive symptoms appeared.[75] Later Bowlby noted a higher incidence of delinquency in boys who had lost a parent by death. This finding added a dimension to the relationship between parental loss and psychopathology. Bowlby warned that other factors besides loss might predispose a person to depression.[76] Many authors have attempted to relate childhood loss (bereavement) to adult depression and other psychiatric conditions, but as yet the relationship remains unproven.[77]

The behaviorists postulate loss as a prime condition for the depressive response. The patient loses either an important positive reinforcer or an important source of reinforcement; hence, responses that were previously reinforced become extinguished and depression results. Further, the low rate of response-contingent reinforcement results not only in a low rate of behavior in a depressed person but acts as a stimulus for other depressive behaviors such as fatigue, somatic symptoms, other depressive mood feelings, and so forth. The net result is that the patient is less capable of eliciting positive reinforcement from the environment and resorts to depressive symptoms as a means of attracting attention and sympathy. A vicious circle of stimulus, response, stimulus is established.[78]

The emphasis on stress as a precipitating cause of certain types of depression has led to controversy. Psychiatrists, whose predilection is towards a psychosocial orientation, invariably find that stressful environmental events and intrapsychic conflict explain depressed states. In fact, even with manic-depressives, involutional melancholics, or patients with an organic brain syndrome, these psychiatrists find psychological explanations for the depressed state. Simply stated they think that the "loss" can be either a fantasy which is given up or, in the case of organic brain syndrome, the psychological perception of the loss of brain tissue. In contrast, biologically oriented psychiatrists pay little attention to environmental factors, but even most of them would agree that stress is a factor in neurotic depression.

Neurotic-depressive reactions may be a stage in the process of unsuccessful biosocial adaptation. The first stage is called an alarm reaction and is part of the general adaptation syndrome. Anxiety, fear, and anger are the major characteristics. The second stage results when the stress continues for a prolonged period of time and a conditioning response develops. This is called the state of resistance and is characterized by anxiety, obsessive compulsive, or phobic neurotic types of reactions. These chronic states may remain stable, resolve, or progress to the third stage of adaptation, called the state of exhaustion. This state is characterized by inhibition and loss of adaptive reserve. In acute depression psychomotor immobilization is complete; in subacute or chronic depression immobilization varies. The state of exhaustion can also be manifested by anxiety, panic, hysteria, or somatizations that inhibit functioning to varying degrees and upset the homeostatic equilibrium or steady state.[79]

Akiskal and McKinney, in an attempt to present an integrative model of depression, posit the importance of the *interrelationship* of anatomical, physiological, chemical, experiential, and behavioral systems for the appearance or nonappearance of a depression. They consider that portions of the diencephalon represent the anatomical substrate of reinforcement and establish connections with other systems. Thereby, a disturbance in one system would lead to a disturbance in another system. The stress neuroendocrine system (hypothalamo-pituitary) has positive and negative feedback connections with the arousal system (reticular activating) and psychomotor system (pyramidal-extrapyramidal). The arousal system has positive and negative feedback connections with the reinforcement system (medial forebrain bundle and periventricular areas), psychomotor system, and stress neuroendocrine system. These authors say:

Melancholic and manic behaviors, according to our scheme, result from a failure in the homeostatic mechanisms that maintain these systems in negative feedback when physiochemical alterations in these systems produce increasing levels of positive feedback in the reinforcement system. Stress or frustration beyond the coping ability of the individual—together with their psychic (anxiety, hopelessness) and neuroendocrine (increased cortisol, sodium retention) correlates—are expected to produce heightened arousal and could disrupt the functional integrity of the reinforcement system. The resultant decline in vegetative and psychomotor functions and the perception of oneself as losing control in an impending state of decompensation serve as novel sources of stress with additional increments in arousal and additional decrements in coping mechanisms. Thus a vicious cycle of more arousal, more hopelessness, and more evidence of purposeless psychomotor activity. In a system's scheme like this, the controversy whether altered catecholamine metabolism is a cause or effect of depression can be easily resolved. Lowering of norepinephrine in the reinforcement system would contribute to functional impairment whether it is primary or secondary. In other words, norepinephrine depletion can be an effect that, in its own right, can then serve as a cause in the pathogenetic chain of events. Besides, it is not necessary to postulate norepinephrine depletion for all types of depressive illness. The final common pathway of derangement in the homeostatic mechanisms, that normally maintain the reinforcement system in optimal balance, may result from a variety of causes . . . . [80]

The etiology of depression is not known. The foregoing attempt is merely a synopsis regarding some of the etiological hypotheses of depression. The literature on this subject is extensive and readers interested in elaboration and details are encouraged to go beyond the references listed at the end of this chapter.

DIAGNOSIS

Depression itself is the most common symptom. It may vary from mild sadness to a feeling of complete nothingness and even stupor in severe cases. Patients say they feel miserable, utterly miserable, more miserable than ever, dreadful, helpless, abandoned, hopeless, lonely, low-spirited, broken-hearted, run down, worried, irritated, frightened, discontent, unhappy, melancholy, awful in myself, dazed, dizzy, muddled, and so forth. In the mild forms the patient expresses feelings of sadness, discouragement and loses interest in his usual activities. It is, however, possible to distract him for short periods of time and he will feel and behave like his usual self. Because of the absence of any striking disturbance and the apparent ability to enjoy life for periods of time these patients are frequently not recognized as depressed.

The moderately depressed patient expresses feelings of constant discomfort. All experiences are painful and he cannot even get temporary relief. He becomes preoccupied with a few subjects, usually of a morbid nature, and usually related to the precipitating event. Bodily complaints—headaches, backaches, chest and abdominal pains, muscle weakness, fatigue, etc.—are very common. He experiences anxiety, irritability, and complains that his memory is going. Yet, he still manages to go to work although he claims his performance is horrible. He attends family functions but does not enjoy them.

The severely depressed patient feels annihilated and wants to be left alone. He complains of confusion, and an inability to sleep. Although the mildly and moderately depressed patient may have difficulty in eating, sleeping, and performing sexually, the severely depressed patient has these same complaints in an exaggerated form. Whereas some mildly and moderately depressed patients resort to excessive eating and sleeping; the severely depressed not only loses interest in food but frequently cannot eat, and suffers from insomnia—early awakening is usual. Ideas of worthlessness and self-accusations are expressed and he reinterprets his past in light of the present mood. Decisions are difficult, replies to questions are delayed and short, and movement becomes difficult. Although in normal as well as in mildly and moderately depressed people the relationship between their appearance and their statements about depressed feelings may appear contradictory, in the severely depressed person the discrepancy is gone. They look the way they say they feel.[81]

Neurotic depression rarely extends to the severe state. It usually varies from day to day, from circumstance to circumstance, and from interest to interest. Neurotic depression differs from the more established category of psychotic depression in that there are no delusions, hallucinations, loss of contact with reality, ideas of reference, or bizarre somatic complaints. Yet neurotic depression can be a very debilitating disease and the distinction between it and psychotic depression is often difficult to discern.[82]

Neurotic depressives usually show only a graver degree of the changes that are observable in the normal person who is temporarily down; and self-reproach is less marked than in the psychotic. The most prominent feature is mood itself and somatization is next in importance. Although the patient can tell his examiner what is making him unhappy, he feels helpless to do anything about it. Sometimes the patient may not attribute his depression to the precipitating cause even though the examiner considers the reaction appropriate to the situation. Of course, the opposite can also be true; that is, the patient reacts to trivialities which the examiner does not consider important.

Neurotic-depressive patients can be unreasonable and demanding. They have been described as greedy or as "love addicts." They plead, demand, and force their family and friends to give them what they want. They can keep people close to them under constant threat and in this sense negate what they say they want, namely, love. It is indeed difficult to love them with these aggressive, obnoxious, pleading, demanding ways. In fact, they often feel self-hatred because of their excessive wants, needs, and demands. Ambivalence is a good descriptive term for their behavior. They want love but reject it. Guilt feelings have a role in their behavior. They feel guilty about minor things or issues. When this occurs a deepening of the depression may be near and it can occur quite suddenly.

Mourning, grief, and bereavement reactions are generally considered synonymous terms. These terms can describe the experiences an individual normally undergoes following the loss of a loved person or the loss of something meaningful, e.g., neighborhood, country, social structure, political system, cultural mores, and so on. Reality dictates that the lost object or ideal no longer exists, yet the mourner at first is unable to give up this attachment. A series of changes occurs, which begin with the denial of the loss and progress to tears and anger. Recent experiences that the mourner had with the deceased are recalled as well as the circumstances of the death and an attempt is made to determine if anything else could have been done to save the person's life. Afterward comes a painful review of the life of the deceased and the relationship between the bereaved and the dead person. Memories keep coming back, incidents recurring, and the gradual process of accepting the reality of the death takes place. The process from death to a more or less realistic acceptance usually takes about nine to twelve months to complete, with the most painful period being the first 30 to 60 days. If grief or mourning goes much beyond one year, the bereaved may then be considered in the realm of abnormal depression. Normal mourning can be viewed as an adaptive process in which the mourner changes to an altered reality. Some have compared this process to any significant change that takes place in an individual's life. For instance, during normal growth and development the individual is in constant change, giving up previous modes of thinking, feeling, and adjustments for new ones. These changes, which lead to new adaptations, are considered to be the basis of the creative process.[83, 84]

DIFFERENTIAL DIAGNOSIS

Distinguishing primary from secondary affective disorders is the first step in differential diagnosis. All nonpsychological causes should be eliminated by proper physical and appropriate laboratory tests. This is not as easy as it may at first seem since many nonpsychological causes of depression may not be demonstrable and the patient's first response to these causes may be depression rather than physical signs or symptoms. It may, therefore, be necessary to periodically check and recheck the patient for nonpsychological etiological factors. Only the psychiatrist's knowledge of general medicine and his willingness to forcefully pursue his medical judgment—even in the face of hostile internists and general physicians—will enable him to competently treat the depressed patient.

Many depressed patients have vague or specific somatic complaints which may be caused by an underlying or "masked" depression. The problems posed by masked or disguised depression—also called depressive equivalents—cover a wide range of somatic symptoms. First, there are the gastrointestinal complaints. These complaints can mimic all the physical conditions that produce cachexia, i.e., a marked degree of malnutrition or ill health. Panhypopituitarism (Simmond's cachexia, Sheehan's syndrome), congestive heart failure, anorexia nervosa, cancer, metabolic and malabsorptive disease, operative myxedema (cachexia strumipriva), and chronic liver disease should all be considered in differential diagnosis. Other gastrointestinal complaints that are possible symptoms of a masked depression are glossalgia, bad breath, lump in the throat, difficulty in swallowing, gagging, choking, grinding of the teeth with resulting tempero-mandibular pain, throat clearing, food intolerances resulting from texture and consistency, air swallowing resulting in abdominal fullness, distention and bloating, peptic ulcerlike symptoms and pain, discomfort, and disorders of defecation. Second, there are symptoms that are referrable to the central nervous and musculoskeletal systems. These symptoms include pains and paraesthesias resulting in scratching or rubbing, headaches with associated hypertonia of cervical muscles, backaches, dizziness, and light-headedness. Third, there are the cardiovascular symptoms which include left chest pain, skipped beats, shortness of breath, heaviness in the chest, and paroxysmal auricular tachycardia. Fourth, are respiratory symptoms, similar to those listed with cardiovascular symptoms, but hyperventilation is most prominent. Obviously, the spectrum of symptoms is wide and diagnostic possibilities endless.[85]

Narcolepsy and depression are easily confused. Narcolepsy is a disease characterized by hypersomnia that may develop at any age but is usually reported in the second and third decades and is often associated with catalepsy (a transient loss of muscle tone), sleep paralysis, and hypnagogic hallucinations. Usually narcolepsy precedes the onset of catelepsy although, rarely, catalepsy may appear first. Sleep paralysis is characterized by inability to move the body while in a state of mental alertness. It occurs on awakening from sleep, lasts for seconds or minutes, and the patient feels as though it will never end. Statistics reveal that 25% of the patients have narcolepsy alone, 68% of these patients develop catalepsy, 24% have associated sleep paralysis, and 30% further suffer with hypnagogic hallucinations. Frequently, other members of the patient's family have symptoms of this tetrad. Narcolepsy is considered a disorder of rapid eye movement (REM) sleep. REM sleep is associated with hypotonia, dreaming, and a desynchronized electroencephalogram that resembles the alert state. A cause for misdiagnosis of this condition is that the patient may not complain of excessive sleeping or drowsiness but of fatigue or tiredness. Hence, the diagnosis of depression is made and narcolepsy is missed. A depression can be a reaction to the narcoleptic disturbance and this further complicates the diagnosis. Also patients who suffer from mild narcolepsy and mild drowsiness, but never experience sleep attacks, could be misdiagnosed as depressed.[86]

Neurotic depression, secondary to other psychiatric conditions, can also be difficult to differentiate since other conditions may either mask the depression or have depression as a complication. As previously noted depression frequently cannot be distinguished from anxiety neurosis; however, depressive feelings, somatization, psychomotor retardation and a history of past depressions may aid in the differentiation from anxiety. In addition anxious patients seem to begin having symptoms earlier in life and more gradually; show early difficulties in school adjustment and in their relationship with their parents; have a greater incidence of psychiatric disorders in their relatives; and tend to persist with their illness for longer periods of time than depressed patients.[87] The problem with all other neuroses is that depression can be associated with each of them as either the primary or secondary disease. Only evaluation of the total clinical picture and the psychiatrist's clinical judgment will enable him to determine which is the predominant entity. In neurasthenia, where fatigue and loss of energy are the cardinal symptoms, this can be especially difficult; and in hypo-chondriasis the transient nature and multiplicity of the somatic complaints may be significant.   Abnormal thought and behavior dominate the clinical features in schizophrenia and in psychophysiological disorders there is usually a demonstrable organic lesion. To emphasize again, depression can be associated with any psychiatric state.

In sum, normal fluctuations in mood are distinguished from neurotic de-pression by the latter having prolonged persistence of depressive symptoms beyond what is expected by existent circumstances. The difference between psychotic and neurotic depression depends on whether reality testing or functional adequacy are impaired enough to be considered a psychosis. Both psychotic and neurotic depressions are precipitated by some circumstance which stimulates the patient's reaction. Manic-depressive illnesses and involutional melancholia do not have an observable precipitating stress. Involutional melan-cholia is distinguished from the manic-depressive illnesses by lack of previous episodes and its occurrence during the involutional period. Schizoaffective disorder shows a mixture of schizophrenic symptoms with elation and depression. These distinctions are artificial and have misleading etiological implications. If one considers the classification as primarily descriptive it helps limit and define the various syndromes. For present purposes the emphasis on the pre-cipitating event is acceptable as a means of differentiating different types of depression. Perhaps for the researcher this division is unacceptable but it works well for the clinician, student, and teacher.

COURSE AND PROGNOSIS

The neurotic depression almost always remits in due course: the patient recovers from physical illness, circumstances change, or passage of time allows him to work through his problems and forget the loss or disappointment. He usually returns to his premorbid personality state. The possibility of chronicity is very real and this is even more true when the personality is unremittingly depressive and pessimistic. As a rule, however, two to four months sees the patient through the worst of his trouble. Much depends on circumstances.

Suicide as a possible resolution of depression must always be kept in the forefront of the psychiatrist's mind. Preventive measures must be taken such as hospitalization, frequent visits with the physician, drugs, family consultation, or any other step to stop its occurrence. It is essential to identify high-risk patients. All suicidal threats and gestures should be taken seriously. It is often hard to distinguish those patients who are serious about wanting to die and seriously attempt to do so, from those who do not want to die but threaten to kill themselves and make feeble suicidal gestures. Clinical judgment based on a knowledge of the patient, his environment, and family background can be helpful. Statistics may help to decide whether a patient is a high- or low-risk suicidal candidate. Statistics, however, should be evaluated with caution as many suicidal attempts and even suicides are never reported. Accidents, especially those occurring while driving an automobile, may in fact be suicidal if not homocidal; overdosage of drugs may never be detected, and if detected could have been taken not for suicidal purposes, but rather for sleep or relief of pain; and knife or gun wounds may just as easily be accidentally as intentionally self-inflicted. At times the underlying motive may even be unknown to the patient. Feelings of nothingness and hopelessness are perhaps better clues to suicidal intent than any of the other components of depressive illness.[88]

Suicide is a term that was introduced into the English language in 1651[89] and still the best treatment psychiatrists have been able to devise in all of these elapsed centuries is to identify high-risk patients. The hope is that a knowledge of the following statistics will serve as a preventive measure. Suicide is more often:

(1) Threatened than actually attempted.
(2) Attempted by women than men but men are more successful.
(3) Attempted by persons under 30 but more successful in those over 30 and increases in rate with age.
(4) Attempted and successful in those who are schizophrenic, depressed, suffering from a chronic physical illness, or alcoholic.
(5) Attempted and successful with single, widowed, and divorced than with married people; and with those living alone and unemployed than with those living with another person and employed.
(6) Attempted and successful in those whose parent, parents, or close relatives committed suicide.

Other statistics reveal that in 1973 in the United States there were 25,000 suicides and 200,000 attempted suicides; in addition suicide was the tenth leading cause of death in all age groups and second in the college age group. Physicians had a higher suicide rate than the overall population—psychiatrists, opthalmologists, otolaryngologists, and anaesthesiologists had the highest rate among physicians. Common methods of suicide are an overdose of pills, lacerations, gunshot wounds, jumping from heights, suffocating, burning, and automobile accidents. The high-risk suicidal patient can be typified as a male diabetic, over 40, depressed, unemployed, and living alone.[90,91]

TREATMENT

The treatment of a patient with neurotic depression begins with a comprehensive examination. Since many depressed patients have somatic and visceral complaints these must be investigated. Questions should be directed towards clarifying the complaint or complaints emphasizing description, duration, circumstance under which the symptoms began, and subsequent course or progression. A proper physical examination should be followed by appropriate laboratory testing. Once the physician is as certain as he can be that the somatic and visceral complaints are on a depressive basis, further treatment can be instituted.

The lack of definite boundaries between the various types of depression and the use of signs and symptoms as the major criteria for diagnosis makes an improper diagnosis a definite possibility. Hence, treatment, at least initially, should be based on trial and error with common sense as the major guideline. If one approach does not work, another approach should be tried.

If the circumstances that precipitated the illness can be remedied, this should be done. If this does not work, some form of supportive, directive, or dynamic psychotherapy may be started. This type of therapy should be directed toward increasing the patient's ability to work and his capacity for social relationships. During the acute phase of the depression it is advisable not to concentrate on interpretation of behavior but rather to assist the patient in adapting to circumstances. If the depression becomes chronic, intensive psychotherapy may be essential with, when possible, family participation.

Psychotherapy—individual, family, or group—may be used in conjunction with pharmacotherapy. There are four major classes of antidepressant drugs. Since neurotic depressions can become chronic and be extremely incapacitating these drugs can be just as useful in the neurotic as in all other types of depression. The four classes of antidepressant drugs are the following: (1) central nervous system stimulants, such as dextroamphetamines (Dexedrine), methamphetamine (Desoxyn), and methylphenidate (Ritalin); (2) tricyclic derivatives, such as imipramine HCL (Tofranil, SK-Pramine, Presamine, Imavate, Janimine), desipramine HCL (Norpramin, Pertofrane), amitriptyline HCL (Elavil, Endep), doxepin HCL (Adapin, Sinequan), nortriptyline HCL (Aventyl), protriptyline HCL (Vivactil), and imipramine pamoate (Tofranil-PM); (3) monoamine oxidase inhibitors, such as tranylcypromine (Parnate), phenelzine sulfate (Nardil), isocarboxazid (Marplan), iproniazid and nialamide (Niamid); (4) lithium carbonate (Lithane, Eskalith). There is some controversy regarding the effectiveness of central nervous system stimulants in the treatment of depression. Since the other antidepressants can take from one to three weeks before their effects are evident, it is often helpful to use the stimulants for this period of time in conjunction with one of the antidepressants. The usual effective dose of the stimulants is around 5 to 15 mg per day, given in two or three divided doses. The major side effects are—these drugs are sympathomimetic, can increase blood pressure, heart rate, pulse, and so on. They can also simulate the signs and symptoms of acute anxiety.

Drugs used for depression, like all drugs, should have specific clinical indications and be used judiciously. The following guidelines may be helpful. First, a proper diagnosis is essential. Second, the general physical status, especially cardiac, of the patient should be known. Third, a drug history should include what drug worked in previous attacks and whether or not other family members were treated with antidepressant drugs. Families often respond to medications in a similar manner. Fourth, the physician should not stick with a drug that does not help. If after an appropriate trial a drug seems to be a failure, another drug should be used. Fifth, if the side effects are intolerable to the patient, discontinue the drug. The drugs are not so specific that patients should be subjected to additional suffering which the side effects can inflict.

The tricyclics are the drugs of choice when antidepressive drugs are used. Since they all act more or less similarly, there is little reason to select one drug over another. Thus the choice of drug usually depends on which allows the specific patient to endure undesirable side effects. The most sedative tricyclics are doxepin and amytriptyline. Protriptyline might increase psychomotor activity or act as a stimulant. Amitriptyline, imipramine, and doxepin are thought to have the highest degree of anticholinergic reactions. It is possible to mix the drugs—doxepin in the P.M. and protriptyline in the A.M. This would give maximum sedation in the evenings and maximum stimulation during daytime hours. Drugs with the greatest degree of sedation are not for pilots, automobile drivers, or steeplejacks. The age of the patient is also important. In the elderly, where little supervision is available, care must be taken since accidents can occur.

Antihistaminic (sedative) and anticholinergic (dryness of mouth, difficulties with urination, visual accommodation, constipation, and other atropinelike actions) side effects should be considered before prescribing tricyclics to patients with prostatic hypertrophy, untreated glaucoma, or intestinal obstruction. However, there are other side effects and cardiovascular complications are the most hazardous. These include orthostatic hypotension, cardiac arrhythymias, heart blocks, exacerbation of preexisting arrhythmias, and myocardial infarction. Doxepin HCL has the least effect on cardiac conduction and is the drug of choice in the elderly and in those with known heart disease. Another side effect is convulsive seizures that occur on rare occasions.

The dosage range of the tricyclics is usually between 75 to 300 mg per day except for protriptyline where the range is 30 to 60 mg per day. The drugs are given three times a day with meals or in the case of long action drugs such as imipramine pamoate, the drug is administered in one dose at bedtime. Plasma levels of some of these drugs can be measured and the therapeutic range seems to be between 50 ng/ml to 150 ng/ml. It is wise to start with low dosages and to build up gradually to an optimum level. Once this level is reached the dosage may be gradually reduced. It is usual to maintain the patient on medication for three months after clinical recovery is evident.[92]

Drug combinations are used in treating depression. Patients who are anxious and depressed may benefit from either a major tranquilizer sedative or antianxiety drug used alone or in combination with a tricyclic. Hypnotic drugs are frequently helpful when the tricyclic does not alleviate insomnia. However, barbiturates by increasing liver microsomal enzyme activity can decrease the plasma level of tricyclic antidepressants.   In contrast, benzodiazepines do not affect the plasma levels of the tricyclics, and hence a flurazepam HCL (Dalmane) may be more beneficial. Thyroid, thyroid stimulating hormones (TSH), and triiodothyronine (T_3) may increase the action of the tricyclics, especially in women. With thyroid releasing hormone (TRH), however, the patient does not improve.[93, 94] There are cardiovascular dangers with this combination.   Methylphenidate decreases liver microsomal activity and increases plasma levels of tricyclics. Monoamine oxidase inhibitors, tricyclics, and lithium may be used in combination and produce good therapeutic results. However, at this time the Federal Drug Administration has not approved the usage of tricyclics in combination with MAOI—so it should be eliminated. Combinations of drugs are indicated more for other types of depression than for the neurotic.[95, 96]

The MAOI are used in the United States usually after a two or three week medication-free interval when patients are switched from one MAOI to another or from a tricyclic to an MAOI. The two or three week interval is recommended because hypertensive crises and death can result when the combinations are used. The contraindications to MAOI are many. They should not be given to patients over 60 or to those with cardiovascular disease, hypertension, or a history of headaches.   Once on the medication, patients should avoid the following: strong or aged cheese, chocolate, raisins, sour cream, pickled herring, red wines, canned figs, avocados, beer, the pods of broad beans, yeast extracts, chicken livers, and all foods with a high tyramine content. These substances can precipitate a hypertensive crisis. The indication for MAOI is that they do bring about improvement in patients who do not respond to tricyclics or other types of medication. The nonhydrazine monoamine oxidase inhibitor tranylcypromine (Parnate) is probably safer than the hydrazine MAOI isocarboxazid (Marplan), phenelzine dihydrogen sulfate (Nardil), and so on.[97, 98]

The role of lithium carbonate in depressive illness, either for prophylactic maintenance or for its value in treatment of the depressive phases, is still not known.   This is especially true for neurotic depression. Caution should be observed in the use of lithium since the FDA only sanctions its use for bipolar disease. However, there are other precautions that should be taken when this drug is used. The plasma level of lithium should be maintained between a narrow range usually around 1 m Eq/liter. Toxicity is indicated by anorexia, gastric discomfort, diarrhea, vomiting, thirst, polyuria, and hand tremor. The tremor does not respond to antiparkinsonian medication. At plasma levels above 1.5 m Eq/liter muscle fasiculation, twitching, hyperactive deep tendon reflexes, ataxia, somnolence, confusion, dysarthria, and epileptiform seizures may occur. There is no specific antidote for severe lithium intoxication. With chronic ingestion of lithium the side effects are a diabetes-insipiduslike syndrome, blood sugar elevation, thyroid disturbance, and elevated white cell count. Lithium should not be used in patients with impaired renal function, cardiovascular disease, brain damage, or with patients on diuretics or low salt diet. In neurotic depression the dangers encountered by using this drug may far outweigh the expected benefits.[99]

There are many other methods to treat depression, besides those mentioned above. First, intravenous sodium amytal used alone or in combination with amphetamines has been recommended.[100] Second, electroconvulsive treatment (ECT), until the discovery of the antidepressant drugs, was the standard and most effective method for treating acute and chronic depressions throughout the world. For suicidal patients ECT is probably still the best preventative and in comparative studies of ECT, tricyclics and placebos, ECT was found to be most effective for treatment of depression. Recently unilateral ECT applied to the nondominant hemisphere has been found to produce results equal to those with bilateral ECT. The unilateral treatments can be given daily whereas bilateral treatments are usually three times a week; and unilateral ECT does not produce the memory impairment so prevalent with bilateral ECT. The disadvantages to ECT treatment are that hospitalization is necessary, anesthetic complications, frequent relapses, memory disturbances (which are usually temporary), and fractures can occur. ECT should be reserved for the most serious depressions and for those patients who are suicidal. It is usually not recommended for neurotic depressions but it is recommended when other methods fail.[101] Third, psychosurgery using stereotactic procedures such as orbital tractotomy and cingulotomy are not often recommended except as a last resort. The results of these operations still need more documentation.[102, 103]

Neurotic depression is a self-limiting disease. Irrespective of the treatment modality, it has a definite onset and end. Time is important. A depression reaches a lowest point and then recovery begins. Environmental change, psychotherapy, drugs, ECT or psychosurgery merely hasten the natural process. For some, depression lasts for weeks or months, with others for years, and for a few patients a lifetime. Irrespective of the treatment modality, the physician who treats depressed patients should recognize the importance and value of time. Not only does the recovery process require time but it is essential that the physician possess qualities of patience, understanding, and kindness which are so vital if he is to remain with the patient and sustain him during his illness until the inevitable recovery arrives.[104]

REFERENCES

1. Katz, M., "The classification of depression: normal, clinical and ethnocultural variations," in *Depression in the 1970's: Modern Theory and Research* (edited by Fieve, R.). The Hague: Excerpta Medica, 1971, p. 31.

2. Pollitt, J.D., Suggestions for a physiological classification of depression. *Brit. J. Psychiatry* **111**:489–495 (1965).
3. Costello, C.G., *Anxiety and Depression: The Adaptive Emotions.* Montreal: McGill-Queen's University Press, 1976, pp. 47–64.
4. Macfayden, H.W., The classification of depressive disorders: I. A review of statistically based classification studies. *J. Clin. Psychol.* **31**:380–394 (1975).
5. Beck, A.T., "Introduction," in *The History of Depression* (Consultants: Beck, A.T. and Brady, J.P., Technical Adviser: Quen, J.M.). New York: Psychiatric Annals, 1977, p. 7.
6. Editors, "Depression in Ancient Times," in *The History of Depression* (Consultants: Beck, A.T. and Brady, J.P., Technical Adviser: Quen, J.M.). New York: Psychiatric Annals, 1977, pp. 9–13.
7. Lewis, A.J., Melancholia: A historical review. *J. Mental Sci.* **80**(328):1 (1934).
8. Ibid., pp. 2–3.
9. Madden, J.R., Melancholy in medicine and literature: Some historical considerations. *Brit. J. Med. Psychol.* **39**:125–126 (1966).
10. Ibid., pp. 127–128.
11. Jelliffe, S.E., Some historical phases of the manic-depressive synthesis. *Assoc. Res. Nerv. Ment. Dis.* **11**:24–25 (1931).
12. Burton, R., *The Anatomy of Melancholy* (edited by Dell, F. and Jordan-Smith, P.) New York: Tudor, 1948.
13. Veith, I., Elizabethans on melancholia. *J. Amer. Med. Assoc.* **212**(1):127–130 (1970).
14. Lindsay, J.H., Fashions in psychiatry, melancholia 1621 and depression 1961. *Can. Psychiatric Assoc. J.* **8**:150–161 (1963).
15. Lewis, A.J., op. cit., pp. 5–11.
16. Jelliffe, S.E., op. cit., pp. 30–38.
17. Lewis, A.J., op. cit., pp. 6, 7.
18. Veith, I., English Melancholy and American Nervousness. *Bull. Menninger Clinic* **32**:301–317 (1968).
19. Lewis, A.J., op. cit., p. 12.
20. Ibid., pp. 12, 13.
21. Jelliffe, S.E., op. cit., p. 38.
22. Lewis, A.J., op. cit., pp. 20–22.
23. Jelliffe, S.E., op. cit., p. 42.
24. Ibid., pp. 4–8.
25. Ibid., p. 8.
26. Meyer, A., The problems of mental reaction-types, mental causes and diseases. *Psychol. Bull.* **5**:245 (1908).
27. Muncie, W., *Psychobiology and Psychiatry: A Textbook of Normal and Abnormal Human Behavior.* Saint Louis: Mosby, 1939, p. 242.
28. Lewis, A.J., op. cit., pp. 27–30.
29. Abraham, K., "Notes on the psycho-analytical investigation and treatment of manic-depressive insanity and allied conditions (1911)," in *Selected Papers of Karl Abraham* (transl. by Bryan, D. and Strachey, A.), 4th impression. London: Hogarth Press, 1949, pp. 137–156.
30. Freud, S., "Mourning and melancholia (1917)," in *Collected Papers,* vol. 4 (edited by Jones, E. and transl. by Riviere, J.). London, Hogarth Press, 1950, pp. 152–170.
31. Abraham, K., "A short study of the development of the libido, viewed in the light of mental disorders (1924)," in *Selected Papers.* op. cit., pp. 418–501.

32. Rickman, J., The development of the psychoanalytical theory of the psychoses, 1894-1926. *Brit. J. Med. Psychol.* 6:270-294 (1926).

33. Rado, S., The problem of melancholia. *Int. J. Psychoanal.* 9:420 (1928).

34. Rado, S., Psychodynamics of depression from the etiologic point of view. *Psychosom. Med.* 13:51 (1951).

35. Zubin, J., "Presidential address: Biometric methods in psychopathology," in *Depression* (edited by Hoch, P. and Zubin, J.). New York: Grune & Stratton, 1954, pp. 123-143.

36. Zubin, J. and Fleiss, J., "Current biometric approaches to depression," in *Depression in the 1970's: Modern Theory and Research* (edited by Fieve, R.). The Hague: Excerpta Medica, 1971, pp. 7-8.

37. Beck, A.T., *The Diagnosis and Management of Depression.* Philadelphia: University of Pennsylvania Press, 1973, p. 69.

38. Ibid., p. 70.

39. Ibid.

40. United States War Department, *Nomenclature and Methods of Recording Diagnosis,* Tech. Bull. Med. 203. Washington, D.C.: United States Printing Office, October 19, 1945.

41. *Diagnostic and Statistical Manual,* Mental Disorders. Washington, D.C.: American Psychiatric Association, 1952, pp. 33-34.

42. Provisional classification: Published as a looseleaf manual entitled *DSM-III Draft, 4/15/77.* DRAFT OF AXES I and II of DSM-III CLASSIFICATION as of March 30, 1977.

43. Kendell, R.E., *The Role of Diagnosis in Psychiatry.* Oxford: Blackwell Scientific Publications, 1975, pp. 106-118.

44. Wulff, H.R., *Rational Diagnosis and Treatment.* Oxford: Blackwell Scientific Publications, 1976, pp. 152-175.

45. Macfayden, H.W., op. cit., p. 385.

46. Ibid., p. 391.

47. Macfayden, H.W., The classification of depressive disorders: II. A review of historical and physiological classification studies. *J. Clin. Psychol.* 31:396 (1975).

48. Ibid., pp. 396-401.

49. Robins, E. and Guze, S.B., "Classification of affective disorders; the primary-secondary, the endogenous-reactive and the neurotic-psychotic concepts," in *Recent Advances in Psychobiology of the Depressive Illnesses* (edited by Williams, T.A., Katz, M.M. and Shield, J.A.). Washington, D.C.: United States Government Printing Office, 1972, p. 283.

50. Kupfer, D.J., Pickar, D., Himmelhoch, J.M. and Detre, T.P., Are there two types of unipolar depression? *Arch. Gen. Psychiatry* 32:866 (1975).

51. Foulds, G.A., The relationship between the depressive illnesses. *Brit. J. Psychiatry* 122:533 (1973).

52. Pollitt, J.D., op. cit., pp. 489-490.

53. Ibid., p. 491.

54. Mendels, J. and Frazer, A., Alterations in cell membrane activity in depression. *Amer. J. Psychiatry* 131(11):1240-1246 (1974).

55. Frazer, A. and Stinnett, J.L., "Distribution and metabolism of norepinephrine and serotonin in the central nervous system," in *Biological Psychiatry* (edited by Mendels, J.). New York: Wiley, 1973, pp. 35-36.

56. Ibid., pp. 37-40.

57. Ibid., pp. 40-64.

58. Hullin, R.P., Metabolism of indole amines in depression. *Postgrad. Med. J.* 52 (suppl. 3):18-24 (1976).

59. Schildkraut, J., The current status of biological criteria for classifying the depressive disorders and predicting responses to treatment. *Psychopharmacol.* **10**:5-25 (1974).
60. Ridges, A.P., The potential value of biochemical parameters in the diagnosis and mediation of affective disorders. *Postgrad. Med. J.* **52** (suppl. 3):9-17 (1976).
61. Mendels, J., Stern, S. and Frazer, A., Biochemistry of depression. *Dis. Nerv. Syst.* **37**(3):5 (1976).
62. Antelman, S.M. and Caggiula, A.R., Norepinephrine-dopamine interactions and behavior: A new hypothesis of stress-related interactions between brain norepinephrine and dopamine is proposed. *Science* **195**:646-653 (1977).
63. Carroll, B.J., Curtis, G.C and Mendels, J., Neuroendocrine regulation in depression: I. Limbic system-adrenocortical dysfunction. *Arch. Gen. Psychiatry* **33**(9):1039-1044 (1976).
64. Carroll, B.J., Curtis, G.C and Mendels, J., Neuroendocrine regulation in depression: II. Discrimination of depressed from nondepressed patients. *Arch. Gen. Psychiatry* **33**(9):1051-1058 (1976).
65. Nyström, S. and Lindegård, B., Predisposition for mental syndromes: A study comparing predisposition for depression, neurasthenia and anxiety state. *Acta. Psychiat. Scand.* **51**(2):69-76(1975).
66. Videbech, T., The psychopathology of anancastic endogenous depression. *Acta. Psychiat. Scand.* **52**:336-373 (1975).
67. Allen, M., Twin studies of affective illness. *Arch. Gen. Psychiatry* **33**(12):1476-1478 (1976).
68. Weissman, M.M. and Klerman, G.L., Sex differences and the epidemiology of depression. *Arch. Gen. Psychiatry* **34**(1):103-104 (1977).
69. Spicer, C.C., Hare, E.H. and Slater, E., Neurotic and psychotic forms of depressive illness: Evidence from age-incidence in a national sample. *Brit. J. Psychiatry* **123**: 535-541 (1973).
70. McDonald, G., An age-specific analysis of the neuroses. *Brit. J. Psychiatry* **122**: 477-480 (1973).
71. Kline, N.S., Incidence, prevalence and recognition of depressive illness. *Dis. Nerv. Syst.* **37**(3):10-14 (1976).
72. Bibring, E., "The mechanism of depression," in *Affective Disorders: Psychoanalytic Contributions to Their Study* (edited by Greenacre, P.). New York: International Universities Press, 1953, pp. 13-49.
73. Akiskal, H.S. and McKinney, W.T., Overview of recent research in depression: Integration of ten conceptual models into a comprehensive clinical frame. *Arch. Gen. Psychiatry* **32**:293-295 (1975).
74. Spitz, R.A., "Anaclitic depression: An inquiry into the genesis of psychiatric conditions in early childhood," in *The Psychoanalytic Study of the Child,* vol. 2. New York: International Universities Press, 1946, pp. 313-342.
75. Bowlby, J., The nature of the child's tie to his mother. *Int. J. Psychoanal.* **39**:350 (1958).
76. Bowlby, J., The Adolph Meyer lecture: Childhood mourning and its implications for psychiatry. *Amer. J. Psychiatry* **118**:481 (1961).
77. Akiskal, H.S. and McKinney, W.T., op. cit., pp. 294-295.
78. Lewinsohn, P.M., "Clinical and theoretical aspects of depression, innovative treatment methods," in *Psychopathology* (edited by Calhoun, S., Adams, H.E. and Mitchell, K.M.). New York: Wiley, 1974, pp. 63-120.
79. Cammer, L., Antidepressants as a prophylaxis against depression in the obsessive compulsive person. *Psychosomatics* **14**:201-202 (1973).

80. Akiskal, H.S. and McKinney, W.T., op. cit., p. 299.
81. Lewis, A.J., Melancholia: A clinical survey of depressive states. *J. Mental Sci.* 80:277-378 (1934).
82. Kiloh, L.G., Andrews, G., Neilson, M. and Bianchi, G.N., The relationship of the syndromes called endogenous and neurotic depression. *Brit. J. Psychiatry* **121**: 183-196 (1972).
83. Pollack, G.M., On mourning, immortality, and utopia. *J. Amer. Psychoanal. Assoc.* **23**(2):334-362 (1975).
84. Pollock, G.M., "The mourning process and creative organizational change." Post-Presidential Address, December 20, 1975, Mid-Winter Meeting of the American Psychoanalytic Association (in publication).
85. Rome, H., Depression: Unmasking the symptoms. *Medical Opinion,* May 1975, pp. 16-20.
86. Fail, L., Narcolepsy and neurosis. *Med. J. Aust.* **2**:223-225 (1973).
87. Costello, C.G., op. cit., p. 108.
88. Wetzel, R.D., Hopelessness, depression, and suicide intent. *Arch. Gen. Psychiatry* **33**(9):1069-1073 (1976).
89. Cohen, E., Melancholy and suicide. (Letters to the Journal) *J. Amer. Med. Assoc.* **212**(12):2121 (1970).
90. Fabian, J.J., Maloney, M.P. and Ward, M.P., Self-destructive and suicidal behaviors in a neuropsychiatric inpatient facility. *Amer. J. Psychiatry* **130**(12):1383-1385 (1973).
91. *American Medical News,* December 17, 1973, pp. 11-14.
92. Hollister, L.E., Clinical use of antidepressants. *Dis. Nerv. Syst.* **37**(3):17-21 (1976).
93. Hollister, L.E., Davis, K.L. and Berger, P., Pituitary response to thyrotropin-releasing hormone in depression. *Arch. Gen. Psychiatry* **33**(11):1393-1396 (1976).
94. Mountjoy, C.Q., The possible role of thyroid and thyrotrophic hormones in depressive illness. *Postgrad. Med. J.* **52** (suppl. 3):103-109 (1976).
95. Spiker, D.G. and Pugh, D.D., Combining tricyclic and monoamine oxidase inhibitor antidepressants. *Arch. Gen. Psychiatry* **33**(7):828-830 (1976).
96. Ban, T.A., Pharmacotherapy of depression—A critical review. *Psychosomatics* **16**(1):17-20 (1975).
97. Berger, F.M., Depression and antidepressant drugs. *Clin. Pharmacol. Ther.* **18**(3): 243-244 (1975).
98. Johnson, W., A neglected modality in psychiatric treatment—The monoamine oxidase inhibitors. *Dis. Nerv. Syst.* **36**:521-525 (1975).
99. Davis, J.M., Overview: Maintenance therapy in psychiatry: II. Affective disorders. *Amer. J. Psychiatry* **133**(1):1-13 (1976).
100. Kraines, S.H., Therapy of the chronic depression. *Dist. Nerv. Syst.* **28**:578-580 (1967).
101. d'Elia, G. and Raotma, H., Is unilateral ECT less effective than bilateral ECT? *Brit. J. Psychiatry* **126**:83-89 (1975).
102. Culliton, B.J., Psychosurgery: National Commission issues surprisingly favorable report. *Science* **194**(4262):299-301 (1976).
103. Shevitz, S., Psychosurgery: Some current observations. *Amer. J. Psychiatry* **133**(3): 266-270 (1976).
104. Kraines, S.H., op. cit., pp. 577-584.

9
NEURASTHENIA

The diagnostic status of neurasthenia has been a cause of debate and confusion since the term was coined in 1869. Its definition has changed many times since its conception and even varies from country to country. This has led to so much confusion that some American psychiatrists believe that the term should be discarded. But since neurasthenia is widely used in countries other than the United States, its use in America would help to coordinate an international classification, particularly if a worldwide definition could be agreed upon. It is therefore, recommended that neurasthenia be retained in the United States Classification System.[1, 2]

Neurasthenia is defined as a condition with the following essential components: chronic weakness, easy fatigability, sporadic exhaustion, and genuine distress. There may be other components (vegetative, somatic, psychic, or behavioral) but these components are not essential for the definition. Additionally, neurasthenia differs from chronic anxiety, depression, hysterical neurosis, and other types of illnesses in which somatic symptoms predominate such as psychophysiological disorders or hypochrondriasis. In short, neurasthenia is a disease entity which is reasonably delineated from all other diseases.

The keystone in defining and understanding neurasthenia depends upon the meaning of energy and fatigue. From a practical point of view, everyone knows that the amount of energy available for functioning varies from minute to minute, hour to hour, day to day, and year to year. All of us have high and low energy days, feel more or less "alive" on different days, and are aware of energies that on this or that day are or are not called forth. All people habitually live both mentally and physically below their highest level of awareness, lucidity in reasoning, certainty in deciding, and potentiality in performance. Yet no one knows exactly what the term energy implies, which probably explains why so little is written or known about it. Energy must have anatomical, chemical, and physiological connections within the central nervous system, which still remain untranslated into measurable terms. Psychic energy presents itself as a quantity, yet its ebbs and flows can represent different qualities and its relationship to the soma is unknown.

The existence of reserved untapped energy is familiar in the phenomenon of "second wind." One usually stops activity upon encountering the first effective layer of resistance or fatigue. One has worked or played enough and stops. There can be no doubt that fatigue is an effective obstruction to further activity. Nevertheless if necessity forces one to press onward, something happens. Fatigue worsens to a critical point; then suddenly or gradually it passes away and leaves the person refreshed. One evidently reaches a new energy level that was masked by fatigue and this experience may be repeated layer after layer. Both mental and physical activities demonstrate this phenomenon. For instance, by pushing enough one can find amounts of power that he never knew he possessed but generally individuals do not push through the early critical points. Unusual circumstances, excitements, incentives, and needs or necessities induce a person to push to higher levels of energy. Wars, shipwrecks, earthquakes, marriage, religious conversions, compelling ideas, strong emotions, sex, power, love, and so forth enable one to attain periods of rejuvenated energy. Besides, the normal tasks of everyday life should place a person's deeper levels of energy on tap, i.e., accessible as a ready reserve. If this is not so, then life's circumstances are deleterious to health or the individual has an illness. Normally, drive and will open the person to deeper levels of energy.[3]

Fatigue or exhaustion is a condition characterized by a reduction of energy, a diminished capacity for mental or physical effort, and a lack of initiative for goal-directed activities. Fatigue itself is not unpleasant and is normal toward the end of day. Rest overcomes fatigue and energetic people benefit from short naps and sleep well, but the neurasthenic tends to be insomniac and will not recover his energy after rest. Fatigue, in contrast to boredom or monotony, is not relieved by a change in activity. An understanding of the mechanism of fatigue could be the key to neurasthenia.[4]

HISTORY

In the nineteenth century, the rational and mechanistic tradition in medicine prevailed and each clinical entity was thought to have a distinct etiology and pathology. Therefore, to the psychiatrist of that day, it seemed quite logical to describe syndromes that would be caused by an atonic, weakened, or exhausted nervous system. In 1869 George Miller Beard, an American psychiatrist, coined the term "neurasthenia" from the Greek "neuro" (nerve) and "asthenia" (weakness).[5] This condition was thought to be a weakness of the nervous system, not the mind. However, he thought the weakness was a functional disturbance, i.e., a disease without a demonstrable lesion. He equated nervousness with neuroses (Cullen's term) and within a short period of time the term gained wide acceptance.   In fact, neurasthenia became known as the American disease, Americanitis, or American nervousness.[6]

Beard wrote extensively on neurasthenia. By 1881, he thought that nervousness "is nervelessness—a lack of nerve force."[7]   Further, he posited that it resulted at least in part from rapid industrialization, primarily from developments such as: steampower, dissemination of printed material, telegraph, science, and mental activity of women.[8] The following are some of the symptoms that Beard listed:

> Insomnia, flushing, drowsiness, . . . dilated pupils, pain, pressure and heaviness in the head, changes in expression of the eye . . . noises in the ears, atonic voice, mental irritability, tenderness of the teeth and gums, nervous dyspepsia, desire for stimulants and narcotics, abnormal dryness of the skin, joints and mucous membrane, sweating hands and feet with redness, fear of lightning, or fear of responsibility, of open places or of closed places, fear of society, . . . fear of contamination, fear of everything, deficient mental control, lack of decision in trifling matters, hopelessness, . . . tenderness of the spine, and the whole body, . . . coccyodynia, pains in the back, heaviness of the loins and limbs, . . . cold hands and feet, pain in the feet, localized peripheral numbness and hyperaesthesia, tremulous and variable pulse and palpitation of the heart, . . . local spasms of muscles, difficulty of swallowing, convulsive movements, especially on going to sleep, cramps, a feeling of profound exhaustion unaccompanied by positive pain, coming and going, . . . attacks of temporary paralysis, pain in the perineum, involuntary emissions, partial or complete impotence, . . . certain functional diseases of women, . . . rapid decay and irregularities of the teeth, . . . vertigo or dizziness, explosions in the brain at the back of the neck, dribbling and incontinence or urine, frequent urination, ...[9]

This is not Beard's complete list and he seemed to include symptoms of physical illnesses as well as anxiety, depression, hysteria, hypochondriasis, obsessions and compulsions, phobia, and psychosomatic disorders. To Beard neurasthenia was a functional nervous disease and encompassed almost all mental symptoms except insanity, mental deficiency, and certain types of melancholia.[10]

Beard's syndrome within three or four decades of its inception became a popular everyday household word and replaced hypochondriasis as the prevalent diagnostic label.   Subdivisions and divisions of these subdivisions appeared. There were congenital, acquired, cerebral, spinal, digestive, and sexual neurasthenia.   Traumatic neurasthenia followed a shock or injury and was referred to as "railway spine" or "railway brain" from the frequency with which it occurred during railroad accidents. In all types of neurasthenia, the subjective symptoms were numerous and varied but the objective signs were few and slight.[11]

Why did this disease become so prominent an entity? The first explanation of it as a natural consequence of the eighteenth century rational and mechanistic "scientific" philosophy was not enough. Beard interpreted neurasthenia as a disease of civilization related to industrialization. Beard's view of neurasthenia reflected a theory of man in an urban setting. As industrialization evolved, a new type of individual came into existence—"the brain worker"—who found himself subject to nervous diseases: the brain worker suffered from neurasthenia, not the housewife, peasant, laborer, or the black. This rationalization for the etiology of the disease supported an interpretation of evolutionary theory in which the upper and middle white collar classes were superior to all other classes. The "American disease" became a badge of honor. To suffer from neurasthenia meant one was higher in the evolutionary scale. Beard looked upon the blacks and the Indians of North and South America as just immature children living by their senses and emotions, incapable of coping with the problems of complex civilized society.[12]

As for nervous exhaustion in white women, physicians at that time were divided into two opposing factions: those who claimed that white women had allowed their lives to become too much of a dull habit and others who claimed that nervous exhaustion in white women resulted from woman's natural inferiority in attempting the work and duties of men. Women, like the "inferior races," were damned no matter what they did. Nevertheless, Jane Addams (1860-1935)— an American social worker, humanitarian, founder of Hull House, and Nobel Peace Prize winner—was a neurasthenic who gave the impression that it was a distinction to have this disease and that society thought her a better woman for it. But she also remarked that newly emancipated women, by giving up the life that their grandmothers and great-grandmothers led, paid too high a price.[13]

Neurasthenia, Beard and his successors postulated, resulted from factors other than the complexities of advanced civilizations exhausting the vitality of inherited nerve cells by depleting their stored nutriment. Beard stated that:

> The greater prevalence of nervousness in America is a complex resultant of a number of influences, the chief of which are dryness of the air, extremes of heat and cold, civil and religious liberty, and the great mental activity made necessary and possible in a new and productive country under such climatic conditions.[14]

Beard thought that dephosphorization of central nervous system cells caused neurasthenia. S. Weir Mitchell thought that neurasthenia was caused by the depletion of lipoids in the brain and developed the rest cure treatment as a means of restoring the lost substance.[15] Neurasthenia was also attributed to infection, toxins, poor nutrition, hormone imbalances and so forth. Neurasthenia, therefore, from its very beginning was viewed as a holistic disease with constitutional, physical, psychological, social, and environmental components.[16]

By 1913, Dejerine and Gauckler maintained that neurasthenia was not a neurosis but rather a psychoneurosis. They summed up the two prevalent organic theories of their day—the theory of intoxication and autointoxication, and the theory of exhaustion—and concluded that the evidence for both theories or a combination of these theories was inadequate to account for the reality of the clinical facts. In refuting the exhaustion hypothesis they said:

> First of all, in the etiology of neurasthenia, it is the role of physical, intellectual, or moral overwork which has probably been the important starting-point of this conception. Now, this role seems to us doubtful, at least. Overwork in itself has never created neurasthenic conditions . . . . This is because when one is overworked there is generally some special reason for it . . . . As one of us had already written in 1886, 'It is brain work doubled by worry and anxiety which creates neurasthenia.' In one case it may be the future which comes into play. There it is one's *amour propre*. In another case it is the family fortunes, the bread for one's children, that one is striving for. There is always added to overwork such psychological elements of preoccupation.[17]

They claim that in many neurasthenics no amount of rest will help or alleviate the condition and that neurasthenia is wholly caused by psychological factors. Emotion, to them, is the primary factor that causes the disease.[18]

Dejerine and Gauckler believed that the cause of neurasthenia was the association of emotion with overstrain, not the overstrain itself. In addition they believed that the emotional factor was constitutionally predisposed in such a way that the patient became preoccupied, not obsessed, with feelings. He took things to heart. With this predisposition, an entity developed in which a group of phenomena appeared that were the result of the patient's inability to adapt to some emotional cause. The phenomena that appeared might be psychic, somatic, visceral, or behavioral. They considered the disease as progressing through several stages as follows:

(1) Phenomena of simple emotional fatigue and psychic and physical disturbances in direct and immediate relation to emotional excitation.
(2) By reason of these disturbances, manifestations due to auto- and hetero-suggestion by deficient and disharmonic attitudes.
(3) After a greater or less length of time, symptoms of all kinds which are the immediate or remote results of functional troubles previously created.[19]

They spelled out a specific disease category, separated neurasthenia as a psychoneurosis, and differentiated it from hysteria, hypochondriasis, psychasthenia, cyclothymic constitution, depression, organic diseases with secondary psychological reactions, etc.   Besides, they attributed to neurasthenia a sub-conscious component, i.e., a subconscious memory of fatigue and autosuggestion of the memory of fatigue.[20]   This attempt at classification, although admirable, was still too broad a concept, and did not meet with general acceptance. The fact that Freud considered neurasthenia an actual neurosis and not psychoneurosis may be one of the reasons that the preceding classification was not widely accepted.   Another factor may be that Dejerine considered that the only true psychoneuroses were hysteria and neurasthenia.

Psychiatric nosology in the latter half of the nineteenth and early part of the twentieth centuries gave neurasthenia a very prominent position.   Since the term became so all-inclusive, refinements in terminology obviously had to be made. The French psychiatrists prepared the way for the change.   Bernheim introduced the term psychoneurosis.[21]   In 1893, Hecker first described anxiety neurosis.[22] In 1903, Janet coined the term "psychasthenia" to include phobias, anxiety, obsessions, compulsions, and certain types of depressions.   This stripped neurasthenia of some of its symptomatology; however, the term psychasthenia never really caught on and it is not used frequently today.   In 1895, Freud included anxiety, neurasthenia, and hypochondriasis as parts of the actual neurosis and separated actual neurosis from the psychoneurosis-conversion hysteria, anxiety hysteria (phobia), obsessions, and compulsions.   To Freud, symptoms of the actual neurosis had no meaning or significance for the mind and were the direct somatic consequences of sexual disturbances.[23]   Stekel and other psychoanalysts disagreed with Freud and thought that neurasthenic patients did have unconscious psychic conflicts.   Federn confirmed Freud and thought that the actual neuroses were all chronic disturbances of either the sexual discharge or else accumulations of undischarged sexual libido.   He writes:

Anxiety neurosis originates as a result of the detension of the sexual wave of satisfaction from the psyche.   The etiology of hypochondria is as yet not sufficiently clarified.   It is the narcissistic actual neurosis; considered from the libido-economic point of view, it rests upon an overcathexis of the bodily ego with narcissistic libido.[24]

Neurasthenia results when pregenital libido components prevent genital satisfaction.[25]   As noted in a previous chapter Kraepelin included depression as part of the manic-depressive synthesis and Meyerian terminology considers depression in several categories including meregasia (neurotic).   Neurasthenia was stripped to the symptoms of excessive fatigue and exhaustion.

Treatment for neurasthenic patients in the heyday of its popularity consisted of the use of different types of electrical gadgets.   The use of electrical gadgets was based on the notion of the positive relationship between electrical and nervous system energy.   Electrical appliances were applied to or into muscles, nerves, head, back of the neck, spine, stomach, liver, bowels, urethra, etc. Other treatments consisted of rest, isolation, psychotherapy, drugs (ergot, arsenic, caffeine, coca, zinc, chloral, strychnia, opium, mineral acids, cod liver oil, etc.), and many individual remedies. One such remedy consisted of macerated sheep brain and glycerine injected into the abdomen of the patient. Other treatments also were administered—some fanciful and some in accordance with the prevalent medical practices of that time.[26]

Various names were used to describe the somatic symptoms associated with autonomic nervous system activity. These include Da Costa's syndrome, effort syndrome, soldier's heart, war neurasthenia, irritable heart, vasomotor instability, vasomotor neurosis, cardiac neurosis, and cardiovascular reaction. Today these labels are synonymous with neurocirculatory asthenia.[27] Other names for neurasthenia include nerve exhaustion, tropical asthenia, and war neurosis. The term war neurosis, popularized during World War I, chiefly categorized soldiers and veterans rather than citizens, and the British Army trained physicians as neurasthenic experts.[28] How multiple were the aspects of neurasthenia!

CLASSIFICATION

While theoretical differences existed between what entities should be subsumed under neuroses or psychoneuroses, standard classifications were proposed. But these classifications made very little difference to what the leaders were writing and teaching. For instance, in 1935 so outstanding a textbook as *Diseases of the Nervous System* by Smith Ely Jelliffe and William A. White listed the classification[29] adopted by the American Psychiatric Association and published in the Standard Classified Nomenclature of Disease[30] in 1933 but did not use the Psychiatric Association's classification. The Psychiatric Association's classification used the term psychoneurosis and subsumed under that designation the following:

(1) Hysteria (anxiety hysteria, conversion hysteria and subgroups)
(2) Psychasthenia or compulsive states and subgroups
(3) Neurasthenia
(4) Hypochondriasis
(5) Reactive depression (simple situational reaction, others)
(6) Anxiety state
(7) Mixed psychoneurosis

Smith and White used the Freudian classification which had the divisions of Psychoneuroses and Actual Neuroses. Neurasthenia is one of the Actual Neuroses.[31] This was confusing and played havoc with psychiatrists attempting to communicate with each other not only about neurasthenia but other entities as well. Besides, statistical analysis was impossible.

Neurasthenia remained in the official classification until 1952 when, in the DSMI, it was removed from Psychoneurotic Disorders, and placed under Psychophysiologic Autonomic and Visceral Disorders. There neurasthenia was subsumed under Psychophysiologic nervous system reaction and called psychophysiologic asthenic reaction. DSMII (1968) subsumed Neurasthenic neurosis under Neuroses; Asthenic personality under Personality Disorders and Certain Nonpsychotic Mental Disorders; and neurocirculatory asthenia under Psychophysiologic cardiovascular disorder. The proposed DSMIII (March 30, 1977) makes no mention of the term neurasthenia.[32] With all the changes of and confusion over this term, it is understandable why its use in recent years has been very limited. But, within the limits of its present definition, it can become a useful term and concept.

ETIOLOGY

The definition of neurasthenia has changed from the term's inception to the present. Besides this, the definition varies from country to country. It is, therefore, impossible to get any comparative cross-cultural studies. In fact different investigators in the same country often differ in their diagnostic criteria of the entity. This leaves the basis for studying the causes of this disease at the level of testimonial reports; hardly, a solid basis for valid conclusions.[33] Yet, fatigue and fatigue states are common enough conditions that psychiatrists as well as all other persons concerned with these phenomena should give them serious consideration.

Laughlin, a contemporary psychiatrist, offers a classification and explanation for neurasthenia or fatigue states: fatigue (tiredness or weariness) results from either physical or mental exertion and when normal, is proportionate to the degree of expended effort; organic fatigue is the consequence of illness; and emotional fatigue results from psychic conflict. The distinguishing feature of the latter is that the degree of weariness or tiredness is out of proportion to the effort. Excessive psychic conflict causes fatigue.[34] Such reasoning implies that one has at his disposal a means of measuring either the amount of energy expended or the degree of fatigue. In truth, the only instrument of observation and evaluation is the patient who is complaining, and that certainly is not an objective evaluation. Furthermore, the notion of equivalency in the physical, mental, organic, and emotional types of fatigue is subjective, i.e., so much physical or mental activity will lead to so much fatigue in a certain individual at a specific time under certain circumstances. Fatigue is as qualitative a notion as the concept of energy and is not a purely quantitive phenomenon. Such an impediment forces the psychiatrist to search for other approaches to understanding and explaining normal fatigue and neurasthenia. The basic principles of multiple causation are as valid here as in all other forms of neuroses and should be applied without undue emphasis on one or another factor. Any fatigue state, including those in which a primary factor is a known organic illness, must include constitutional, psychological, and stress factors.

No scientific studies prove either a hereditary or an environmental basis for fatigue or neurasthenia yet it is known that some people tire more easily than others and a reflex may be fatigued by rapid and repeated stimulation.[35] Since the major site of fatigue in a reflex arc takes place at the synapse and the greatest number of synapses are in the brain and spinal cord the assumption of some thinkers is that the central nervous system is the principal organ of fatigue. Another assumption of these thinkers is that fatigue could be explained on the basis of stimuli—the more stimulation the more fatigue. Some behaviorists capitalizing on these notions would therefore claim that fatigue as well as all behavior could be explained in terms of environmental stimuli; thus denying the existence of an inner "will" within the tissues of the organism itself. Skinner says:

> The extension of the principle of the reflex to include behavior involving more and more of the organism was made only in the face of vigorous opposition. The reflex nature of the spinal animal was challenged by proponents of a "spinal will." The evidence they offered in support of a residual inner cause consisted of behavior which apparently could not be explained wholly in terms of stimuli . . . . As more and more of the behavior of the organism has come to be explained in terms of stimuli, the territory held by inner explanations has been reduced. The "will" has retreated up the spinal cord, through the lower and then the higher parts of the brain, and finally, with the conditioned reflex, has escaped through the front of the head. At each stage, some part of the control of the organism has passed from a hypothetical inner entity to the external environment.[36]

In contrast to this extreme position Herrick says:

> There are two components in what is commonly called fatigue . . . . One component is an objectively demonstrable impairment or exhaustion of the tissues, the other is a subjective feeling of tiredness. These are independent variables. There may be considerable impairment without the feeling of tiredness, and conversely one may feel very tired when there is no demonstrable impairment of any functions . . . . Both components ordinarily are present, but they should be separately investigated . . . . But, however the problem is studied, it is clear that fatigue results from bodily work of some kind, and it is the whole body that gets tired, not the muscles only, or the brain only, or a disembodied ego.[37]

The total pattern of behavior including both environmental stimuli and the state of the organism are involved in the appearance of fatigue and neurasthenia. Most important is the interrelationship between organism and environment.

Some laboratory studies comparing fatigued individuals with those who are not fatigued are of interest. Fatigued persons have a flat glucose tolerance test and the insulin tolerance test shows that after two hours the blood sugar level of normals returns to fasting levels while the fatigued person's blood sugar level is below the fasting level.[38] Investigators claim that neurasthenics do not perform as well under stress or exercise, have lower physical work capacity and demonstrate sympathicotonic EKG changes.[39] Musculoskeletal pain and tenderness, and fatigue resulted when patients were deprived of stage 4 (non-REM) sleep.[40] Undoubtedly these data suggest a biochemical, physiological, endocrine, metabolic basis for fatigue but there is no definitive proof.

Claims are made that associate neurasthenia with certain types of body habitus and personality. The physique usually associated with neurasthenia is the leptosome (asthenic) type of Kretschmer or the ectomorph of Sheldon. These types are tall, slender, thin-boned people with flaccid muscles, small heart, and infantile appearance. Although this association may be of interest, it is not proven; many psychiatrists deny that any such connection exists. Personality types that are associated with neurasthenia are asthenic, sensitive, and psychasthenic types. The asthenic personality embodies a lifelong, deeply ingrained pattern of easy fatigability, low energy level, lack of enthusiasm, marked incapacity for enjoyment, plus an oversensitivity to physical and emotional stress. European classification systems divide the insecure personality into two types, the sensitive and compulsive (anancastic, psychasthenic). The sensitive personality refers to persons of increased impressionability to all stimuli with little ability or capacity for discharge of their emotional tension. They tend to ruminate on the meaning of any experience and, being insecure, they are inclined to look upon themselves as the possible cause of all sorts of unfortunate occurrences. They possess a strict conscience and subsequently have conflicts over sex, ethics, and aggression. These individuals are sensitive to the feelings of others. Besides transient depressions, they develop ideas of reference and believe that others regard them askance. Although other physical and personality types are associated with neurasthenia these are the main ones.[41-43]

The relationship of tiredness or weariness to physical illness is well known. Practically all chronic illnesses and many acute diseases have fatigue as one of the complaints. Special attention should be paid to such diseases as myasthenia gravis, cerebral arteriosclerosis, renal failure, tuberculosis, hypothyroidism, adrenal insufficiency, diabetes mellitus, anemias, avitaminosis, viral disease, and so on. At times the physician places too much emphasis on these illnesses as a cause of fatigue and this can lead the patient in the direction of an exaggerated tiredness. The danger of suggestion is always present, and the physician should be on guard to avoid this pitfall. Conversely, claims are made that fatigue predisposes the individual to infectious illnesses, particularly poliomyelitis. Animal studies indicate that exercise before and after inoculation with poliovirus or pneumococcus results in increased rates of infection and death. Also, latent Salmonella infections appear to be activated by fatigue. Speculation exists that the mechanism of increased infection by fatigue is related to lactic acid or other metabolites.[44]

Confusion over the symptomatology of neurasthenia makes a psychoanalytic evaluation especially speculative. Freud's original explanation as a toxic effect from undischarged libido has been changed to include psychological dynamics. Today neurasthenia is explained as resulting from frustration of the sexual instinct, inhibition of aggression, a struggle over unconscious dependency needs, a reinforcement of repression, and other unresolved infantile conflicts. Neurasthenia is considered as having preoedipal roots. Analysts think that the fear of rejection which interferes with social relationships between those of the same sex has its basis in latent homosexuality. Guilt, hypochondria, and paranoid elaborations of the oedipal problem disrupt heterosexual relationships. Consequently, these individuals are left with a constricted social life.[45, 46]

Psychoanalysts who attempt to explain neurasthenia by relating personality types and ego psychology emphasize the tension that develops between the patient's ego ideal and his realistic ability. This is an experience that undermines self-esteem and might release the neurasthenic reaction. It is viewed as a moral defeat which leads to or results from feelings of shame and failure. Tiredness and weariness of the neurasthenic can reflect a lack of self-esteem, a feeling of insufficiency, and an inability to accomplish anything of value. But such patients also believe others recognize their ineffectual nature and think little of them, whereas in fact, they are often conscientious, dutiful, and respected. Their commitments to high ideals that they cannot reach create a cyclic conflict with chronic disappointment and eventual exhaustion. Perhaps one of their main problems is the inability to express overt aggression. It places these patients in a paradoxical situation. How can the aggressive, hostile individual be dutiful and self-sacrificing at the same time?[47]

Neurasthenia may be a stress-intolerance syndrome since it can occur following a trauma. Posttraumatic syndromes (railway spine, Da Costa's syndrome, tropical asthenia, war neurosis) are included in this category. To one author, posttraumatic syndromes refer not only to those personal stressors such as family, work, money, and personal relationships but also to adverse social condition stressors, such as war, periods of national instability, decreased group cohesion, and major disruptive social issues.[48] External stress is undoubtedly a factor in the etiology of neurasthenia. To consider adverse social conditions, however, as more of an etiological factor in neurasthenia than with other neuroses is a very imaginative speculation. This speculation is reminiscent of Beard's undue emphasis on industrialization as the prime cause of neurasthenia because it exhausted the nervous system by draining its energy like an electric current discharges a battery.

DIAGNOSIS

The core symptoms are clear enough—easy fatigability, chronic weakness, exhaustion, and genuine distress. "Typically" these patients are thin and under-weight, have poor muscle tone with slight tremors of the hands, eyelids and tongue, and suffer from either cold or flushed extremities. They are usually polite, sensitive, submissive, introspective, quiet, orderly, but can be restless, oversensitive to noise and light, and easily irritated by others. Neurasthenics tend to avoid being with people and live a solitary, carefully regulated life. They tediously exist on a low level of social adjustment and can become incapable of following a regular occupation. Any exertion is too great. They complain of overwhelming exhaustion and are distressed at their limited ability to function.

Although neurasthenics are constantly tired, they complain that they cannot sleep. Usually they awaken exhausted but feel less tired as the day progresses. However, they are always tired to some extent. They never admit to feeling vigorous, are easily distracted, cannot concentrate or sustain any prolonged mental or physical effort, lack will and are convinced that they suffer from poor memory. In addition, they complain of sexual disturbances, gastric dis-comfort, constipation, diarrhea, belching, abdominal cramps, chest pains, and generalized muscle aches and pains. With the least effort they may get short of breath, dizzy, faint, or be unable to walk. They are "weak." Occipital tension is common and may extend down the nape of the neck. These and other symptoms can be mixed with transient episodes of hypochondriacal, obsessional, or depersonalization symptoms. In sum, they may resemble a low grade anxiety neurosis with depressive features but the overall clinical manifestations present a fairly typical picture. To the neurasthenic, life is just one big drag.[49]

DIFFERENTIAL DIAGNOSIS

Neurasthenia is a neurosis which usually develops some time in the course of adult life, whereas the asthenic personality develops gradually from childhood and is deeply ingrained by adolescence. Both conditions are distinguished from psychophysiologic cardiovascular disorder (neurocirculatory asthenia) by a major emphasis on somatic symptoms such as shortness of breath, palpitations, and tachycardia after slight effort; chest pains; and coldness, sweating, or flushing of the skin. All three conditions present the major manifestations of neurasthenia.

Neurasthenia must be differentiated from organic illness, anxiety, and depression. Patients who complain of exhaustion and fatigue deserve a careful physical evaluation before making a diagnosis of neurasthenia. Besides the innumerable diseases that mimic neurasthenia, there are also many drugs which have tiredness or weariness as a side effect. Special attention should be paid to diuretics (such as mercurials and carbonic anhydrase inhibitors) which lower body potassium and sodium, to antihypertensives (reserpine) which deplete norepinephrine stores, and to central nervous system depressants (sedatives, tranquilizers, and hypnotics). Chronic anxiety neurotics have more spirit, are not as persistently tired, and complain more of nervousness than neurasthenics. Depression is very difficult to distinguish and at times only the past history of previous attacks and the precipitating events can be of help. In addition depressives have a better prognosis; neurasthenics have a persistent continuity in their clinical conditions that need to be differentiated.

Neurasthenia is also distinguished from other conditions. It is unlike hysteria in that neurasthenics are weary and show less evidence of secondary gain, i.e., the advantage the patient gains from sickness such as gifts, attention, and release from responsibility. This contrasts with the primary gain of illness, i.e., the reduction of tension or conflict. Hysterics are thought of as pretenders; neurasthenics as spiritless, lifeless, and grouches. Because of their conscientiousness and dutifulness the neurasthenics will sometimes be called obsessive compulsive neurotics but they usually are not as rigid as obsessives. Hypochondriacs have more preoccupation with organ disability, may not be of the same physique or personality type, and more often interweave and alternate with paranoia.[50] It is the total configuration that ultimately will determine the diagnosis.

COURSE AND PROGNOSIS

Neurasthenia is a chronic disease. Rarely is it seen in children or adolescents and it usually begins to make its appearance in adult life; although, the personality characteristics may be evident in childhood. The illness increases in incidence throughout middle life and into senescence when degenerative changes in the brain take place.[51]

As a rule the disease is a slowly progressive one with a gradual onset. Neurasthenia can, however, have an acute onset when it is associated with a traumatic event. But once started it usually progresses into a long-term, persistent chronic condition. In very severe cases the patient may become completely exhausted or may commit suicide. Such states of exhaustion insidiously lead to conditions in which the patient does not eat, sleep, or rest. This ultimately can lead to physical collapse and death, a rare occurrence.

TREATMENT

As with all conditions, treatment depends first on proper evaluation and diagnosis. Where neurasthenia is a secondary symptom, the primary condition should be dealt with first. In the chronic neurasthenic treatment depends on the patient's willingness and ability to change. The change involves both the personality and environmental stresses that contribute to the incapacity. Where possible it is important to remove the stressor since some cases are not accessible to psychotherapy. Some may be helped by amphetamines and antidepressive drugs; and in others, where desire is strong, a new life can be established by general rehabilitation and psychotherapy.

Restoration of energy may be accomplished through proper nourishment, rest, moderate exercise, sleep, and relaxation therapies. Certainly these old and reliable methods should be tried but they are, by themselves, usually not enough and psychotherapy is usually necessary. On this note, the words said almost 100 years ago by the father of the rest cure treatment, S. Weir Mitchell, seem appropriate. Referring to treatment of psychiatric patients, he said:

> The position of the physician who deals with this class of ailments, with the nervous and feeble, the painworn, the hysterical, is one of the utmost gravity. It demands the kindliest charity. It exacts the most temperate judgements. It requires active, good temper. Patience, firmness and discretion are among its necessities. Above all, the man who is to deal with such cases must carry with him that earnestness which wins confidence. None other can learn all that should be learned by a physician of the lives, habits and symptoms of the different people whose cases he has to treat. From the rack of sickness sad confessions come to him, more, indeed than he may care to hear. To confess, is, for mysterious reasons, most profoundly human, and in weak and nervous women this tendency is sometimes exaggerated to the actual distortion of facts. The priest hears the crime or folly of the hour, but to the physician are oftener told the long, sad tales of a whole life, its faraway mistakes, its failures, and its faults. None may be quite foreign to his purpose or his needs. The causes of breakdowns and nervous disaster, and consequent emotional disturbances and their bitter fruit, are often to be sought in the remote past. He may dislike the quest, but be cannot avoid it. If he be a student of character, it will have for him a personal interest as well as the relative value of its applicative side. The moral world of the sick-bed explains in a measure some of the things that are strange in daily life, and the man who does not know sick women does not know women.[52]

Multiple forms of treatment—psychotherapy, environmental readjustment, drugs, rest, exercise, proper nutrition, etc.—were and still are the best approach.

REFERENCES

1. Chatel, J.C. and Peele, R., The concept of neurasthenia. *Int. J. Psychiatry* 9:38–39 (1970–1971).
2. Chrzanowski, G., An obsolete diagnosis. *Int. J. Psychiatry* 9:54–56 (1970–1971).
3. James, W., The energies of men. *Phil. Rev.* 16(1):1–20 (1907).
4. Dejerine, J. and Gauckler, E., *The Psychoneuroses and Their Treatment by Psychotherapy,* 2nd English ed. (transl. by Jelliffe, S.E.).   Philadelphia: Lippincott, 1915, p. 216.
5. Beard, G.M., Neurasthenia or nervous exhaustion. *Boston Med. Surg. J.* 3:217–220 (1869).
6. Veith, I., English melancholy and American Nervousness. *Bull. Menninger Clinic* 32(5):311–317 (1968).
7. Beard, G.M., *American Nervousness: Its Causes and Consequences. A Supplement to Nervous Exhaustion (Neurasthenia),* reprint ed.   New York: Arno Press, 1972, p. 5.
8. Ibid., Preface, p. vi.
9. Ibid., pp. 7, 8.
10. Bunker, H.A., From Beard to Freud: A brief history of the concept of neurasthenia. *Med. Rev. of Reviews* 36:108–110 (1930).
11. McGrew, F.A., Overstimulation neurasthenia. *J. Amer. Med. Assoc.* 232(10):1076 (1975). (Reprinted from *J. Amer. Med. Assoc.* June 9, 1900, p. 1467.)
12. Haller, J.S., Neurasthenia: Medical profession and urban "blahs." *N.Y. State J. Med.* 1:2489–2497 (1970).
13. Haller, J.S., Neurasthenia: The medical profession and the "new women" of late nineteenth century. *N.Y. State J. Med.* 15:473–482 (1971).
14. Beard, G.M., *American Nervousness: Its Causes and Consequences. A Supplement to Nervous Exhaustion,* op. cit., p. vii.
15. Mitchell, S.W., The evolution of the rest-treatment. *J. Nerv. Ment. Dis.* 31:368–373 (1904).
16. Chatel, J.C. and Peele, R., A centennial review of neurasthenia. *Amer. J. Psychiatry* 126(10):1406–1407 (1970).
17. Dejerine, J. and Gauckler, E., op. cit., pp. 216–217.
18. Ibid., pp. 214–240.
19. Ibid., p. 256.
20. Ibid., pp. 241–262.
21. Noyes, A.P., *Modern Clinical Psychiatry,* 2nd ed.   Philadelphia: Saunders, 1939, pp. 334–335.
22. Brill, A.A., Diagnostic errors in neurasthenia. *Med. Rev. of Reviews* 36:125 (1930).
23. Freud, S., *A General Introduction to Psychoanalysis* (transl. by Riviere, J.).   New York: Garden City Publishing, 1943, pp. 336–339.
24. Federn, P., The neurasthenic core in hysteria. *Med. Rev. of Reviews* 36:140 (1930).
25. Ibid.
26. Haller, J.S., Neurasthenia: Medical profession and urban "blahs," op. cit., pp. 2494–2495.
27. Chatel, J.C. and Peele, R., A centennial review of neurasthenia. op. cit., p. 1406.
28. Berger, D.M., The return of neurasthenia. *Compr. Psychiatry* 14(6):557–558 (1973).
29. Jelliffe, S.E. and White, W.A., *Diseases of the Nervous System: A Text-Book of Neurology and Psychiatry,* 6th ed. thoroughly revised.   Philadelphia: Lea & Febiger, 1935, p. 896.

30. *Diagnostic and Statistical Manual: Mental Disorders.* Washington, D.C.: American Psychiatric Association, 1952, p. v.
31. Jelliffe, S.E. and White, W.A., op. cit., p. 18.
32. Provisional classification. Published as a looseleaf manual entitled *DSM-III Draft, 4/15/77.* DRAFT OF AXES I and II of DSM-III CLASSIFICATION as of March 30, 1977.
33. Chatel, J.C. and Peele, R., A centennial review of neurasthenia. op. cit., pp. 1405-1406.
34. Laughlin, H.P., *The Neuroses.* Washington, D.C.: Butterworths, 1967, pp. 381-384.
35. Skinner, B.F., *Science and Human Behavior.* New York: The Free Press, 1965, p. 48.
36. Ibid., pp. 48-49.
37. Herrick, C.J., *The Evolution of Human Nature.* New York: Harper Torchbooks, 1961, p. 281.
38. Laughlin, H.P., op. cit., pp. 418-419.
39. Taylor, M.A., Letters to the Editor. *Amer. J. Psychiatry* 127(3):390 (1970).
40. Moldofsky, H. and Scarisbrick, P., Induction of neurasthenic musculoskeletal pain syndrome by selective sleep stage deprivation. *Psychosom. Med.* 38(1):35-44 (1976).
41. Slater, E. and Roth, M., *Clinical Psychiatry,* 3rd ed. Baltimore: Williams & Wilkins, 1969. p. 83.
42. Nyström, S. and Lindegård, B., Predisposition for mental syndromes: A study comparing predisposition for depression, neurasthenia, and anxiety state. *Acta. Psychiat. Scand.* 51(2):69-76 (1975).
43. Kuiper, P.C., *The Neuroses: A Psychoanalytic Survey.* New York: International Universities Press, 1972, pp. 169-170.
44. Utz, J.P., "Factors predisposing to infectious disease," in *Pathologic Physiology: Mechanisms of Disease,* 4th ed. (edited by Sodeman, W.A. and Sodeman, Jr., W.A.). Philadelphia: Saunders, 1968, p. 208.
45. Chrzanowski, G., "Neurasthenia and hypochondriasis," in *American Handbook of Psychiatry,* vol. 1 (edited by Arieti, S.). New York: Basic Books, 1965, pp. 261-263.
46. Kuiper, P.C., op. cit., pp. 170-171.
47. Ibid., pp. 167-173.
48. Berger, D., op. cit., pp. 559-562.
49. Anderson, E.W. and Trethowan, W.H., *Psychiatry,* 3rd ed. Baltimore: Williams & Wilkins, 1973, p. 210.
50. Kuiper, P.C., op. cit., pp. 165-170.
51. Slater, E. and Roth, M., op. cit., p. 84.
52. Mitchell, S.W., *Doctor and Patient.* Philadelphia: Lippincott, 1887, pp. 9-10.

10
DEPERSONALIZATION NEUROSIS

Depersonalization is a complex phenomenon with so many components that even defining it is difficult. Different investigators emphasize different groups of phenomena. In fact, it not only eludes accurate definition by psychiatrists, but even patients are unable to accurately describe and communicate what is disturbing them. In no single patient, however, are all the possible symptoms of depersonalization ever found. Therefore, definition must be based on the presence of certain leading features.[1]

Depersonalization is a condition in which a patient notices some change in his consciousness. An alteration in consciousness can be manifested in innumerable ways. To name some, there are changes in: (1) sensory characteristics of the external world (seeing glowing lights at the edge of things); (2) perception of the body image (change in size and shape), of physiological parameters (increased or decreased heart rate, respiration, muscle tone), of special bodily feelings not normally present (energy either overall or localized as in the spine); (3) emotion (not reacting, overreacting, underreacting, or reacting in a different way); (4) memory (incongruities between present and past experiences); (5) time sense (moving slower or faster); (6) sense of identity (alienation, detachment, unusual role); (7) evaluation of cognition (rate, sharpness, clarity, logic); (8) motor activity (quantity or quality of self-control, restlessness, tremors); and (9) interaction with environment (consensual validation or lack of it, voice quality, orientation to or contact with environment).[2] There are other changes that can take place in consciousness but these are enough to render some idea why such divergence exists in defining this entity.

Ackner posits the following definition:

> The leading features, then, are a subjective feeling of internal and/or external change, experienced as one of strangeness or unreality; an unpleasant or even highly distressing quality to the experience; the retention of insight and lack of delusional elaboration of the experience; and an

affective disturbance characterized often by the complaint of loss of affective responsiveness.[3]

These features, although without clear boundaries, do delineate a disease entity within a holistic framework.

Further clarification of this definition is necessary and each feature needs detailed consideration.

(1) Patients often describe their inner and outer worlds during a depersonalization experience as being dead, unfamiliar, strange, detached, and so forth. They often do not use the word unreal. Psychiatrists may apply the label "feelings of unreality" to describe a patient's depersonalization experience. Actually what the patient is describing is a change in his awareness which he recognizes as not belonging to his normal experience. In another patient this may be within his normal range of experience, not abnormal, and even within the same patient at different times it may be viewed as a normal occurrence. It is therefore up to the psychiatrist to determine the nature of the experience and to apply "unreality" as a generic term for purposes of definition.

(2) Reactions to symptoms vary and an unpleasant quality, especially fear of dying and insanity, is a common feature of the depersonalization experience. The degree of unpleasantness varies from person to person and attack to attack. One patient may feel restful or peaceful, another uncomfortable, and yet a third may become anxious, fearful, or depressed. Unpleasantness, although often present, is not always present, therefore, this feature is not an absolute essential for defining the entity.

(3) Patients with depersonalization do not suffer from delusions. Since perceptual and thought disturbances of the body, self, and the outer world are involved it becomes incumbent upon the psychiatrist to differentiate among illusions, hallucinations, delusions of somatic depersonalization, and hypochondriacal delusions. In depersonalization the patient retains insight into his condition. In patients with schizophrenia, depression, or organic brain syndromes perceptual and thought disturbances can fluctuate but are usually not recognized as abnormal by the patient. Boundaries may not be sharp between depersonalization and these other conditions and borderline cases are often found. It seems proper, therefore, to exclude all cases with a delusional quality from depersonalization neuroses.

(4) Patients with depersonalization complain that they lose their ability to feel and yet *feel* distressed at this inability. A paradox exists. Psychiatrists should not be disturbed by this paradox since normally people are capable of living with two or more contradictory feelings or thoughts without apparent disturbances. In addition, a loss of feelings does not have to be complete, i.e., present in all areas of existence. The fact remains that a change in feelings in one area of psychic functioning does not negate the possibility that feelings

are present in other areas. This is so, even though, the patient says "I lost my feelings for everything." Besides feelings of unreality involve, at least in part, a disturbance of affect.

The criteria that must be fulfilled by all patients suffering from depersonalization neuroses include a change in the way reality is experienced and an affective disturbance. It excludes delusions and may or may not include the presence of unpleasantness. Within these limits a definite disease entity is defined which has biopsychosocial components.[4]

Many terms characterize the various aspects of this disease. Derealization describes external changes: the environment may appear like a two-dimensional stage set, color changes; objects may appear smaller or larger, closer or farther away, cloudy or dreamlike. Sounds may be exaggerated—running water from a faucet sounds like a waterfall. Desomatization describes bodily changes in which the individual or his parts seem enormous, tiny, detached, hollow, without sensation, or deformed. Deaffectualization describes a lost capacity to feel so that the individual is unable to love, hate, cry, laugh, or worry. Perceptual cognitive aberrations may occur. The patient thinks he is weightless, believes he can float or fly without assistance, and can lose a sense of time. Such individuals may confuse past, present, or future. Time seems speeded up or slowed down and present action seems to occur simultaneously in the past or future. *Déjà vu* describes a subjective sensation in which an experience which is actually happening for the first time seems to have occurred on a previous occasion. Depersonification describes the individual who perceives himself as somebody other than what in fact he is, viz., a distortion of identity or self. He thinks that he is no longer himself, or even that his voice does not belong to him. He is different, strange, or to varying degrees, someone else. Although these terms spell out some particular area of pathology, depersonalization is used here to cover all of the above conditions.[5]

Normal persons may have transient episodes of depersonalization symptoms, lasting from seconds to hours, but these episodes are not considered as prodromal to either depersonalization neuroses or any other psychiatric illnesses. These transient episodes, however, can become persistent but usually do not. If symptoms persist a neurosis may be present. In normals, the symptoms occur most frequently under conditions of fatigue, drug intoxication, or hypnagogic state, appearing with the same frequency in either sex and between the ages of 12-35. The incidence approximates one-third to one-half of the normal individuals in this age group.[6]

HISTORY

Depersonalization was delineated as a mental illness in the nineteenth century. Johann Christian Reil (1759-1813) and Esquirol described cases of depersonalization.[7, 8] Following these early descriptions, interest in the disease did not reappear until the latter half of the nineteenth century. The interest centered around its definition, classification, and etiology. Different writers stressed different aspects of the phenomenon. Taine (1870), Krishaber (1872), and Ribot (1882) attributed it to a disturbance in sense perception. Krishaber described a syndrome characterized by a loss of sense of external or internal reality and the feeling that the world was a dream. He classified it under cerebrocardiac neurosis. In 1898 Dugas coined the term "depersonalization." Janet (1903) considered hyperactivity of memory, narrowed consciousness, fatigue, and constitution as the major etiological factors. Pick (1904), Oesterreich (1910), and Loewy (1908) stressed emotional disorder as the essential element. No agreement existed regarding definition, etiology, and even whether or not depersonalization was an independent entity or a secondary symptom of other illnesses, especially manic-depressive psychoses.[9-11]

In 1914 Paul Schilder wrote a paper in which he separated depersonalization from all other psychiatric conditions and described it as a state in which the person experiences a change in self and outer world. He thought it was due to a shift of the libido, an increase in self-observation, and a disturbance of body image. In 1935 Mayer-Gross adapted Mapother's term derealization which referred to the changes in the environment and retained depersonalization for changes of the self. Mayer-Gross thought that depersonalization was not an independent entity but rather a nonspecific syndrome that occurred with other illnesses. He viewed the whole syndrome as a preformed functional response of the brain. Mayer-Gross thought that depersonalization was a characteristic built-in brain reaction that could be triggered by many causes.[12] The controversy over definition, classification, and etiology continues to this day.

CLASSIFICATION

With so little agreement regarding the nature of depersonalization it should come as no surprise that the DSMI (1952) merely considered it as a symptom of Dissociative Reaction. But in 1968 the DSMII listed Depersonalization Neurosis under Neuroses. Here the term becomes all-inclusive and does not separate such forms as derealization, desomatization, etc. The draft (March 30, 1977) of the DSMIII subsumes Depersonalization under Dissociative Disorders.[13]

ETIOLOGY

Since most studies dealt with depersonalization as a phenomenon in association either with normal subjects, medical illnesses, or other psychiatric conditions and not simply with the depersonalization disease entity, it is assumed that whatever applies to depersonalization as an experience is also valid for depersonalization as a neurosis. The prevalent theories conceptualize depersonalization along organic, psychological, psychoanalytic lines, or as a form of schizophrenia.

There is no evidence of a hereditary basis for this entity. But, as noted, Mayer-Gross thought that the organization of the brain itself accounted for this phenomenon. He followed the work of Hughlings Jackson (1835-1911) who in 1884, applying Darwinian principles, considered nervous system diseases as a reversal of the evolutionary process. Jackson called this reversal dissolution. He thought mental symptoms resulted from disturbances of brain function by removing (dissolution) the higher levels of cerebral functioning. Higher levels exert an inhibiting or controlling influence over the lower levels. To Jackson, the central nervous system was seen as a hierarchy of interacting levels of organization. He defined these levels in functional or physiological rather than anatomical terms. The lowest levels (the spinal cord and brain stem) were the most automatic, least voluntary; the highest levels (anterior and posterior association areas of the cerebrum) were the least fixed, most complex, and least committed to one or only a few special and predetermined functions; the intermediate levels (motor and sensory cortical areas and several subcortical areas) were somewhere between the other two levels in regard to being fixed, automatic, and organized. Jackson's conception of organic brain disease, representing a retreat from higher to lower levels of performance, led to the doctrine of the duality of symptoms. When dissolution occurred the symptoms presented two aspects: positive mental symptoms which showed the amount of remaining mental capacity and which resulted from a release of the lower level functioning; negative mental symptoms which showed what was lost and resulted from the higher level of functioning.[14]

Transient depersonalization experiences are not uncommon in normal persons in states of fatigue, ill health, hypnagogic period, toxic conditions, sleep and sensory deprivation, or under the influence of hallucinogenic drugs. These observations led some to modify the organic hypothesis of Mayer-Gross and to postulate that an alteration of consciousness is the common factor necessary for the appearance of the depersonalization. Changes in consciousness occur during any 24 hour period. The continuum from full awareness through tiredness, hypnagogic state, sleep, dreaming, hypnopompic period, and return to full awareness happens daily. Depersonalization may occur during any phase of the sleep-wakefulness cycle and an alteration of consciousness should refer to deviation from full awareness but is often used synonymously with clouding of consciousness. Fatigue, sleep and sensory deprivation, or psychotomimetic drugs (LSD, mescaline, etc.) induce a clouding of consciousness similar to the hypnagogic state. Pathologic conditions (encephalitis, epilepsy, toxins, traumatic head injuries, space occupying brain diseases—tumors, abscesses, hemorrhages, metabolic disturbances, cerebral arteriosclerosis, etc.) may or may not induce either a clouding of consciousness or depersonalization. The incidence, however, of depersonalization with pathological conditions is amazingly not high. Depersonalization occurs without an apparent alteration of consciousness in the normal as well as in persons with affective illnesses. Also a large number of individuals never suffer from depersonalization irrespective of the circumstances. Clouding of consciousness as a precondition for the appearance of depersonalization, therefore, does not appear to be essential.[15] Sedman summed up the data as follows:

> These facts seem to indicate: (a) that there may be a 'built in' or 'preformed' mechanism in approximately 40 per cent of the population to exhibit depersonalization; (b) that the factors which initiate such a response are not specifically those associated with clouding of consciousness; or (c) where clouding of consciousness appears to be playing a part it may well be the presence of another common factor that is more relevant.[16]

Yet the relationship between clouding of consciousness and depersonalization cannot be entirely disregarded.[17]

In normal development, breadth and depth of experiences increase from infancy to maturity. Even with advancing age the individual is constantly changing. Changes are taking place within the brain and total biological organism as well as in levels of conscious awareness and in the development of self-concept. Alterations of consciousness, not necessarily clouding of consciousness, take place.

In this sense, an alteration of consciousness can be a precondition for depersonalization. Each person would be in a constant state of depersonalization but to such a small degree that it is not apparent to himself. Depersonalization with its subsequent reintegration can be viewed as essential for growth. New equilibriums are constantly being established. This process may be the mechanism by which the conscious self is capable of being in contact with its deepest being and the external world or else, if it fails, being alienated from both. Therefore, the organic hypothesis, which holds that an alteration of consciousness is an essential ingredient for the depersonalization phenomena, could just as well claim that concepts of self are equally dependent on alterations of consciousness. This then suggests that the status of self ultimately depends upon the state of organic or biological substrata. It establishes the importance of the relationships among internal and external stimuli, the experiential self, and brain structure . This is a holistic hypothesis.

In sum, the difficulty in proving the holistic hypothesis may be partially due to the insensitivity of present methods of psychological testing as well as the undue emphasis placed on clouding of consciousness as the necessary alteration. Resorting to concepts such as organic substrata being responsible for a lowered self-awareness are metaphysical and vague yet they do offer clues to understanding depersonalization. Certain criteria support the organic hypothesis. Over one-third of the population experiences transient depersonalization at sometime in their lives; attacks last anywhere from seconds to months; attacks increase with increasing age, and psychiatrists and patients are unable to find words to adequately describe the condition.

The personality factor is controversial. Personality types reported include: introverted, anxious, obsessional, and cyclothymic.[18, 19]   In studying the personality of depressed, anxious, and depersonalized individuals one investigator could not demonstrate any personality differences among any of these three groups.[20]   Yet it appears that many investigators posit an association between obsessive compulsive personality and depersonalization.[21]

Psychological theories as noted relate depersonalization to perceptual, memory, thought, and emotional disturbances as well as distortions of the body image. Those theories follow the general scheme of faculty psychology and place emphasis on a particular "function of the mind" as not performing properly. This assumption is unacceptable. Man cannot be broken into his parts and must be viewed not from an isolated part position but from the total structure in an environment position. One attempt to relate these various components of mind starts with depersonalization as an impairment in perceptual development. This impairment limits the patient's ability to develop appropriate emotional responses which in turn leads to disturbances in thinking and other faculties such as memory, judgment, will, etc. Selecting from various subtypes of depersonalization, derealization (dr) is chosen as the model and most unambiguous type. Further, it is thought that the patient interprets perceptions according to a preconceived self-image.[22] This is explained by Roberts who attempted to integrate the faculties as follows:

'Emotion' is a substantive derived from many adjectives used to denote a state of mind. It does not exist as an entity, any more than a word coined from the adjectives used to describe states of matter would label an entity. A particular emotion is said to be present as and when the mind alters its state, and to persist until this state alters. If the mind alters its state upon perception of an object, sentimental emotion is said to exist. A two-way traffic is felt to be present in such a case. The object is said to evoke feeling in the perceiver, and feeling is considered to flow towards or into the object. It is this sense of flow to the object which has probably led to the belief that emotion directly effects perception. The author now suggests that (if his account of perceptual development is correct) sentimental emotion must necessarily depend upon the presence in the precept of a representation of the observer. Or, in other words, that in dr, where this component of perception is lacking, sentimental emotion must fail.[23]

This viewpoint conflicts with others which consider emotions, especially those connected with anxiety, depression, and phobia, as the most important factor and starting point of depersonalization.[24]

Several points regarding emotions and depersonalization are important. First, it is thought by some that feelings attune individuals to the actual circumstance of their lives and that interest is a necessary precondition to interpret reality properly. In depersonalization both emotion and interest are not in adequate balance; hence, reality is misinterpreted.[25] Of course, one should not confuse this with the fact that one can entertain "right" or "wrong" feelings about a situation dependent on judgment and sensitivity, not on interest or emotional state. Second, in agoraphobics who suffer from a high anxiety level, the onset of depersonalization can be quite abrupt. An interesting example of a sudden onset occurred with a patient during the galvanic skin response test. The patient complained for some minutes of severe anxiety and suddenly changed the complaint to one of feeling strange and unreal. It was noted that at the point the strange and unreal feelings appeared (depersonalization) the GSR tracing displayed a more relaxed pattern. This phenomenon led to speculation that sometimes depersonalization is a switch or cutoff mechanism which is triggered when anxiety reaches a critical level.[26] Yet other studies fail to support any important association of anxiety with depersonalization but do in fact find that depression is an important concomitant of depersonalization states.[27] Still a more recent study views the patient who depersonalizes as one with chronic anxiety, depression, and a thinking disturbance.[28] The issue is far from settled. Third, phobic anxiety-depersonalization syndrome is proposed as a well-defined entity that occurs under stress and follows a predictable course and outcome. It begins with symptoms of acute anxiety, progresses to a phobic stage in which fear of loss of control or insanity and agoraphobic symptoms predominate and finally reaches a third stage when depersonalization symptoms appear.[29, 30] Whether or not such a definitive entity can be distinguished is debatable. In addition to being associated with calamitous stressful circumstances, depersonalization is thought, by some, to be associated with an alteration of consciousness and temporal lobe disturbance.[31, 32] Marks stated:

> There is no doubt that depersonalization does occur in temporal lobe disturbances, but it would be premature to conclude that agoraphobics with depersonalization have temporal lobe dysfunction. It is also important to note that many agoraphobics do not experience any depersonalization at all. As with depression, the two groups of symptoms are often found together and often are totally separate.[33]

Some consider depersonalization as either a form or precursor of schizophrenia. While it is true that certain schizophrenic disturbances do resemble depersonalization, there are distinctions which can be clinically discerned. Yet many schizophrenics do have depersonalization symptoms. This should not lead to the assumption that depersonalization is anything but an associated phenomenon.[34, 35]

Psychoanalytic hypotheses vary and there is no commonly accepted position. Some psychoanalytic interpretations of depersonalization consider it a shift of libidinal cathexis, primarily a withdrawal of object libido in response to narcissistic wounds. Others view the mechanisms involved as a splitting of the ego, a perceptual problem, or a hysterical phenomenon. Still others deem depersonalization as a regression to the oral phase of development, a withdrawal of cathexis from object and ego, or as a defense against aggressive drives. The lack of clear definitions and of agreement in terminology results in one author's work bearing very little relation to another's; so it becomes questionable whether psychoanalysis has helped our understanding of depersonalization.[36–38]

Stress, internal or external, is a definite factor in precipitating this disease. Excessive physical or mental activity can evoke an attack, usually one of short duration. Acute or crisis situations (death in a family, childbirth, marriage, war, threats to one's life, fainting, automobile accidents, surgery) can provoke a depersonalization experience as can chronic circumstances (pressure on a job, difficulties with personal relations, financial troubles). In life-threatening situations that suddenly appear, the response may be adaptive. During acute situations many persons perform mental and physical feats that under normal conditions they would be incapable of doing. By depersonalizing the person is protected from disorganizing fear that one would expect as a response to life-threatening dangerous circumstances.[39]

DIAGNOSIS

Certain poets, novelists, and mystics who are gifted with a special talent for describing their experiences offer vivid examples of depersonalization. Jean-Paul Sartre writes:

M. de Rollebon was my partner; he needed me in order to exist and I needed him so as not to feel my existence. I furnished the raw material, the material I had to re-sell, which I didn't know what to do with: existence, my existence. His part was to have an imposing appearance. He stood in front of me, took up my life to *lay bare* his own to me. I did not notice that I existed any more, I no longer existed in myself, but in him; I ate for him, breathed for him, each of my movements had its sense outside, there, just in front of me, in him; I no longer saw my hand writing letters on the paper, not even the sentence I had written—but behind, beyond the paper, I saw the Marquis who had claimed the gesture as his own, the gesture which prolonged, consolidated his existence. I was only a means of making him live, he was my reason for living, he had delivered me from myself. What shall I do now?[40]

and William Wordsworth (1770-1850) wrote:

There was a time when meadow, grove,
  and stream,
The earth, and every common sight,
  To me did seem
  Apparelled in celestial light,
The glory and the freshness of a dream.

It is not now as it hath been of yore;
  Turn wheresoe'er I may,
    By night or day,
The things which I have seen I now can
  see no more.[41]

These two examples should convey a sense of what the clinical picture is in depersonalization.

The patient feels that his personality is lost. Sartre expressed this loss as nonexistence. The "me" is not involved in the events of the patient's daily life and he cannot make or has lost contact with his own self (essence?). In contrast to Sartre who finds his own existence so unpleasant, the patient finds this quality of estrangement from or unfamiliarity with self, fearful and uncomfortable. The patient doubts his identity. He, like Wordsworth, searches for the old self. He desires to return to what was, to a knowledge of his feelings, his self, his body, and his environment. The contrast between Sartre's searching to lose self in some other person or thing, and Wordsworth yearning to gain a self he lost, fairly well covers the spectrum that depersonalized patients feel when they observe a sense of change within the self.

This illness can take many forms. The depersonalized patient appears unfamiliar to himself when viewing his image in a mirror, feels a sense of nonrecognition when hearing his name spoken, fears a sudden failure of memory will result in a lapse into blankness and a total loss of identity. He fears insanity. He can have feelings of floating in space and of blunted sensations anywhere in or over the body. This leads some patients to touch, punch, or prick themselves repeatedly in an attempt to "feel real." The experience can be similar to a dream from which the patient cannot awaken. It is as if whatever is happening has no connection to him and he seems like a puppet to himself. It is a weird and uncanny experience.

One should not underestimate how distressed these patients feel. They know what they are supposed to feel but do not feel it. They do not derive pleasure

from what they want to enjoy. Success in business, school, or social relationships brings no gratification only the recognition of their inability to enjoy their
own accomplishments. Even sexual intercourse can be accomplished without
any feeling towards the act but a reaction to this lack of feeling. Most of these
patients suffer, and this they do feel.

Depersonalization is seen in immature adolescents. They have difficulty
in establishing personal relationships and experience an abnormal degree of
self-absorption, withdraw into fantasy and ruminate about fate, time, and
death. Such cases of depersonalization neurosis, though relatively rare, are
not secondary to other psychiatric disorders. But when they do occur, they can
last for long periods of time. Previously, there may have been fleeting attacks of
unreality but the illness is generally of abrupt onset.[42]

There is a folk illness found in Indonesia, Malay, and Southern China known as
"Koro." In this illness there are two elements: (1) the experience that the penis is
shrinking and (2) interpretation of this experience that the penis subsequently disappears into the abdomen and the person dies. The Koro depersonalization
syndrome involves a subjective experience of penile shrinkage usually in association with acute anxiety. Only in the folk illness is there fear that the penis will
retract into the abdomen and this distinguishes it from Koro depersonalization
syndrome which is found throughout the world.[43]

DIFFERENTIAL DIAGNOSIS

Depersonalization in most patients is found in association with other illnesses and
the biggest problem can be to determine which is primary and which secondary.
This is especially important since depersonalization can be an early stage in the development of any other neuroses or psychoses, and in many organic conditions. It
is, however, practically absent in paranoia and rare in children and senile states. In
normals it occurs quite commonly. When depersonalization symptoms are predominant and presenting, the patient is suffering from primary depersonalization.[44]

Depersonalization can easily be missed since many patients do not tell their
physicians about these symptoms for fear of being considered insane. Instead
they present themselves complaining of anxiety, phobic, and depressive
symptoms which are a response to the depersonalization experience and not
primary. Usually these patients complain of one or more somatic symptoms—
headaches, giddiness, palpitations, stomach ache, backache, and so on. Only a
careful examination will aid the physician in discerning which disease is primary.

Recurrent attacks of depersonalization occur in obsessive compulsive, and
hypochondriacal neuroses. These attacks usually appear at the peak of intense
somatization, rumination, or ritualistic behavior and disappear as the intensity of
these symptoms decreases. A similar relationship exists between recurrent attacks
of depersonalization and other neuroses as well as psychoses.

Hysterical neurotics may resemble depersonalization neurotics in personality, age distribution, and complaints regarding feelings. In addition, they too may suffer from anxiety, phobia, and depression. The total picture of the two neuroses must be evaluated and the prominent features discerned. Neurasthenics only pose a problem when they depersonalize but the major symptom picture and the course of the illness (neurasthenics are chronically and persistently tired) will distinguish the two conditions.

Drug intoxications, temporal lobe epilepsy, and other organic conditions can precipitate an acute transient depersonalization reaction. A careful examination plus laboratory tests (blood, urine, EEG, brain scan) will differentiate these conditions.[45] Physicians should be aware that depersonalization can occur in those who practice meditative techniques. Since the number of people joining "consciousness movement" organizations is increasing, it should be expected that more patients will be referred.[46]

A serious risk is that depersonalization may be mistaken for one of the more malignant illnesses or vice versa. Patients may say, "I am not alive" or "I don't have any eyes or body." Such statements can be attributed to a patient with psychotic depression as well as to the depersonalized patient and careful differential diagnosis is necessary. Insight is lacking in delusional patients. When depression is relieved the depersonalization disappears. Similarly, a loss of affect or looseness of associations, or feelings that all actions are automatic, may suggest schizophrenia. But the patient who prefaces his thoughts, feelings, and behavior by an "as if" is more likely to be suffering from depersonalization than schizophrenia or depression. Depersonalization in schizophrenia, is usually fleeting in character, especially when it occurs as a precursor to an overt schizophrenic psychosis. A careful examination of the patient will reveal some of the symptoms of schizophrenia: an affective incongruity, autism, defect in association, marked ambivalence, and peculiar attitude and behavior.

COURSE AND PROGNOSIS

Depersonalization often appears suddenly, without any warning, or any apparent precipitating event. It may last for seconds or minutes, disappear for a short period, only to return again and persist for months or even years. The initial experience can terrify the patient and bring him to the doctor in acute panic. More often, however, unpleasantness occurs, not panic.

Prognosis with depersonalization secondary to other conditions varies with the primary disease. In primary depersonalization the prognosis is variable. Some patients have recurrent attacks and these cycles continue for years, others have one attack that lasts from minutes to months, clears up and never returns, and so on.

TREATMENT

Many patients find relief simply in knowing that this strange but common experience is familiar to the doctor. Reassurance may be all that is required. In other patients the treatment is directed toward the underlying psychiatric disorder. When symptoms of depersonalization are secondary to some other psychiatric disorder, treatment is given for the primary illness. In depersonalization neurosis treatments vary. Psychotherapy, from supportive to psychodynamic exploration and working through, may be indicated. The avoidance of precipitating factors such as fatigue, anxiety, or drugs may be helpful. A wide variety of treatment methods including EST, continuous narcosis, dexedrine, vasodilators, ether abrication, behavior modification, modified insulin therapy, and leucotomy have met with mixed results. Attempts to treat with tranquilizers have not been successful and phenothiazine may even increase depersonalization. Intravenous amphetamines and antidepressives are considered the drugs of choice. Unfortunately, usable data are scarce. The final word on treatment of this neurosis has yet to come.[47, 48]

REFERENCES

1. Lewis, A.J., Melancholia: A clinical survey of depressive states. *J. Mental Sci.* 80:330–337 (1934).
2. Tart, C.T., *States of Consciousness.* New York: Dutton, 1975, pp. 12–13.
3. Ackner, B., Depersonalization: 1. Aetiology and phenomenology. *J. Mental Sci.* 100:845 (1954).
4. Ackner, B., op. cit., pp. 841–853.
5. Editorial, Depersonalization syndromes. *Brit. Med. J.* 4:378 (1972).
6. Roberts, W.W., Normal and abnormal depersonalization. *J. Mental Sci.* 106:478–485 (1960).
7. Zilboorg, G., *A History of Medical Psychology.* New York: Norton, 1941, p. 288.
8. Lewis, A.J., op. cit., p. 334.
9. Ibid., pp. 334–336.
10. Shorvon, H.J., The depersonalization syndrome. *Proc. Roy. Soc. Med.* 39:779 (1946).
11. Sedman, G., An investigation of certain factors concerned in the aetiology of depersonalization. *Acta. Psychiat. Scand.* 48:191 (1972).
12. Mayer-Gross, W., On depersonalization. *Brit. J. Med. Psychol.* 15:103–126 (1935).
13. Provisional classification: Published as a looseleaf manual entitled *DSM-III Draft, 4/15/77.* DRAFT OF AXES I and II of DSM-III CLASSIFICATION as of March 30, 1977.
14. Jackson, J.H., "Croonian lectures on evolution and dissolution of the nervous system," in *Selected Writings of John Hughlings Jackson,* vol. 2 (edited by Taylor, J.). London: Staple Press, 1958.
15. Sedman, G., Theories of depersonalization: A re-appraisal. *Brit. J. Psychiatry* 117:1-6 (1970).
16. Ibid., p. 11.

17. Sedman, G., An investigation of certain factors concerned in the aetiology of depersonalization, op. cit., pp. 209-214.
18. Brauer, R., Harrow, M., and Tucker, G.J., Depersonalization phenomena in psychiatric patients. *Brit. J. Psychiatry* 117:509-515 (1970).
19. Shorvon, H.J., op. cit., pp. 785-792.
20. Sedman, G., An investigation of certain factors concerned in the aetiology of depersonalization, op. cit., pp. 215-216.
21. Videbech, T., The psychopathology of anancastic endogenous depression. *Acta. Psychiat. Scand.* 52:345-348 (1975).
22. Roberts, W.W., op. cit., pp. 485-493.
23. Ibid., p. 489.
24. Sedman, G., Theories of depersonalization: A re-appraisal, op. cit., pp. 6-10.
25. Ibid., pp. 6-7.
26. Lader, M.H. and Wing, L., Physiological measures, sedative drugs and morbid anxiety. Maudsley Monograph No. 14. London: Oxford University Press, 1966.
27. Sedman, G., An investigation of certain factors concerned in the aetiology of depersonalization, op. cit., pp. 193-219.
28. Tucker, G.J., Harrow, M. and Quinlan, D., Depersonalization, dysphoria, and thought disturbance. *Amer. J. Psychiatry* 130(6):702-706 (1973).
29. Ambrosino, S.V., Phobic anxiety-depersonalization syndrome. *N.Y. State J. Med.* 73:419-425 (February 1, 1973).
30. Linton, P.H. and Estock, R.E. The anxiety phobic depersonalization syndrome: Role of the cognitive-perceptual style. *Dis. Nerv. Syst.* 38(3):138-141 (1977).
31. Roth, M., The phobic anxiety-depersonalization syndrome. *Proc. Roy. Soc. Med.* 52(8):587 (1959).
32. Roth, M., The phobic anxiety-depersonalization syndrome and some general aetiological problems in psychiatry. *J. Neuropsychiatry* 1:293-306 (1960).
33. Marks, I.M., Agoraphobic syndrome (phobic anxiety state). *Arch. Gen. Psychiatry* 23:549 (1970).
34. Tucker, G.J., Harrow, M., and Quinlan, D., op. cit., p. 704.
35. Sedman, G., Theories of depersonalization: A re-appraisal, op. cit., p. 11.
36. Levitan, H.L., The depersonalizing process: The sense of reality and of unreality. *Psychoanal. Quart.* 39:449-470 (1970).
37. Lower, R.B., Affect changes in depersonalization. *Psychoanal. Rev.* 59(4):565-577 (1972).
38. Bradlow, P.A., Depersonalization, ego splitting, non-human fantasy and shame. *Int. J. Psychoanal.* 54:487-492 (1973).
39. Noyes, Jr., R. and Kletti, R., Depersonalization in face of life-threatening danger. *Psychiatry* 39:19-27 (1976).
40. Sartre, J.P., *Nausea* (transl. by Alexander, L.). Norfolk, Conn.: New Directions Paperback, 1950, pp. 133-134.
41. Wordsworth, W., Ode: "Intimations of immortality from recollections of early childhood," in *English Poetry and Prose of the Romantic Movement,* revised ed. (edited by Woods, G.B.). Chicago: Scott, Foresman and Co., 1950, p. 329.
42. Rinsley, D.B., The adolescent inpatient: Patterns of depersonification. *Psychiat. Quart.* 45:3-22 (1971).
43. Edwards, J.G., The Koro pattern of depersonalization in an American schizophrenic patient. *Amer. J. Psychiatry* 126(8):1171-1173 (1970).
44. Shorvon, H.J., op. cit., p. 790.

45. Melges, F.T., Tinklenberg, J.R., Hollister, L., and Gillespie, H.K., Temporal disintegration and depersonalization during marihuana intoxication. *Arch. Gen. Psychiatry* **23**:204–210 (1970).

46. Kennedy, R.B., Self-induced depersonalization syndrome. *Amer. J. Psychiatry* **133**(11):1326–1328 (1976).

47. Lehmann, L.S., Depersonalization. *Amer. J. Psychiatry* **131**(11):1221–1224 (1974).

48. Walsh, R.N., Depersonalization: Definition and treatment. (Letters to the Editor). *Amer. J. Psychiatry* **132**(8):873 (1975).

11
HYPOCHONDRIACAL NEUROSIS

A "healthy" person does not dwell unduly upon his body and its functions. This is not to imply that he does not pay attention to his health. He does concern himself about being well and takes appropriate health measures such as eating properly, getting adequate sleep, working reasonable hours, enjoying a compatible social and sexual life, exercising, and so on. In fact if he has a bodily complaint he seeks medical evaluation. A recent study revealed that two out of five patients coming for treatment showed no evidence of physical illness. A follow-up survey of these "undiagnosed" and "untreated" patients showed that, after only one visit, 82% felt better and 11% were not improved. This study shows that a patient can be made to feel better by merely consulting a physician and that people do go through transitory periods of questioning their health.[1] These patients cannot be considered hypochondriacs simply because they had a somatic complaint and sought help. However, with repeated visits to the doctor for physical complaints, in which no basis for the complaints can be found, a different situation exists. Hypochondriasis may be present.

Hypochondriacal neurosis needs to be defined within specific boundaries and by certain essential components or else it becomes a meaningless label. In fact, controversy exists as to whether or not hypochondriasis is a symptom of other illnesses, a personality trait, a mechanism of defense, a disorder of body image, or a primary disease entity.[2] Unfortunately even recent research attempting to prove or disprove whether or not hypochondriasis was a disease entity incorporated a "disease phobia" factor.[3] This factor tends only to further confuse and increase controversy since phobia is in its own right an entity. Separating hypochondriasis into primary and secondary types may help eliminate this problem. Secondary types are part of some other mental or physical condition. Hypochondriasis is most commonly associated with anxiety, phobia, obsession, hysteria, or depression. Patients who suffer with unbased physical complaints and have more than a mild degree of either anxiety or depression are considered as cases of secondary hypochondriasis. Primary hypochondriasis has the following components: (1) persistent preoccupation with health or disease, involving one or more systems, organs or anatomical portions of the body, that is disproportionate to the amount of demonstrable biological damage or disturbance, (2) conviction that biological damage or disturbance exists which responds only temporarily to reassurance even after negative physical and laboratory examination; and (3) constant complaints, regarding the body, of hurt, distress, discomfort, or pain.[4,5] All these criteria are essential for the definition of hypochondriacal neurosis.

Pain, an essential component of hypochondriasis, is a word with various connotations. Among these can be acute discomfort from a laceration, exaggerated hurt following a slight injury, mild irritation towards a companion (pain in the neck), or even profound displeasure. The experience of bodily pain includes: (1) feelings of hurt, (2) presence or absence of a harmful stimulus, and (3) protective and adaptive patterns of response. In so far as bodily pain functions as a signal of current or impending biological damage or disturbance, it is organic. In so far as it functions to help maintain a balance among body, mind, and environment in situations where there is no biological damage or disturbance it may be hypochondriasis. In addition, a hypochondriacal bodily pain response, may develop where biological damage and disturbance do indeed exist, but the patient becomes excessively preoccupied and convinced that the disease is more serious than the facts warrant. Since the central nervous system mechanisms may be operant in hypochondriacal as well as organic pain, some understanding of these mechanisms may be helpful.[6]

Several theories exist regarding the mechanisms of pain. The specificity theory postulates that pain results from stimulation of specific nerves. Nakahama wrote:

> Pain is classified into three types: (1) Pricking pain, or first pain (fast pain), is a sharp pain evoked by a brisk needle stab in the skin, is precisely localized, and subsides quickly after removal of the stimulus. This type of pain does not induce emotional reaction. (2) Burning pain, or second pain (slow pain), is intolerable. It takes 0.5 to 1 second until pain is experienced, and is not distinctly localized. The pain remains for a few seconds after removal of the stimulus and is accompanied by cardiovascular and respiratory changes. The pain momentarily affects the subject and changes his frame of mind. (3) Aching pain is induced from the viscera and somatic deep structures and is sometimes accompanied by a sensation of burning. It is difficult to distinguish the actual site of the pain, because it is perceived as distant from the actual location of the stimulus (referred pain).[7]

Furthermore, it is believed that specific free nerve endings exist for the various types of pain and that specific nerve fibers carry the different types of pain.

For example, pricking and sensation of coolness are mediated by small, rapidly conducting myelinated, a-delta fibers; and burning pain and warmth by slower conducting unmyelinated C fibers. Tissue damage releases pain-producing plasma kinin and spasm seems to play a more prominent role in producing pain from the intestines than neural or chemical mechanisms.[8] After stimulation of the nerve ending, the pain impulse is transmitted into the spinal cord via the lateral spinothalamic tract, goes to the thalamus, and then to the cerebral cortex. The pain center in the thalamus and cerebral cortex interprets the impulse.[9]

The pattern theory postulates that all cutaneous receptors are alike and have a common sensitivity. The information is subsequently encoded by the temperospatial pattern of impulse discharge and perceived as pain through the central pain pathways. Some pattern theories stress central summation rather than peripheral stimulation. Reverberating circuits in spinal internuncial pools can then be triggered by non-noxious stimuli and produce pain sensation centrally.[10]

The gate-control theory of pain, according to Nathan and Rudge, is based on work:

> . . . in which it was shown that stimulation of small afferent fibers resulted in a positive dorsal root potential, whereas stimulation of large afferent fibers caused a negative dorsal root potential. These observations were interpreted as evidence of presynaptic facilitation and presynaptic inhibition of the cutaneous input. According to the gate-control theory, the output of a group of first central transmission (T) cells in the posterior horn depends upon the balance of large and small afferent fibre activity of the posterior roots. If this balance is such that small fibre activity predominates, there will be presynaptic facilitation and a large increase in T cell activity; this results in pain phenomena (gate open). The converse applies if large fibre activity predominates (gate closed). This is a quantitative theory of pain; the number of impulses in a given time reaching the relevant parts of the brain determines the occurrence of pain. The implication of the theory . . . is that exciting large afferent fibers will cause a reduction of the local input to the spinal cord and thus pain will be reduced or stopped.[11]

These three theories are primarily concerned with the anatomical and physiological basis of pain and do not mention the relationship of the patient's psychological state to pain. Yet, pain can be influenced by the mind. This applies equally to pain that has an organic basis as it does to pain for which no demonstrable organic basis can be found.

Pain thresholds vary from individual to individual and even within the same individual at different times. No strict relationship exists between the amount of noxious stimulus (tissue damage, etc.) and the experience of pain. Some patients are more immune to pain than others and these people complain less. Some specific data exists: elderly persons experience less pain than younger persons who suffer from the same disorder; women tend to have lower pain thresholds than men; pain increases in the presence of anxiety, depression, poor health, resentment, lack of confidence in the doctor; and so forth.[12] Yet some physicians persist in believing that pain is a specific sensation directly proportional to the extent of tissue damage. Of course, the overwhelming amount of evidence disputes this assertion.[13]

Pain clearly involves the emotional state of the individual. One study attempts to evaluate in patients with carcinoma of the cervix, the relationship of pain, its communication to others, personality, physical symptoms, and attitudes towards illness. The psychological tests used for this study were: the Eysenck Personality Inventory, Cornell Medical Index, and Whiteley Index of Hypochondriasis. The Eysenck Personality Inventory measures two dimensions of personality, neuroticism and extraversion–introversion. It defines neuroticism as emotional lability, over-responsiveness, and a tendency for neurotic breakdown under stress. The higher neuroticism (N) score implies a greater degree of emotional instability. Extraversion (E) means an outgoing personality with uninhibited social tendencies. A higher E score reflects a greater degree of outgoing tendencies. This study attempts to determine the influence personality structure has on awareness of pain and ability to communicate this information. Findings are divided into three groups: first, those patients who were pain free and had a low N, high E score indicating a low degree of emotionality with an ability to freely communicate; second, those who felt pain but did not complain and had a high N and low E score, indicating increased emotionality with a tendency not to communicate; third, those who felt pain, had high N and E scores, complained, and received analgesic drugs. This study concluded that the presence of pain and other symptoms was related to the N score, but the E score determined whether or not the patient would communicate distress to others. Evidence shows that perception and expression of pain are related to specific personality factors and may have relevance for etiology in hypochondriacal neurosis.[14]

In sum, pain is the most common complaint of patients who seek medical attention. It is associated with either bodily or mental disturbances and can occur in the absence of demonstrable biological damage or disturbance. The pain experience, its perception and interpretation, as well as the person's response to pain, depends upon the state of the body (especially the nervous system) and the psychological predisposition of the individual. Factors such as an intact consciousness, emotions, cognition, personality, memory, and so forth are important considerations. Likewise, hypnosis, suggestion, electrical stimulation, autosuggestion, psychotherapy, acupuncture, drugs, surgery, etc. can affect the intensity of pain experienced by individuals.[15]

An essential component of hypochondriacal neurosis is the persistent conviction these patients maintain regarding physical illness—even in the face of negative physical and laboratory examinations. Reassurance that no physical illness exists is resisted. In this one sense, the hypochondriac has a false belief or delusion. Conviction regarding bodily complaints varies with time. It can begin with a normal concern for one's body, progress to an exaggeration of insignificant complaints, develop into an unjustified and constant involvement, and finally lead to a state of true delusion. It therefore behooves the psychiatrist to decide whether hypochondriacs are neurotic, psychotic, or borderline. Except in those cases where hypochondriasis is part of another mental condition and hence psychosis might be present, the patient with primary hypochondriasis has no formal thought or affective disorder. Their thought disturbance only refers to bodily complaints; hence, these patients are neurotic. The DSMII takes the position that only cases without delusions are cases of hypochondriacal neurosis. But since these patients have preoccupations and convictions that are in themselves false beliefs, where does one draw the line? The DSMII definition, therefore, leaves too much room for personal interpretation and is too hazy. The lack of response to reassurance, itself, implies a delusion. It seems, then, that the definition proposed in this book is not in agreement with the DSMII definition. That is, even with delusion a condition may, under certain circumstances, be considered neurotic. This position is maintained because hypochondriacs do not suffer from an overall personality disintegration nor do they have formal thought disorder, emotional blunting, hallucinations, generalized delusions, organic brain disease, and so on. On balance, therefore, primary hypochondriasis is a neurosis. To place it into the borderline category solves nothing and only adds to the confusion surrounding that category.[16]

HISTORY

Hypochondria (singular: hypochondrium) are anatomical regions of the body. They are the regions of the abdomen, below the ribs and on either side of the epigastrium, which contain the liver on the right and the spleen on the left. Hypochondriasis, from the time that the ancient Greeks originated the term until the eighteenth century, was thought to be a disease or derangement of one or more of the abdominal viscera located in the hypochondria. Over the centuries the definition of the term changed as new concepts of pathology developed and, in pre-eighteenth century times, it was known by such names as the spleen, the vapours, melancholy, atrabilious, and valetudinarian.

The description and etiology of hypochondriasis has, from the beginning, been in constant flux. Hippocrates referred to the hypochondrium, described some symptoms of hypochondriasis, and in Aphorisms 73, said the following:

When the hypochondriac region is affected with meteorism and borborymi, should pain of the loins supervene, the bowels get into a loose and watery state, unless there be an eruption of flatus or a copius evacuation of urine. These things occur in fevers.[17]

Hippocrates divided melancholy into three types according to the seat of the disease: head, body, and hypochondria. Apparently he did not localize hypochondriacal melancholy to any organ in that region but did view it within the context of the humoural theory as a disturbance of black bile.[18] Galen, however, did localize the disease as being caused by heat and obstruction of the mesenteric veins which caused the passage of chyle from the stomach to the liver to be detained, stopped, corrupted, and turned into rumbling and wind.[19] So the disease became known as windy hypochondriacal melancholy. Both the symptoms and the seat of this disease were ambiguous. Burton (1621) did not feel that fear and sorrow are general symptoms of windy melancholy but as will be shown he did think that they could be present at some stage of the disease. Burton wrote:

> . . . some fear and are not sad; some are sad and fear not; some neither fear nor grieve. The rest are these, beside fear and sorrow, *sharp belchings, fulsome crudities, heat in the bowels, wind and rumblings in the guts, vehement gripings, pain in the belly and stomack sometimes, and moist spittle, cold sweat unseasonable sweat all over the body* . . . . Their ears sing now and then, vertigo and giddiness come by fits, turbulent dreams, dryness, leanness; . . . . Some again are black, pale, ruddy, sometimes their shoulders and shoulder-blades ache, there is a leaping all over their bodies, sudden trembling, a palpitation of the heart, and that grief in the mouth of the stomack, which maketh the patient think his heart itself acheth, and sometimes suffication, short breath, hard wind, strong pulse, swooning . . . .[20]

These symptoms were attributed by different authors to disturbances in stomach, spleen, liver, mesenteric veins, and heart, and Burton went on to say:

> And from these crudities windy vapours ascend up to the brain, which trouble the imagination, and cause fear, sorrow, dullness, heaviness, many terrible conceits . . . . one, by reason of those ascending vapours and gripings rumbling beneath, will not be persuaded but that he hath a serpent in his guts, a viper; another frogs.[21]

Thus the connection between hypochondriasis and melancholia was well established by the seventeenth century. Hypochondriasis was a type of melancholy.

In 1610 Smollius allied hypochondriasis with hysteria. He attributed the relationship of the hypochondrium to hypochondriasis similar to that of the uterus to hysteria.[22] Yet women do suffer from hypochondriasis, and men from hysteria. An apparent paradox existed. Sydenham (1624-1689) got around this paradox by considering hypochondriasis and hysteria as the same disease but called by different names. Thus by the end of the seventeenth century hypochondriasis was very broadly defined and became a popular diagnostic label. Etiology of this disease, however, was still in dispute.[23]

During the eighteenth century hypochondriasis not only became a very prevalent diagnosis but it attained status. It was considered an honor to be afflicted with this disease since hypochondriasis, which was earlier subsumed under melancholy, was thought to be a disease of civilization. Hence, as noted in the chapter on depression, those who were the most cultured, those in the highest socioeconomic strata were vulnerable, and had the greatest risk of contracting it. Hypochondriasis as a diagnostic label had snob appeal. Englishmen of that day were proud to refer to the disease as the English Malady, a name that evolved as a result of a book published in 1733, called *The English Malady* which was written by George Cheyne (1671-1743).[24] Hypochondriasis had assumed the symptomatological burden of most of melancholy and hysteria.

Hypochondriasis blossomed in the eighteenth century. New names appeared to describe the entity: nervous disorders, maladies, nerveuses, hystero-hypochondriasis, and so on. Etiological debates centered around which hypochondriac organ was responsible for the disease, or was the disease a disturbance of the central nervous system, or a combination of both? Naturally, boundaries were not set or agreed upon in defining the disease and etiological considerations were based on the theories and speculations of the day.[25] Even literary men got into the act. Jean Baptiste Poquelin (Molière, 1622-1673), wrote *The Imaginary Invalid* (1673) and Bernard Mandeville (1670-1733) wrote *A Treatise of the Hypochondriack and Hysterick Passions* (1711). Both are delightful books dealing with hypochondriacs and their relationship to physicians.[26]

By the third quarter of the eighteenth century the nervous etiology of hypochondriasis gained ground. The humoural theory was nearly discarded. In 1777 Cullen classified hypochondriasis under neuroses and he among others considered the brain to be the seat of the disease. In 1777 James Boswell regarded hypochondriasis as a mental rather than a nervous disease and thus contrasted sharply with most other thinkers of his day.[27]

Changes continued throughout the nineteenth century. Étienne Jean Georget (1795-1828), emphasizing the cerebral origin of the disease, suggested the name cerebropathie. Jean Pierre Falret (1794-1870), described hypochondriasis as a morbid condition of the nervous system characterized by depression and false beliefs regarding an impaired state of health.[28] Things were beginning to churn but it was George Miller Beard and his concept of neurasthenia which finally displaced hypochondriasis. From 1880 onward hypochondriasis decreased in importance as a nosological entity. Of course the same fate awaited neurasthenia which in its turn was replaced by neuroses.[29]

The term hypochondriasis in the latter half of the eighteenth and on into the nineteenth century continued to change its definitions and its position in psychiatric nomenclature. Some considered it synonymous with melancholia and lypemania,[30] others renounced the idea of hypochondriasis completely or considered it a symptom within the greater concept of nervous disease. Still others retained the term but only as a clinical syndrome without any etiological implications. In 1904 Robert Wollenberg considered hypochondriasis as part of some other disease and not a distinct clinical entity.[31] J. Raecke thought that hypochondriasis was a disease entity and this debate—both for and against an entity—had its proponents and antagonists.[32] The nosological problem was far from settled.

Hypochondriasis was not considered a syndrome, by some, but rather a symptom of conditions such as melancholia, depression, neurasthenia, and so forth. But it did become associated with a group of characteristic symptoms. Thus in 1923, Bleuler said:

> The picture of the condition of *hypochondria* consists in continuous attention to one's own state of health with the tendency to ascribe a disease to oneself from insignificant signs or also without such. It occurs in dementia praecox, in depressive and neurasthenic conditions, in initial stages of organic psychoses (arteriosclerosis, paresis), and in psychopathic states of all kinds. We no longer recognize *hypochondria as a disease.*[33]

Thus, Bleuler considered hypochondriasis as a personality trait and was in agreement with Kraepelin who considered it as a symptom of other conditions. Freud in his early formulation included hypochondriasis as one of the actual neuroses. There were many others who participated in the discussion surrounding hypochondriasis. Their thoughts centered around definition, etiology, classification, and dynamic understanding.[34] However, it was not until Gillespie (1928, 1929) developed a definition of hypochondriasis and declared it a disease entity that modern-day views began to take shape. In 1936 Felix Brown said that Gillespie:

> . . . defines hypochondriasis as (1) a mental preoccupation with a real or suppositious physical disorder; (2) a discrepancy between the degree of preoccupation and the grounds for it; (3) an affective condition of interest with conviction, but not of anxiety or depression. The latter criterion narrows the scope of hypochondriasis considerably . . . . For the purpose of the present paper, hypochondriasis will be taken to be a physically

unjustified or exaggerated body complaint. This is essentially an attempt to bring together all the psychogenic body complaints without any distinction into hypochondriacal delusions or attitudes.[35]

Here in synoptic form are the problems that plague us till this day. Whereas Gillespie limits the definition of hypochondriasis and describes a disease entity, he presumes that it is "an affective condition of interest." In so doing he implies that the disease is one of mood disturbance. Brown, on the other hand, proposes no such etiological implication but considers hypochondriasis as a psychobiologic reaction of the individual to difficulties rather than a disease entity. He, therefore, accepts hypochondriasis as an accompaniment of other mental conditions. Similar arguments continue to this day.

In sum, hypochondriasis, in the early part of the twentieth century, was considered under the name neurasthenia by Kraepelin and Beard, psychasthenia by Janet, cerebropathie by Georget, actual neurosis by Freud, and a type of self-love or narcissism by Paul Schilder (1886-1940). Bleuler considered it a symptom of depression and schizophrenia or as a personality trait, and the Meyerian school believed it to be a psychobiological reaction (meregasia). Hypochondriasis has been considered a disease of the visceral organs, black bile, nervous system, stomach muscles and fermentation, organic body structure, psyche, caused by God, and failure of adaptation. The fact that it has survived in the face of so much adversity should tell psychiatrists that the phenomenology is real and that this entity should not be neglected.

CLASSIFICATION

Workers continue to struggle with the problem of taxonomy and are divided as to whether or not hypochondriasis is a symptom, personality trait, or disease entity. One area of agreement, that all recognize, is that bodily symptoms without a demonstrable organic basis are an extremely common phenomena. The problem is to organize these phenomena into meaningful groups and correlate them with physiochemical mechanisms, experience, intrapsychic conflict, or here and now existent situations. Classifications are proposed. Sociological models are based on patients' complaints of somatic disturbances without a known physical cause and are referred to as disease-claiming behavior, sick-role behavior, abnormal-illness behavior, or dispensary-attenders. Likewise, medical models are based on patients' complaints about bodily symptoms without a known physical cause in which the phenomena are viewed as part of some other disease or else as a primary or true hypochondriasis.[36-38]

Alistair Cooke, British literary critic, historian, and commentator, wrote a delightful article in which he classified hypochondriacs according to their interpersonal relationships. He proposed the following classification. (1) The folklore hypochondriac, i.e., one who believes in certain unproven causes and cures for disease. Some believe drafts cause pneumonia or sitting on wet steps cures piles. (2) The fatalistic hypochondriac who instinctively believes in instant cures and instant damnation. (3) The smart-Aleck hypochondriac who keeps up with the latest in medical knowledge and knows the proper treatment for innumerable illnesses. Of this type Cooke said:

> There is a new drug, and in acquiring it he conveys that medicine has been floundering in a dark tunnel since Hippocrates and has at last seen the light. He usually has a passionate belief in vitamins, following their miraculous progress through the alphabet. One year it is C, the next D, now E. He ridicules the doubts of any layman; and his doctor, if he is wise, does not tell him that he cannot build up an inventory or storage battery of vitamins, that if he takes 400 units a day of vitamin C he will use five of them and pee 395 away. These smart-Alecks are often very healthy people but only, they assure you, because they religiously observe a regimen: fifteen minutes jogging, two dozen deep breaths, two sets of vitamin pills at intervals and honey from a special farm in Canada or Norway. And they have discovered a pharmacopoeia all their own.[39]

(4) The supportive hypochondriac, i.e., the husband who tenderly takes his wife to the doctor week after week, year after year, and is as much concerned about her headache when she does not have it as when she does have it. A variation of this type (5) the martyr hypochondriac, often a wife who is devoted to her family but who is never free from several chronic ailments. Cooke stated:

> Suddenly, if she's lucky, she becomes a widow. Her symptoms vanish, she takes off; she, who had been a housebound housewife, takes up the cello, goes to the theatre, rustles up old female companions and goes to the mountains, or the West, or Europe. She blooms, she puts on weight or takes it off, according to whichever she had regarded as her lifelong problem. I have only very rarely known a widow who did not take a new lease on life. I have never known a widower who did. This may go to show that inside every devoted wife is a women's liberationist struggling to get out.[40]

(6) The Siamese hypochondriacs, the mutual martyrs, who struggle through a stormy marriage for most of their lives. Yet, both have protective attitudes towards each other when it comes to their bodily complaints. And they totter down the twilight years happy in their mutual protection. They would love to go to the theatre, but—they will have to call off the dinner because he, poor man, she, poor old girl, is not up to it.[41] (7) The happy hypochondriac who enjoys the symptoms as well as the attention that the complaining begets.[42]

Although Cooke's classification system is too broad and uncritical for scientific purposes it does send a loud and clear message that bodily complaints are a means of communication. It emphasizes the role of social, cultural, and interpersonal relations as factors that have classificatory and etiological significance for hypochondriasis.

There are many others whose work on classification, with special attention to social and cultural aspects, could be cited but basically for the medical taxonomist the issues revolve around whether or not hypochondriasis is an independent entity, or part of another syndrome. Collecting cases in which body complaints are predominant and using psychological tests and analyzing them according to factor analytic techniques, has not resolved the differences.[43-46] The leading opposing exponents of disease entity versus nondisease entity concepts are Kenyon and Pilowsky. Kenyon stated:

> It would now seem best to drop altogether the terms hypochondria and hypochondriasis, but to retain hypochondriacal as a descriptive adjective. If this usage is accepted, it would be proper to refer to hypochondriacal traits, symptoms, ideas, fears, and so on, with the added implication that there is a morbid preoccupation with mental or bodily functions or state of health. This would leave the options open as to the precise psychopathology and mechanisms involved. 'Somatic' would still be used in a much more general sense, as synonymous with physical or bodily, as in such terms as psychosomatic or somatic pathology.[47]

Pilowsky stated:

> It has been demonstrated that a number of clinical differences exist between patients diagnosed as suffering from "primary" hypochondriasis and patients with "secondary" hypochondriasis. Patients in whom it was felt that no other diagnosis but hypochondriasis could be made. This meant eliminating patients with obsessional or hysterical illness and in particular those in whom anxiety or depression were present in more than a mild degree. The results of the statistical comparison of the two groups provide additional evidence for maintaining that anxiety and depression were associated with "secondary" rather than "primary" hypochondriasis. Thus the patients designated as having "secondary hypochondriasis" tended to have a shorter history when first referred, were more likely to have made a suicidal attempt, to have had previous psychiatric illness treated and more likely to be treated with electroconvulsive therapy and antidepressants. In addition, patients, with "secondary" hypochondriasis tended to be anxiety-prone personalities, to have fears of illness and to be treated with sedatives.[48]

The answer to this debate will ultimately rest upon finding definitive methods of testing that are scientifically reliable and valid.[49, 50]   Since there are clinical cases in which the criteria as set forth in this chapter are available, the position posited here is that hypochondriasis can be classified into primary and secondary types. Further it may be divided on the basis of duration. Acute hypochondriasis lasts from days to months, semiacute lasts from one to two years, and chronic lasts longer than two years.[51]

The official classification of the American Psychiatric Association during the 1920's and 1930's, did list hypochondriasis as a diagnostic category,[52] however, in the DSMI (1952) this term disappeared. Such patients might then have been classified under Psychophysiologic Autonomic and Visceral Disorders. It returned as one of the neuroses in the DSMII (1968) only to disappear again as an official diagnostic category in the proposed classification for DSMIII. Here, it is considered as Atypical somatoform disorder.[53]

ETIOLOGY

Comparative studies of hypochondriacal neuroses are difficult since there is no general agreement regarding definition or classification. Hence, any attempt to determine causation is highly speculative. Even so, it is necessary to examine the etiological factors because hypochondriasis is one of the diseases in which the relationship between mind and body has particular relevance.

Constitution is one factor. Twins have not yet been adequately evaluated. Family studies are not conclusive, although they do find several members of the same family suffering from the disease; especially hypochondriacal fathers of males with primary hypochondriasis.[54, 55]   Personality studies of hypochondriacs are not definitive but several types are described: (1) body-sensitive or body-conscious personalities who, beyond their concern with somatic symptoms, have nothing else in common;[56] (2) inadequate personalities with behavioral patterns of passivity, self-pity, and complaining;[57] (3) egocentric, selfish, or persons who lead solitary and subjective lives; (4) persons with traits such as orderliness, parsimoniousness, and obstinacy;[58] (5) paranoid, obsessional, immature; and so forth.[59]   There is no general agreement regarding the relationship between personality type and hypochondriasis; even though claims are made that male hypochondriacs begin as anxiety neurotics with an obsessional personality and females with "chronic hypochondriacal symptoms are often associated with a relatively bland or complacent affect and the personality background reveals more hysterical traits although motives for escaping into illness may be difficult to define."[60]

Burns and Nicols evaluated the association between obsessive compulsive personality, lifelong excessive preoccupation with health, family morbidity of chest disease, and certain life events. They tried to determine the relationship between these groups of factors and whether or not somatic complaints referable to the chest would or would not occur in depressed patients. These investigators correlated respiratory symptoms during episodes of depression and evaluated them over and above the fact that depression itself intensifies respiratory symptoms. Their study was well controlled and used two types of depressed patients: those who did not somaticize and those who did. They interviewed patients and their families, and did psychological testing. The authors concluded that all the above factors contributed to localized chest symptoms during a depressive episode; however, they noted that the predominant premorbid personality type found in conjunction with somatic complaints referable to the chest was the obsessional.[61]

If the mechanism of pain were understood it would greatly enhance the understanding of hypochondriasis. Unfortunately, as previously noted, several hypotheses are offered to explain pain and hence the physiological speculations regarding hypochondriasis are even more tentative. Hypochondriacal preoccupation with an organ or functional system is seen, from a physiological viewpoint, as a disturbance or distortion of body image which occupies an increasing and disproportionate position of consciousness.[62] In the normal there is a constant stream of sensations from all parts of the body. By some mechanism, probably in the limbic or reticular activating system, the majority of these sensations never register in consciousness. It is as if a grid or gate-control were acting selectively. In hypochondriasis selectivity is broken down and an abnormal amount of impulses get past the grid, and sensations are consciously appreciated that cause discomfort. Perhaps there is a breakdown in the information, communication, or excitation–inhibition arousal systems of the central nervous system such as may occur in causalgia or phantom limb.[63, 64] Yet more clarification of what constitutes distorted body image or scheme is necessary. Does hypochondriacal preoccupation result from a distorted body image, a pathological experiencing of sensations, or a morbid perception of self? The physiological basis of hypochondriasis has yet to be discovered. In any event hypochondriasis is a morbid condition whether it is caused by a disturbance of sensation, perception, body image, or conviction and it differs from anxious or fearful preoccupation.[65]

Other factors may enter into the complex balance of mind and body that result in body concerns and hypochondriasis. Bodily complaints occur frequently and for the most part are transitory. Estimates, however, indicate that three out of four persons take action for somatic complaints during any month and use medicines, see a physician, resort to bed rest, or limit their activities. Yet many with symptoms do not take action, hence, no reliable statistics are available regarding the true incidence or prevalence of somatic symptoms.[66]

Changes of internal and external environment tend to promote bodily symptoms. It is, therefore, to be expected that an increased incidence of hypochondriasis begins around age 45 and becomes progressively higher as people get older. This may be related to biological changes connected with the involutional period of life, changing marital relationships since children usually leave home by the time parents reach that age, a lack of replacements for time spent with the children, and a progressive withdrawal from competitive business and social life. Friendships become fewer and more limited.[67] Changes—biological, psychological, social—in those at the other end of the life cycle (children) are constantly and relatively rapidly occurring; hence, a higher incidence of bodily complaints is expected and found during this period. Complaints by children such as bellyaches, headaches, sore muscles, and so on can be endless. Stability and security are lacking during the earlier and latter parts of life. One assumption that can be drawn from these observations is that somatic complaints and/or hypochondriasis, in part, are a response of a poorly automatized functioning of the motor and vegetative apparatus. Conversely, individuals with highly organized and strongly automatized behavior would be less vulnerable to concerns involving bodily complaints or even health.[68]

Automatized behavior is the routine daily activities which all people perform with a minimum of physical or mental effort. These are well practiced, repetitive activities such as walking, talking, reading, perfunctory decision making, sleeping, eating, routine work activities, daily social relationships, and so forth. Strong automatizers seem to get more done during a day, suffer from less fatigue, and have higher level occupations than those weak automatizers of comparable age, education, and intelligence. Comparing these two groups, evidence supports the hypothesis that patients with strong automatized behavior express less concern over body health or have less bodily complaints and hypochondriasis than those with weak automatized behavior.[69]

Departing from routine, which is a form of change, is a factor in hypochondriasis whether the departure is due to new learning, or deviation in one's biological cycle. Thus medical students and psychiatric residents frequently develop the complaints of their patients. This, however, may not only be due to the new knowledge gleaned from the study of the patient but also results from an educational system which is geared to promote, produce, or exaggerate emotional or physical problems of the student or resident.[70] Improper education cannot be understated as a factor that can precipitate a hypochondriacal illness in students or patients. The physician, as an educator of his patients, can be guilty and aid in predisposing his patient to a hypochondriacal neurosis (iatrogenic illness). He can accomplish this by focusing too much on healthy organs or by exaggerating the degree of disease in an unhealthy organ. Mechanic aptly stated:

As an initial formulation, it appears that persons tend to notice bodily sensations when they depart from more ordinary feelings. Each person tends to appraise new bodily perceptions against prior experience and his anticipations based on the experiences of others and on general knowledge. Many symptoms occur so commonly throughout life that they become part of ordinary expectations and are experienced as normal variations. Other experiences, such as a young girl's first menstruation, might be extremely frightening if prior social learning has not occurred, but would ordinarily be accepted as normal if it had. In analyzing responses to more unusual symptoms it is instructive to examine situations in which normal attribution processes become disrupted as a consequence of special kinds of learning, and in this regard hypochondriasis among medical students is an interesting example.[71]

The wrong words or experience received by a receptive individual can be a factor in hypochondriasis.

Social and cultural factors are important. Jews and Italians respond emotionally to pain, the Irish deny it, and white Anglo-Saxon Americans react stoically to pain. Various cultural groups even emphasize pain in certain parts of the body more than others. The person with the pain that is acceptable to his cultural group gets more attention.[72] Social and cultural studies leave no doubt that somatic complaints, their frequency and type, have a direct relationship to and vary with background.

Psychoanalysts make one cardinal error in attempting to explain hypochondriasis. They lump together all patients who have somatic symptoms as a predominant part of their clinical picture and then offer psychodynamic explanations for all. The net result of this neglect of strict diagnostic criteria is a potpourri of diverse explanations.

To review in detail the contributions of various analysts from Freud to the present would accomplish little since there is no certainty that any one of them is discussing the same clinical entity. Yet, an overview of the various ideas that psychoanalysts have proposed may be of value, but it must be kept in the forefront of the reader's mind that the analysts are discussing somatic symptoms and not a clearly defined entity termed hypochondriacal neurosis.

Freud, as noted, originally considered hypochondriasis as one of the actual neuroses. It had no psychological significance since it was caused by a damming up of the libido into bodily organs. Freud later proposed three character traits—orderliness, parsimoniousness, and obstinacy—to be associated with anal eroticism. Ferenczi considered anal eroticism as the underlying cause of hypochondriasis. It was an unconscious unsublimated coprophilic interest from the original objects to other organs of the body. Further, the commonly found association of paranoid conditions and melancholia in patients with hypochondriasis suggested that all three conditions were fixated at a similar stage of psychosexual development with slight differences. Hypochondriasis resulted from a narcissistic or autoerotic preference for one's own body. Hypochondriacs withdraw libido from external objects into their body, therefore, a change occurs in the external libidinal cathexis of the ego. Another interpretation of this withdrawal of ego cathexis was that it was a masochistic compensation. In sum, earlier analytic theory included a narcissistic regression of the libido with masochistic compensation, anal eroticism, and direct physical excitation of an organ homologous with sexual excitation of the turgid genital.[73]

Fenichel referred to hypochondriasis as an organ neurosis and in 1945 he wrote:

> The term object cathexis means that the sum total of the ideas and feelings a person has in regard to another person constitutes an "intrapsychic object representation," and that this representation is cathected with a special amount of mental energy. In an analogous way, an individual's own body and its organs are represented intrapsychically by means of a sum of memories of sensations and their interrelations. The "body image" thus created has great significance for the constitution of the ego. It is not simply identical with the real body. Clothes, amputated members, or even one's automobile may be included in the body image, whereas "alienated" organs are excluded from it. Hence there are also "intrapsychic organ representations." "Narcissistic withdrawal" means a transfer of libido from object representations to organ representations.[74]

Fenichel also recognized the role guilt played in hypochondriasis:

> Among the impulses that are withdrawn from object to organ representations in hypochondriasis, the hostile and sadistic impulses appear to play a particularly pronounced role. The original hostile attitude toward an object is turned against the ego, and hypochondriasis may serve as a gratification of guilt feelings.[75]

This interpretation represents the more orthodox analytic viewpoint of some 30 years ago.

More liberal psychoanalytic viewpoints are also available. One such interpretation considers the initial event to be frustration of the wish to be loved. Frustration in actual life leads to a turning inward for love. This narcissistic withdrawal of interest from external sources to the self permits the patient to concentrate his attentions upon his bodily organs and complains to others about his discomfort and suffering. In this manner, he gets others to give him more attention and concern. Although this is not the love he originally sought, it does serve several purposes. It defends him from openly declaring how much he loves himself and brings him attention. Frustration not only creates narcissistic withdrawal, it also produces hostility. Hostility, excessive self love, and attention seeking lead to guilt and shame. This in turn produces suffering that relieves the feelings of guilt and shame. A vicious circle is established in which hostile impulses revive earlier conflicts of family, oedipal, and sibling rivalry and this creates more guilt and more suffering.[76] Alexander considered anxiety a major component of the psychodynamics of hypochondriasis:

> The displacement of anxiety is a defense against castration fear. Neurotic guilt arouses the infantile fear of retaliation, the fear of castration. The hypochondriac displaces this fear to another organ as if he would offer his guilty conscience a less highly cherished organ as a substitute for his genitals. Essentially this is a mechanism similar to that seen in phobias.[77]

The obvious haziness of terminology and broad simplified generalizations make this formulation more confusing than amusing.

Other psychoanalysts have elaborated and modified these formulations. These modifications include: (1) an attempt to fill the gap from the conversion of mental conflict into body language; (2) an attempt to clarify the concept of organ language, somatization, hysterical conversion, and psychosomatics; (3) a noting of the relevance of early body ego, regression, conversion, and repression and their relationship to the development of somatic complaints; (4) a profile of the "bellyachers" that consists of repressed hostility directed at the real object and bad introject, of physical symptoms having symbolic significance that are a partial solution of a neurotic conflict, of somatic symptoms as a means of expiating deep-seated guilt, etc.; and so on. No generally agreed upon position regarding hypochondriasis exists or existed among psychoanalysts.[78]

In summary, hypochondriasis affords the psychiatrist one of the best opportunities that he has to study the mind-body problem. He can approach it from multidisciplinary viewpoints. Biochemical and physiological mechanisms of pain can be investigated. How do brain and other organs of the body operate to maintain the individual in a state of painless equilibrium? What happens when this mechanism breaks down? Is there a change in tissue or function? Why? The same questions—what, how, and why—can be asked regarding the psychosocial environmental factors that enter into any consideration of hypochondriasis or the even bigger problem of bodily complaints. The tiger has psychiatrists by the tail and it will not let them go. The fact remains that the mind-body problem, best exemplified by hypochondriasis, has troubled thinkers in innumerable disciplines since the beginning and it is not likely to go away even if the DSMIII eliminates the term hypochondriasis.

DIAGNOSIS

Chronic hypochondriacs are frequently called by such pejorative names as "crock," "doctor shopper," "grunt," "clinic rotator," and so forth.[79] These patients are a source of distress, frustration, and resentment to doctors whose thick files are a testament not only to their lack of treatment success but also to the degree of unhappiness or mental pain from which these patients suffer.[80] The mutual dislike, disdain, and distrust that invariably develops between hypochondriacs and their physicians can become as much a part of the clinical picture of hypochondriasis as the essential components incorporated in the definition of this entity.

Trying to analyze this nonproductive relationship between doctor and patient reveals some interesting insights. To begin, some psychiatrists who write about hypochondriasis for the general physician attribute to doctors both a conscious and an unconscious attitude of wanting to help patients. The purity of the physicians' motives and goals is unquestioned. They are available, affable, and knowledgeable. The burden, therefore, of this unpleasant relationship between doctor and patient falls upon the patient. Most physicians concede that most patients want to get well and that doctors have the goal of wanting to help them get well. However, Rittelmeyer stated:

> The hypochondriac's goal is different. He clings to his symptoms with such tenacity that it becomes apparent, sooner or later, that he neither expects nor desires relief from his physical discomfort. Rather, his goal is to maintain a relationship with his doctor that will provide him with the care and understanding he so desperately needs. Unless the physician understands this, and acts accordingly, he and his patient will be working at cross-purposes. It is no wonder that these patients' encounters with physicians often end in mutual frustration and bitterness.[81]

That not only diagnoses the patients' goals and motives, and in a nutshell explains the etiology of hypochondriasis, but also instructs the "understanding" physician in the psychological message behind hypochondriacs' complaints. In essence the patient does not want to be cured but wants to visit doctors, and an unpleasant doctor–patient relationship apparently is an essential feature in the etiology and treatment of hypochondriasis. Cowan viewed the doctor–patient relationship in an entirely different manner. He saw it as a defiance by the patient towards the doctor:

> You begin to wonder if this sort of patient isn't in fact setting up a situation of challenge. He is in effect saying, "I've got something physically wrong somewhere. I defy you to find it. You may think you are a clever doctor, but I am more clever than you because I can prevent you from ever finding it." The patient is not coming to you to be healed, or for a final diagnosis. He comes to you to pit your skills as a learned professional against his own fantasies that he can outsmart you. The patient, in fact, is taunting the doctor.[82]

Psychiatrists writing in this manner are supporting the general physicians' pejorative attitudes towards hypochondriacs. In effect, psychiatrists view physicians and themselves as all-knowing and as having the ability to explain everything. The patient, on the other hand, is viewed as an arrogant person who dares challenge the almighty authority of the doctor. Hence, general physicians resort to pejorative names for hypochondriacs; and psychiatrists, in the guise of "understanding," either by pat explanations or direct accusations, view these patients as using Machiavellian tactics.[83] In either case such physicians' attitudes are patronizing and only cover up their ignorance. It does nothing toward helping hypochondriacs nor toward revealing the true nature of hypochondriasis. This unessential characteristic (mutual hostility) of the clinical picture can only be corrected by a change in the physician's attitude.

Clinical manifestations of hypochondriasis are varied. The complaints can be referable to one part, many parts, or the whole body; can be mild such as a slight headache, or severe such as a disabling backache which confines the person to bed; and can last for relatively short periods of time (acute, subacute) to a lifetime (chronic). Further, the manifestations can be divided according to their incidence and form.

The most common form of primary hypochondriasis is a simple preoccupation and false belief (conviction) regarding overall physical health. These patients complain that they suffer from some illness for which no basis can be found. Next, the disease takes the form of preoccupation and conviction in which these patients are experiencing pain or discomfort from some bodily organ or system. Again, no amount of physical or laboratory examination convinces them that they are well. The last, most serious and least common form, called monosymptomatic hypochondriasis, is usually confined to one organ or body system, and the symptoms are delusional or near delusional. Yet outside of this one delusional area the patient shows no evidence of mental deterioration or illness. Monosymptomatic hypochondriasis includes many diverse conditions such as intolerable pains in an organ or part of the body, unpleasant or offensive smells (olfactory paranoid syndrome), parasitic or other types of infections in the intestines, brain or other organs, dermatological hypochondriasis, dysmorphophobia and so forth. Dysmorphophobia is a term that describes patients who are convinced that in some respect they are physically misshapen and need corrective surgery.[84-87] All cases of hypochondriasis can be divided into one of these three forms.

In hypochondriasis, the most common bodily regions involved are—in descending order of occurrence—head and neck, abdomen, and chest. In bodily systems, the musculoskeletal is most commonly involved, followed by gastrointestinal, and central nervous systems. Incidentally, with those patients who have only unilateral symptoms (16%) one study found that 73% were left-sided.[88] Kenyon summarizes:

Although symptoms are mostly diffuse or generalized, one particular symptom or area of concern such as pain or disturbed sleep can present as the only complaint, and may well occupy the patient's whole attention and dominate his life. It can also be used to explain all the patient's difficulties, thus playing down any personal inadequacies. This monosymptomatic form can vary from a mild preoccupation to a frank delusion.[89]

The content of hypochondriacal complaints is also diffuse and varied with pain as a prominent symptom in about 70% of the cases. These pains can be in any part of the body and the vague muscular pains frequently are labeled "growing pains," "rheumatism," or "fibrositis." Other pains such as headaches, atypical facial pain, abdominal pain especially in children, and right iliac fossa pain in women are particularly common.[90]

The list of symptoms is endless and the extent to which these patients will go to remove them is legend. Those who suffer from disturbances in smell, be it smelling feces or urine, halitosis, or body odor, not only run to doctors for help but also support such commercial industries as advertising and cosmetics. They buy perfumes, body and vaginal deodorants, mouth washes, and so forth. Those who develop notions about their body appearance—the term dysmorphophobia is not recent, since it was introduced in 1886—not only support commercial enterprises by buying powders, facial creams, and what not but are also frequent patients of dermatologists and plastic surgeons. These physicians should be careful since performing certain procedures on a patient for cosmetic purposes when the problem is primarily psychiatric may lead to symptom substitution, suicide, or even the death of the physician at the hands of a dissatisfied patient. It should, however, be stressed that correction of skin blemishes, acne scars, nose, eyelids, neck, chin, face or some other part of the body such as baldness, or abnormal breasts can help certain individuals. It is the patient who has the problem that is important, not the problem or abnormality by itself; hence psychiatric consultation for these patients should be a common, instead of a rare referral by plastic surgeons or dermatologists. Those who suffer from disturbances in the sexual area such as undue concern for virility, sexual potency or adequacy, small size of penis, sexual orientation, menstrual difficulties, and so forth may also be more suitable for the psychiatrist than the endocrinologist, urologist, gynecologist, or plastic surgeon. Those complaints referable to the gastrointestinal or cardiovascular systems, ear, nose, throat, and eyes need no further elaboration since it would merely be repetitive of what was said regarding the other organ or bodily systems.[91]

In sum, hypochondriasis should be, more than any other disease, the meeting ground of physicians with different types of expertise. Instead physicians often use hypochondriasis as a wastebasket diagnosis, covering their ignorance while deprecating patients. This disease requires that psychiatrists know medicine, and that all other medical specialists including the general practitioner, know psychiatry. Since neither group exerts the effort necessary to acquire this knowledge, a gap exists. If this gap can be filled, medical and psychiatric practitioners would be taking a major step toward enhancing their fields and offering their patients better care. Respect among physicians and between physicians and patients would increase and all would benefit.

DIFFERENTIAL DIAGNOSIS

Hypochondriasis presents many problems to the physician. Distinguishing between complaints in which the major component is physical or psychogenic is difficult in itself and a hypochondriacal reaction to a physical illness compounds the problem immeasurably. Classifying hypochondriasis into primary and secondary groups, however, does help clarify not only diagnosis but also differential diagnosis.

Primary hypochondriasis has previously been distinguished from normal concern for health, and from secondary hypochondriasis. Normal individuals do have transitory periods of hypochondriacal symptoms. Since these symptoms disappear with medical evaluation and reassurance, the differential diagnosis offers little difficulty. Likewise with secondary hypochondriasis, the overall clinical picture will reveal whether or not the hypochondriacal symptoms are part of some other condition. In addition, primary hypochondriasis may exist in association with another condition but yet exist as an independent entity. Only clinical judgment can make these determinations.

Hypochondriasis is found in association with the following:

(1) Acute and chronic organic brain syndrome. In the former some toxic substance such as alcohol, cocaine, LSD, etc. has been ingested and in the latter hypochondriacal symptoms are associated with arteriosclerosis, senile dementia, trauma, tumors, central nervous system infections (syphilis, tuberculosis) and so forth. In the elderly, the relationship of the hypochondriac to his environment is particularly important. One study found that primary hypochondriasis was precipitated by a change in everyday routine in people who were relatively healthy. Secondary hypochondriasis was also precipitated by a change in the environment but these patients suffered from previous psychiatric illness usually neurotic depression, and an inhibited personality disorder. The authors thought that in secondary hypochondriasis the patients used hypochondriacal symptoms as an indirect way of communicating or signaling their distress and hostile feelings; hence, to them it is a disorder of interpersonal relationships.[92]

(2) Chronic pain syndrome (CPS). In this condition pain starts from a somatic illness, persists for at least six months, and is associated with environmental changes. Black says:

The victim of CPS suffers intractable, often multiple pain complaints, which are usually inappropriate to existing somatogenic problems; multiple physician contacts and many nonproductive diagnostic procedures; excessive preoccupation with the pain problem; and altered behavior pattern with some features of depression, anxiety, and neuroticism, and, in particular, no realistic plans for the distant future. This syndrome in its later stages is accompanied by excessive use of analgesic medication and multiple surgical procedures often demonstrating no clear organ pathology.

Chronic pain leads its victims to despair at the seeming uselessness and endlessness of this suffering. Sleep patterns are altered suggesting a primary disturbance of the circadian rhythm. Progressive physical and mental disability follow. Since pain is an acceptable affliction in our society and one especially worthy of sympathy, friends and family may act to sustain or even increase invalid behaviors by their well-meaning attention.

The chronic pain patient in search for help is exposed to the high risk of iatrogenic complications at the hands of well-meaning physicians.... Analgesic abuse, including narcotic addiction, is common .... surgery is a likely consequence .... some patients with CPS, in frantic desperate search for help, turn to quackery.[93]

The similarity to hypochondriasis is remarkable yet there are differences such as an initial physical illness and the presence of depression, anxiety, and neuroticism. In effect CPS starts from a clearly organic origin, e.g., muscle trigger points which lead to responses which are psychogenic in origin, and can result in invalidism.[94]

(3) Affective disorders. The most common condition associated with hypochondriasis is depression and for the most part both conditions are easily distinguishable. But with endogenous (psychotic) and masked depression some difficulty in differentiating the conditions is possible. Essentially psychotic depression may or may not be associated with manic-depressive psychosis and the somatic complaints are dry mouth, constipation, loss of appetite, weight loss, loss of sex drive, early morning awakening, lack of interest and energy, somatic delusions, poor concentration, guilt feelings, self-deprecation, and pessimism.[95] With masked depression, the depressive mood may be negligible and hidden by overt smiling and the appearance of a generalized well-being. Masked depression is manifested by a wide range of symptoms such as vague complaints of general ill-health; autonomic visceral symptoms involving all bodily systems; paraesthesias, altered states of sensation, and itching; various types of algias (headaches, backaches, musculoskeletal aches and pains); grinding teeth that results in temperomandibular joint pain; throat clearing; intolerance to certain foods; aerophagia with bloating; and so forth. The patient who suffers from masked depression can be characterized, in general, as suffering from algias,

belching and bloating, hyperventilation, and cardiovascular manifestations such as paroxysmal ventricular contractions.[96]

(4) Anxiety and phobic neuroses. Since anxiety and phobia are no part of the hypochondriacal neurosis, there should be little problem in distinguishing these conditions. Anxiety neurosis however, is frequently associated with hypochondriacal symptoms but usually anxiety is the primary condition.

(5) Hysterical neurosis, conversion type. Hysterical symptoms can be part of other mental illnesses (depression, hysterical personality trait, depersonalization, etc.) so one must be cautious in making the diagnosis of hysteria. Hysteria is associated with disturbances of voluntary innervation which do not follow known anatomical pathways. It has such symptoms as paralysis and tics, usually characterized by *"la belle indifférence,"* and the hysteric seeks sympathy and attention usually by dramatic displays.[97]

(6) Psychoses with somatic delusions. This includes affective, schizophrenic, and paranoid groupings. Primarily these conditions have to be distinguished from monosymptomatic hypochondriasis and in full-blown cases the differentiation is not difficult; however, hypochondriacal preoccupations can be a prodromal stage of schizophrenia. Yet with the paranoid patient an intriguing question arises. Since basically the conviction of a bodily illness without organic basis is a false belief or a delusion a quandary is present. Is hypochondriasis a form of paranoid psychosis in which the delusion is focused on the body instead of on the outside world? Kenyon posits:

> It is not surprising, with these inherent difficulties in diagnosis and definition, that divergent views exist as to the co-existence and inter-relationship of paranoid and hypochondriacal symptoms. Most authors think their occurrence with paranoid psychosis to be rare, as the essential psychopathology here is based on projection; symptoms are not seen as emanating from the body but as due to external influences.[98]

Although hypochondriasis and paranoid conditions are two distinct entities, they both take the form of delusion but only differ in the content or object of their delusion. There must be more connection between the two than just this and future research will have to find the answer.

(7) Malingering. The only way to differentiate this condition from any disease in which somatic symptoms are a major consideration is to "catch the scoundrel in the act." That is, to observe the malingerer performing an activity for which he claims disability. Hypochondriacs, in contrast, would not attempt to perform an activity which involves the area of functioning that they are convinced is diseased. For instance, the malingerer who claims that he cannot work because of backaches and hip pains, may be seen fully active in a bowling alley. This would not be so with the hypochondriac.

(8)   Psychosomatic or psychophysiological disorders.   These are imprecise synonymous terms for which the definition can be restricted to a limited number of diseases that are mediated through the autonomic nervous system.   This generally includes peptic ulcer, bronchial asthma, essential hypertension, irritable colon (colitis), migraine headaches, and so forth.   If the term is used in this narrow sense differentiation between it and hypochondriasis becomes a simple matter.   However, in the broad sense of mind-body, psychosoma, or psycho-physiological the problem becomes an extremely complex and debatable issue and beyond the scope of this discussion.

COURSE AND PROGNOSIS

Acute and subacute hypochondriasis have relatively short courses; hence prognosis is good.   Chronic hypochondriasis can lead to invalidism; hence generally the prognosis is bad.   Of course with secondary hypochondriasis the course and prognosis is directly related to the primary condition.   However, in general, the presence of hypochondriasis as part of another syndrome seems to make the prognosis worse for the primary condition.   For example, depressed patients with hypochondriacal symptoms have a poorer prognosis than those without hypochondriacal symptoms.   Not much is really known about prognosis in hypochondriasis.[99]

Some of the isolated data are the following:

(1)   Generally suicide in hypochondriacal patients is low and some claim this even when associated with depression; however, suicide has been found in association with primary and monosymptomatic hypochondriasis.[100]

(2)   In general hypochondriacs have the worst prognosis of any of the neurotic group and males have a worse prognosis than females who suffer from primary hypochondriasis.[101, 102]

(3)   One study with the elderly found that patients with primary hypo-chondriasis had a uniformly good prognosis while those patients with secondary hypochondriasis did not have as uniform nor as good a prognosis.[103]

TREATMENT

Treatment is directed toward the primary condition and diagnosis should be made as soon as possible.   Distinguishing primary from secondary hypochondriasis is an absolute prerequisite and once hypochondriasis is confirmed, the patient should be informed of the physician's findings and further somatic investigation stopped.   With this understanding, both patient and physician are in a better position to proceed with the various types of available treatments.

With secondary hypochondriasis, treatment is directed towards the pri-mary condition and the psychiatrist proceeds accordingly.   With primary hypochondriasis, treatment progresses as a continuous process from the frank discussion of the findings in the diagnostic evaluation to a treatment plan. The plan should outline goals and inform the patient of what possible procedures seem advisable.

A therapeutic relationship begins to develop as the psychiatrist explains his overall approach that begins with the more simple techniques and proceeds to the more complex ones. The psychiatrist should point out to the patient that symptom removal is not the only goal. The psychiatrist aids the patient in understanding his relationships with family, friends, and fellow employees. The psychiatrist's goal is to keep the patient functioning on all these levels and hopefully to engender improvement. In addition the psychiatrist may wish to see the family either alone or with the patient and explain to them his diagnosis, goals, and approach. The hope is to gain family cooperation and to direct them in what approach to take in their dealings with the patient. Another person with whom the psychiatrist must maintain open communication is the family physician. Even hypochondriacs get physically ill and when questions of organicity arise the psychiatrist needs the physician to direct him. Likewise, the family physician needs the psychiatrist so as to be in a better position to handle whatever problems come up. Frequently the family physician's knowledge of the interrelationships within the family is invaluable to the psychiatrist as is the psychiatrist's reporting new or old somatic complaints to the family physician. With all this as ground work, the psychiatrist is in a better position to make such recommendations as environmental changes, be it at home or on the job.

Psychotherapy proceeds and as with all mentally disturbed patients the psychiatrist is prepared for difficulties and hardship. Mistrust and disdain does not have to develop if everything is in the open and both patient and psychiatrist recognize that each is doing his best against a very tough disease and against the odds that symptoms will ever remit completely. But symptoms may decrease. If not, other areas of the patient's life may still improve. Of course the patient wants relief and the doctor cannot offer a cure. Hostility and anger may arise but the psychiatrist must do his best and attempt to develop and maintain a therapeutic environment.

The physician should be accepting of the patient and his disease—not only accepting but also noncritical. He should not mock or deprecate the patient, his complaints, or his attitudes. Certainly, the patient's suffering should not be ridiculed. Within this framework the physician attempts to help the patient to understand himself and others better. An often unrecognized peripheral fringe benefit is that psychotherapy can prevent these patients from becoming victims of quacks and sure cure treatment prophets.

When psychotherapy is ineffective other methods should be tried. Behavior modification techniques can be tried or any other approach that may facilitate the patient's ability to cope. These techniques may help relieve or remove the symptoms. Drugs can be most beneficial: sedatives and hypnotics for anxiety, antidepressants for depression, tranquilizers for schizophrenia, and so on. Where all methods fail, and the case is very severe and of long duration, one of the newer forms of prefrontal leucotomy may be considered. This form of treatment should be considered only in very rare and selected cases.[104, 105]

There are several special situations which need discussion.

(1) Recently reports have been appearing that a neuroleptic drug, diphe-nylbutylpiperidine, Pimozide, whose main value is for treating schizophrenic patients who show marked inertia and apathy, is effective in the treatment of monosymptomatic hypochondriasis. Although this drug has only been tested on a small group of patients, the results are initially encouraging. The dosage is 2–6 mg daily, given in one dose in the morning. The authors' claim that the drug works irrespective of whether the monosymptomatic hypochondriasis is associated with schizophrenia, depression, or some other mental conditions; however, it does not work when dysmorphophobia is based on a neurotic personality and not a psychotic delusion.[106]

(2) In working with elderly hypochondriacal patients one investigator found that those who suffered from primary hypochondriasis responded well to weekly 20 minute structured interviews with a 5 minute telephone call between sessions. Besides this the patients were given one nonthreatening task to accomplish and when accomplished the patient was praised by the therapist. Conversely, with elderly patients with secondary hypochondriasis in which there was significant depression and other mental illnesses this technique did not work. Hospitaliza-tion, EST, antidepressant drugs with or without tranquilizers, structured ward situations, continued day care programs, and family therapy were used. The authors emphasize that hypochondriacs should not be treated in isolation from their families and immediate environment. They think that for treatment to be successful the family should be involved.[107]   In another study with elderly patients who had hypochondriacal symptoms associated with organic brain syndrome, it was found that a regimen of psychotherapy and anticoagulant drugs was effective in treating the hypochondriacal symptoms. The authors concluded that with organic brain syndrome the patient's ability to adapt was impaired and that by decreasing anxiety with psychotherapy and increasing cerebral blood flow with anticoagulants an effective method for treating hypo-chondriasis in the elderly was available.[108]

(3) Hypochondriacs frequently suffer from severe pain and in recent years special pain clinics have been established to evaluate and treat pain from a comprehensive viewpoint, i.e., organic, psychiatric, psychological, cultural, and social. Treatments include psychotherapy, milieu and family therapy, physiotherapy, relaxation exercises, biofeedback, drugs, acupuncture, cold applications, weight reduction, local anesthetics, nerve blocks, sympathetic blocks, other neurosurgical procedures, and so forth.[109–111]   This approach,

developed for those who suffer from chronic pain syndromes and intractable pain, could have applicability for those hypochondriacs whose pain is a persistent and predominant symptom.

REFERENCES

1. Thomas, K.B., Temporarily dependent patient in general practice. *Brit. Med. J.* 1:625–626 (1974).
2. Kenyon, F.E., Hypochondriacal states. *Brit. J. Psychiatry* 129:1 (1976).
3. Pilowsky, I., Dimensions of hypochondriasis. *Brit. J. Psychiatry* 113:89–93 (1967).
4. Pilowsky, I., Primary and secondary hypochondriasis. *Acta. Psychiat. Scand.* 46:274 (1970).
5. Idzorek, S., A functional classification of hypochondriasis with specific recommendations for treatment. *Southern Med. J.* 68(11):1326 (1975).
6. Black, R.G., The chronic pain syndrome. *Surgical Clinics North America* 55(4):999 (1975).
7. Nakahama, H., Pain mechanisms in the central nervous system. *Int. Anesthesiol. Clin.* 13(1):109–110 (1975).
8. Ibid., pp. 110–111.
9. Jerva, M., Zavola, G., and Umoren, D., Transcutaneous neurostimulation. *Proc. Inst. Med. Chgo.* 31(2):35 (1976).
10. Ibid.
11. Nathan, P.W. and Rudge, P., Testing the gate-control theory of pain in man. *J. Neuro. Neurosurg. Psychiatry* 37:1366 (1974).
12. Bond, M.R., The relation of pain to the Eysenck personality inventory, Cornell medical index and Whiteley index of hypochondriasis. *Brit. J. Psychiatry* 119:671 (1971).
13. Pos, R., Psychological assessment of factors affecting pain. *Can. Med. Assoc. J.* 3:1213–1215 (1974).
14. Bond, M.R., op. cit., pp. 671–678.
15. Rangell, L., Psychiatric aspects of pain. *Psychosom. Med.* 15:22–37 (1953).
16. Guze, S.B., "Differential diagnosis of the borderline personality syndrome," in *Borderline States in Psychiatry* (edited by Mack, E.). New York: Grune & Stratton, 1975, pp. 69–74.
17. Hippocrates, *The Theory and Practice of Medicine* (Introduction by Kelly, E.C.). New York: Citadel Press, 1964, p. 307.
18. Burton, R., *The Anatomy of Melancholy* (edited by Dell, F. and Jordan-Smith, P.). New York: Tudor, 1927, pp. 151–153.
19. Ibid., p. 323.
20. Ibid., pp. 350–351.
21. Ibid., p. 351.
22. Veith, I., *Hysteria: The History of a Disease.* Chicago: University of Chicago Press, 1965, p. 144.
23. Fischer-Homberger, E., Hypochondriasis of the eighteenth century–neurosis of the present century. *Bull. Hist. Med.* 46(4):391 (1972).
24. Ibid., pp. 391–392.
25. Ibid., pp. 392–394.

26. Shoenberg, P.J., A dialogue with Mandeville. *Brit. J. Psychiatry* **129**:120–124 (1976).
27. Muncie, W., *Psychobiology and Psychiatry: A Textbook of Normal and Abnormal Human Behavior.* St. Louis: Mosby, 1939, p. 564.
28. "Hypochondriasis," in *The Encyclopaedia Britannica,* 13th ed., vol. 14.   New York: Encyclopaedia Britannica, 1926, p. 207.
29. Fischer-Homberger, E., op. cit., pp. 395–396.
30. Ribot, T., *The Diseases of Personality.* Chicago: Open Court, 1895, p. 53.
31. Fischer-Homberger, E., op. cit., p. 397.
32. Gillespie, R.D., Hypochondria: Its definition, nosology and psychopathology. *Guys Hosp. Rep.* 78:408–412 (1928).
33. Bleuler, E., *Textbook of Psychiatry* (authorized English ed. by Brill, A.A.).   London: George Allen and Unwin, 1923, p. 163.
34. Brown, F., The bodily complaint: A study of hypochondriasis. *J. Med. Sciences* **82**:295–300 (1936).
35. Ibid., p. 300.
36. Pilowsky, I., Abnormal illness behavior. *Brit. J. Med. Psychol.* **42**:347–351 (1969).
37. Dewsbury, A.R., Hypochondriasis and disease-claiming behavior in general practice. *J. Roy. Coll. Gen. Pract.* **23**:379–383 (1973).
38. Bianchi, G.N., McElwain, D.W., and Cawte, J.E., The dispensary syndrome in Australian aborigines: Origins of their bodily preoccupation and sick role behavior. *Brit. J. Med. Psychol.* **43**:375–382 (1970).
39. Cooke, A., Hypochondria: The layman's specialty. *J. Roy. Coll. Phys. London* **7**:285–286 (1973).
40. Ibid., p. 287.
41. Ibid.
42. Ibid., pp. 277–290.
43. Dorfman, W., Hypochondriasis–revisited: A dilemma and challenge to medicine and psychiatry. *Psychosomatics* **16**:14–16 (1975).
44. Idzorek, S., op. cit., pp. 1326–1332.
45. Bianchi, G.N., Patterns of hypochondriasis: A principal components analysis. *Brit. J. Psychiatry* **122**:541–548 (1973).
46. Mayou, R., The nature of bodily symptoms. *Brit. J. Psychiatry* **129**:55–60 (1976).
47. Kenyon, F.E., op. cit., p. 11.
48. Pilowsky, I., Primary and secondary hypochondriasis, op. cit., p. 281.
49. Kenyon, F.E., op. cit., pp. 3–4.
50. Pilowsky, I., Primary and secondary hypochondriasis, op. cit., pp. 282–283.
51. Idzorek, S., op. cit., p. 1327.
52. Nemiah, J.C., "Hypochondriacal neurosis," in *The Comprehensive Textbook of Psychiatry/II,* vol. 1 (edited by Freedman, A.M., Kaplan, H.I., and Sadock, B.J.). Baltimore: Williams & Wilkins, 1976, p. 1274.
53. Provisional classification: Published as a looseleaf manual entitled *DSM-III Draft,* 4/15/77.   DRAFT OF AXES I and II of DSM-III CLASSIFICATION as of March 30, 1977.
54. Bianchi, G.N., op. cit., p. 546.
55. Pilowsky, I., Primary and secondary hypochondriasis, op. cit., p. 276.
56. Brown, F., op. cit., p. 308.
57. Mead, B.T., Management of hypochondriacal patients. *Postgrad. Med.* **52**:109(1972).
58. Gillespie, R.D., op. cit., p. 417.
59. Kenyon, F.E., op. cit., p. 7.

60. Slater, E. and Roth, M., *Clinical Psychiatry*.   Baltimore: Williams & Wilkins, 1970, p. 142.
61. Burns, B.H. and Nichols, M.A., Factors related to the localization of symptoms to the chest in depression. *Brit. J. Psychiatry* 121:405–409 (1972).
62. Slater, E. and Roth, M., op. cit., p. 142.
63. Ibid., p. 141.
64. Kolb, L., Psychiatric aspects of treatment of the painful phantom limb. *Med. Rec. Ann. Houston* 46(12):370–374 (1952).
65. Smith, J., Hypochondriasis: Symptom or entity. *Psychosomatics* 11:413–415 (1970).
66. Mechanic, D., Social psychological factors affecting the presentation of bodily complaints. *N. Engl. J. Med.* 286(21):1132 (1972).
67. Dorfman, W., op. cit., p. 15.
68. Palmer, R.D. and Broverman, D.M., Automatization and hypochondriasis. *J. Personality* 37:592–600 (1969).
69. Ibid.
70. Rockwell, D.A., Psychiatric residents' disease: Social system contributions to residents' emotional problems. *Int. J. Soc. Psychiatry* 19:226–229 (1973).
71. Mechanic, D., op. cit., p. 1133.
72. Ibid., p. 1135.
73. Gillespie, R.D., op. cit., pp. 417–420.
74. Fenichel, O., *The Psychoanalytic Theory of Neurosis*.   New York: Norton, 1945, p. 261.
75. Ibid., p. 262.
76. Alexander, F., *Fundamentals of Psychoanalysis*.   New York: Norton, 1948, pp. 232–234.
77. Ibid., p. 233.
78. Lipsitt, D.R., Psychodynamic considerations of hypochondriasis. *Psychother. Psychosom.* 23:132–141 (1974).
79. Rittelmeyer, Jr., L.F., Caring for the hypochondriac. *Amer. Fam. Physician* 14(3): 99 (1976).
80. Goldstein, S.E. and Birnbom, F., Hypochondriasis and the elderly. *J. Amer. Geriatric Soc.* 24(1):150 (1976).
81. Rittelmeyer, Jr., L.F., op. cit., p. 100.
82. Cowan, J., The hypochondriacal patient in the physician's office. *Ill. Med. J.* 139:68 (1971).
83. Idzorek, S., op. cit., pp. 1329–1330.
84. Riding, J. and Munro, A., Pimozide in the treatment of monosymptomatic hypochondriacal psychosis. *Acta. Psychiat. Scand.* 52(1):23–30 (1975).
85. Bebbington, P.E., Monosymptomatic hypochondriasis, abnormal illness behaviour and suicide. *Brit. J. Psychiatry* 128:475–478 (1976).
86. Reilly, T.M. and Beard, A.W., Correspondence: Monosymptomatic hypochondriasis. *Brit. J. Psychiatry* 129:191–192 (1976).
87. Riding, B.E.J. and Munro, A., Letter: Pimozide in monosymptomatic psychosis. *Lancet* 1(7903):400–401 (Feb. 15, 1975).
88. Kenyon, F.E., op. cit., p. 4.
89. Ibid., pp. 4–5.
90. Ibid., p. 5.
91. Ibid., pp. 5–7.
92. Goldstein, S.E and Birnbom, F., op. cit., pp. 151–154.

93. Black, R.G., op. cit., pp. 1000–1001.
94. Pace, J.B., Commonly overlooked pain syndromes responsive to simple therapy. *Postgrad. Med.* **58**(4):107–113 (1975).
95. Pilowsky, I., Primary and secondary hypochondriasis, op. cit., p. 277.
96. Rome, H., The many faces of depression. *Med. Opinion:* 14–20 (May 1975).
97. Gillespie, R.D., op. cit., pp. 414–415.
98. Kenyon, F.E., op. cit., p. 10.
99. Ibid.
100. Bebbington, P.E., op. cit., pp. 476–477.
101. Pilowsky, I., Primary and secondary hypochondriasis, op. cit., p. 280.
102. Smith, J., op. cit., p. 414.
103. Goldstein, S.E. and Birnbom, F., op. cit., p. 153.
104. Mechanic, D., op. cit., pp. 1138–1139.
105. Kenyon, F.E., op. cit., pp. 10–11.
106. Riding, J. and Munro, A., op. cit., pp. 28–29.
107. Goldstein, S.E. and Birnbom, F., op. cit., pp. 151–154.
108. Walsh, A.C., Hypochondriasis associated with organic brain syndrome: A new approach to therapy. *J. Amer. Geriatric Soc.* **24**(9):430–431 (1976).
109. Black, R.G., op. cit., pp. 999–1011.
110. Pilowsky, I., The psychiatrist and the pain clinic. *Amer. J. Psychiatry* **133**(7): 752–756 (1976).
111. Mennell, J.M., The therapeutic use of cold. *J. Amer. Osteopathic Assoc.* **74**:1146–1158 (1975).

12
TREATMENT

Psychiatric treatment is rooted in such diverse orientations that at times the psychiatrists who espouse one viewpoint do not even share a common language with those who advocate other doctrines. Some view psychiatry totally within the framework of medicine; therefore, to them mental illness is a behavioral disturbance caused by a known or, possibly, suggested biological disturbance. Thus treatment consists primarily of drugs, surgery, and physical methods. To this group, psychotherapy is applicable only for selected patients.[1] Besides, psychotherapy "could be administered just as effectively by a psychologist or social worker either independently or under the physician's direction."[2] This view regarding the role of psychotherapy in psychiatric practice and the administrator of psychotherapy has resulted in endless controversy among mental health professionals. It is reminiscent of the old debates that theologians, philosophers, and physicians carried on as to which group was best qualified to treat diseases of the soul.[3] It reflects a viewpoint opposed to those psychiatrists who are identified with psychological or sociological models of mental illness to whom psychotherapeutic intervention—individual, family, conjoint, group, community, or sociological methods—is the proper role of psychiatry.[4-7]

An intermediary approach to treatment between the "scientific" medical and introspective psychological and social models of treatment is behavior therapy. These therapists use specialized techniques that are not introspective but yet can be administered either through psychological or biological methods.[8] Besides these types of therapy there are those who advocate milieu,[9] biofeedback,[10] electrosleep,[11] general systems,[12] and numerous others.[13] Bertram S. Brown,[14] former Director of the National Institute of Mental Health, who does not deny that he practices "political psychiatry" writes:

The interface between psychiatry and social systems is an area in which psychiatry has in some ways overpromised. This interface is the site of hope for integrating prevention efforts with social concerns, for integrating scientific knowledge with humanistic concerns, and, in my opinion, it is a proper domain of psychiatry.[15]

Yet at the same time (May 1976), Judd Marmor in his Presidential Address before the American Psychiatric Association said:

> I have placed considerable emphasis on the developments that have been taking place in the areas of neurophysiology, neurochemistry, and psychopharmacology. But I would like to add a word of caution: we must not allow our growing awareness of the biological component in mental illness to lead us to a depreciation of psychodynamic and sociocultural determinants, causality is hardly ever lineal and almost always multifactorial. The expectation, so often cultivated in the news media, that some day all mental illness will be curable by drugs is a simplistic fantasy that fails to take into account the multifactorial elements in the genesis of mental illness. Our efforts at the primary prevention of mental disorders . . . will always have to be made on a variety of fronts—genetic, biochemical, familial, interpersonal, and sociocultural.[16]

Marmor expresses the comprehensive viewpoint and seeks to identify the role of psychiatry as a balance between the biological organism on one side and the psychosocial human being on the other side. The treatment methods would then fall within the four aspects of the total person, that is constitutional (hereditary and personality), physical (body type and pathology), psychological, and current life situational stressors.

GOALS AND PRINCIPLES OF THERAPY

The purposes of treatment are to relieve or diminish pain and discomfort, improve function, and remove whatever causes the disturbance. Unfortunately, all these goals cannot often be attained, so physicians compromise. The internist is satisfied to maintain the chronic heart patient in cardiac compensation, to control the hypertensive patient within certain limits of blood pressure, and to regulate the diabetic patient's blood sugar level. The physician knows he cannot "cure" these patients but he can treat them; thereby, helping the patient function within a greater range of normality than would otherwise be true. Even in terminal cancer cases the physician will treat the patient with whatever means he can to relieve the discomfort and pain. Most physicians concentrate on the area of "patient comfort" rather than "patient cure" unless the infectious disease process is involved. Psychiatrists, likewise, direct their efforts toward similar goals. Psychiatry, however, since its results are not easily amenable to scientific investigation, cannot make the same claims of success as other medical specialties.

Therefore, psychiatry is regarded as more of an art than all the others. But psychiatrists, like all medical doctors, combine their personality, morality, and scientific knowledge to treat and prevent disease. Hence, psychiatrists have similar methods, goals, values, and ethics.[17]

There is no known method of altering constitutional diseases once they are established. This refers not only to physical hereditary traits and characteristics, but also to personality traits and characteristics directly transmitted by genes and chromosomes. Hence, therapy is limited to physical and psychological methods, and to environmental readjustments.

Physical methods of treatment include drugs that replace a deficient substance (niacin in pellegra), reduce pain (analgesics or narcotics), ameliorate abnormal behavior (tranquilizers or sedatives), and so forth; surgery; insulin, electroconvulsive treatments, etc. The methods are not mutually exclusive. A disease thought to arise primarily from a psychological etiology does not have to be treated exclusively by psychological methods and, likewise, one arising primarily from organic causes does not have to be treated exclusively by physical methods. Sleepless or anxious patients in the midst of a tumultuous divorce may benefit from tranquilizers and hypnotics as well as from psychotherapy. Patients suffering from ulcerative colitis, organic brain disease, or terminal cancer may benefit from psychotherapy as well as from drugs or surgery. The psychiatrist must be in a position to use or to recommend all or any combination of treatments.

The psychiatrist's evaluation of the patient should include some notion of the patient's pre-illness condition and potential. Treatment cannot provide potentials that were never possessed or replace potentials lost through organic changes. Recognition by the psychiatrist of the patient's limitations, both past and present, is essential. These limitations are carefully evaluated during the planning stage of therapy. The degree of adjustment the patient can be expected to accomplish should be realistically determined.

Prompt attention and symptomatic relief are desirable objectives. Treatment should be started as soon as possible since delays can result in secondary gains, chronicity, or secondary reactions. For example, patients with a myocardial infarction can become psychological cripples who may refuse to work, socialize, or participate in any activity that they feel will strain the heart. Likewise, panic reactions, if not promptly relieved, can develop into chronic anxiety neurosis. These superimposed symptoms can occur in all mental or physical illnesses and the physician should be on guard for such reactions. Immediate care, assisting the patient in maintaining usual routines of life, work and social activities, can often avoid expensive and prolonged hospitalization.

Acutely disturbed, suicidal, or homicidal patients may need hospitalization— possibly a lifesaving procedure. Hospitalization arises most commonly with the following: suicidal depressions; panic anxiety attacks; manic, paranoid, confused, or delirious patients who have lost sufficient contact with the environment; situations in which the home or family mitigates against treatment; and those patients who need extensive physical evaluations for a possible organic basis for mental illness.

As a rule the shorter the hospital stay the better. Hospitalization can hinder and perpetuate rather than alleviate the patient's resolution of his problems. It can increase the complexity of the psychiatrist's work by providing a cocoon for the patient and decreasing the patient's ability to cope with the outside world. Recognizing this, psychiatrists in the past 20 years have made extensive efforts to lower the number of patients in mental institutions.[18]

There is a great deal of confusion and disagreement regarding the basic postulates of psychopathology. Davis writes:

> Psychopathology, a branch of science, is that part of psychology which seeks to explain disorders of behavior, including those of mental activity, in terms of psychological processes. Psychotherapy, a form of treatment, applies psychopathological knowledge in modifying the attitudes and behavior of patients.[19]

This implies that psychopathology is a science and its application by psychotherapeutic methods can be scientific. Karl Jaspers is much more cautious in his assertions and he says:

> *Psychopathology is limited* in that there can be no final analysis of human beings as such, since the more we reduce them to what is typical and normative the more we realize there is something hidden in every human individual which defies recognition. We have to be content with partial knowledge of an infinity which we cannot exhaust, as a person, not as a psychopathologist, one may well see more; and, if others see more which is exceptional and unique, we should refrain from letting this interfere with our psychopathology .... It has often been emphasized that psychiatry is still an 'expertise' and has not yet reached the status of science. Science calls for systematic, conceptual thinking which can be communicated to others. Only in so far as psychopathology does this can it claim to be regarded as a science. What in psychiatry is just expertise and art can never be accurately formulated and can at best be mutually sensed by another colleague.[20]

Jaspers' views reinforce the belief that psychiatric treatment should be pragmatic and utilize multiple, broad, and varied approaches.

Treatment, an art, utilizes as much scientific knowledge as possible. The art is learned in its technical aspects and applied by the therapist within intuitive, experiential, and intellectual limitations. The recognition of these limits serves as a constant reminder of certain facts.   First, history reveals innumerable methods of treatment that were thought to be useful but could not stand the test of time.   Trepanning for epilepsy, bloodletting for mania, magnetism for weak nerves, and animal food for diabetes are several examples.[21]   Second, today's treatment may be tomorrow's curiosity.   Physicians can—as patients do—give testimonials for the efficacy of a type of treatment and be totally wrong.   Caution should be exercised in drawing conclusions based solely on clinical experience.   For example, depressive illnesses when untreated have spontaneous remissions, yet the physician and patient will attribute the "cure" to innumerable treatment methods.   Isolating a specific factor which is responsible for the cure requires the strictest of scientific methods and, in psychiatry, the complexity of behavior does not lend itself to such isolation of variables.   Third, unprejudiced observation and evaluation of successes as well *as failures* need to be reported.   Too often observations are not valid, negative results are not reported, and conclusions are mere speculation.   None of this negates the value of clinical observations, often the initiators of important advances; however, clinical observations need verification by scientific methods of validation before they are accepted.   In summary, psychiatrists must distinguish unproven treatment methods from those which are scientifically proven, and must exercise the utmost of caution during treatment.

Any physician and particularly psychiatrists should be informed of all prevailing methods of treatment and not limit his knowledge to any one specific modality.   This is equally true for biological, psychological, or sociological dogmatists since their limitations may inhibit or prevent the patient's recovery. Yet psychiatrists who limit their practice to a single form of treatment can, at times be helpful and their expertise should be utilized.   But the general psychiatrist is best suited to determine the treatment the patient needs; not the specialized practitioner who lacks a broad base.   The general psychiatrist may treat or refer a patient to the psychoanalyst, hypnotist, psychopharmacologist, behavior therapist, existentialist, and so on.   Only he is in a position to make such referrals since it is difficult for the individual dedicated to a single mode of treatment to make an unprejudiced judgment.   Personal financial gain may also influence judgment.   It seems prudent, therefore, to recommend that psychiatric training be broadly based.   This might help eliminate dogmatism, increase communication among the various schools of psychiatry, and better prepare those psychiatrists who become dedicated to one mode of treatment to appreciate their modality in an overall perspective.

HISTORY

The social aspects of treatment can be divided into four periods.   The first period involved the humane reforms that resulted from man's desire for political freedom.   As a consequence of the spirit of equality, fraternity, and liberty during the French Revolution the mentally ill were given the right to have fresh air, good food, and a clean place to live.   The second period shifted to England around 1837 with the abolition of such mechanical restraints as chains, handcuffs, and other bindings.   The third period, the hospital period, received its greatest impetus in the 1840s from Dorothea Lynde Dix (1802-1887), an American who championed the cause for improved treatment and suitable mental institutions.   In the United States this movement eventually led to a system of state hospitals which, by 1955, housed approximately 550,000 people.   The fourth period, the community period, has been established within the past 20 years.[22, 23]

Within 20 years—from 1955 to 1975—the number of hospitalized patients decreased to an estimated 220,000.   Although drugs were important in bringing about the decrease in hospitalized patients, they were not the only factor.   The social climate in the United States had also changed as people became more tolerant of the mentally ill and psychiatrists and politicians responded to this change in attitude.   Patients were discharged to halfway houses, old hotels, their families, or whatever facilities would accept them.   There are now community outpatient mental health centers, day centers, night centers, rehabilitation centers, and so on.   The return of the patient to the community has unfortunately, not eliminated abuses.[24]   What the future holds is unknown.   Who knows what will happen to psychiatry or medicine with government controls, peer review, and third party payment?   Are we returning to a period of inhumane treatment?[25, 26]

Advances in psychiatric therapy in the twentieth century have been remarkable.   These advances have occurred in every treatment modality and only major contributors and their work can be discussed in this synopsis.   Much progress has been made in the study of genetics in recent years.   Yet, for the most part, treatment is limited to counseling patients regarding heredity and prenatal and postnatal diagnostic techniques.[27]

Sir Francis Galton (1822-1911), a cousin of Charles Darwin, coined the term "eugenics" and in 1904 established the first eugenic laboratory.[28]   Galton believed that the human race could be improved by selective breeding and the unfit could be prevented from reproducing.   Of course this led to moral and ethical difficulties as well as to the problem of determining the exact nature of the "ideal" person.   An individual might have a brilliant mind and a frail body, thereby, offering the eugenicist a dilemma as to which trait to preserve.[29]   The problem of eugenics is a biological, psychological, political, and social one.   It has implications for abortion, euthanasia, and even definitions of life or death.   That, however, is beyond the scope of this discussion.[30]   But, there are certain hereditary diseases that, if left untreated, can cause mental deficiency, and this is our proper concern.

Phenylketonuria, a disease caused by an inborn error in metabolism is an example of a hereditary disease that when treated can prevent the development of mental deficiency. It was first described by Fölling in 1934 when he noticed that the urine of children suffering from this disease had an odd smell.[31] Investigation led to the discovery that these children lacked a liver enzyme, phenylalanine hydroxylase, that converts the amino acid phenylalanine to tyrosine. Phenylalanine hydroxylase is manufactured by a gene. The absence of this gene (enzyme) results in the accumulation of phenylalanine in the blood and spinal fluid. High levels of phenylalanine interfere with the development and functioning of the brain. When this condition is allowed to persist and progress, severe mental deficiency develops.

Phenylketonuria is diagnosed in the nursery by examination of the urine for phenylpyruvic acid and of the plasma for elevated L-phenylalanine. Once the disease is diagnosed, treatment consists of eliminating phenylalanine from the diet by a special protein hydrolysate that lowers the phenylalanine in the plasma and eliminates phenylpyruvic acid from the urine. Mental deficiency can thereby be prevented; hence, phenylketonuria, a genetic disease, accounting for about 1% of institutionalized mental defectives (or one in every 10,000 births in the United States), can be treated.[32] There are inherited diseases that are treatable but Durell, referring to mental illness writes:

It has naturally been the hope of investigations in biological psychiatry that within the syndromes of concern to psychiatry (e.g., schizophrenia) cases would be found that were manifestations of genetically determined enzyme defects. To date, outside the area of mental retardation, simple enzyme defects have not been found; and modern genetic theory would not predict that enzyme defects need necessarily be found in adults manifesting genetic disorders.[33]

The search for diagnosis and treatment by means of hereditary methods continues and offers possibilities and hope for progress toward understanding mental illness.

Those who employ physical treatment for mental illness assume that mental disease is, at least in part, an illness of either the structure or function of bodily tissues. The problem can exist within the molecule, cell, organ, complex neuroendocrine biochemical imbalances, or can result from infection or degeneration. The multiplicity of supposed etiologies has led to the great variety of physical treatments.

Julius Wagner Von Jauregg (1857-1940), a Nobel laureate in medicine (1927), began the malarial treatment of general paresis in 1917. This followed the work of Hideyo Noguchi (1876-1928) and Moore who in 1913 established *Treponema pallidum* as the cause of syphilis and paresis.[34] Von Jauregg demonstrated that patients with general paresis and afflicted with erysipelas, had remissions from their illness. He thought fever was the cause of the remission and administered the old tuberculin injections, typhus vaccine, and malaria tertiana. He found that malaria worked best and that 75% of the general paresis cases diagnosed early were cured. This advance, occurring during a time when general paresis invariably ended in death, encouraged doctors to believe that some other types of psychoses could also be treated. Later, malarial treatment was replaced by electrically induced fever, and today by antibiotics.[35]

Pellegra is a disease characterized by dermatitis on areas exposed to sunlight, inflammation of mucosal surfaces, confusion, hallucinations and other mental symptoms. In 1925 Joseph Goldberger (1874-1929) demonstrated that this disease occurred in patients subsisting on a faulty diet (insufficient supply of niacin and its precursor tryptophan) and that proper diet could effect a cure.[36, 37] The discoveries of the spirochete in general paresis and the deficiency of a vitamin in pellegra are two of the outstanding examples of defining a psychiatric disorder by description, establishing an etiological disease entity, and prescribing specific therapeutic measures that cure or stop the progression of the disease. These diseases also demonstrate that once an organic etiology is determined the psychiatrist ceases to treat these patients.

The history of functional psychoses abounds in diverse treatment methods. In 1921 Jacob Kläsi (1883-?) introduced prolonged sleep. The patient under the influence of barbiturates could be kept sleeping for weeks. Sleep therapy resembled the rest cure treatment of S. Weir Mitchell and at times it showed similar success.[38] In 1927 Manfred Sakel (1900-1957) introduced subcoma insulin for the treatment of morphine withdrawal and shortly thereafter developed insulin coma therapy for the treatment of schizophrenia.[39] He thought the excitement of morphine withdrawal and schizophrenic excitement were both due to an excess of adrenalin; hence insulin, an antagonist of adrenalin, could influence both conditions. In 1933 Sakel published his findings concerning insulin treatment in schizophrenia.[40] In 1934 Ladislas J. Von Meduna (1896-1964) introduced cardiazol (metrazol) shock treatment. He noted that patients during insulin treatment sometimes had epileptic fits and he reasoned, wrongly, that the fits rather than the insulin coma cured the schizophrenic patient. Von Meduna also believed, incorrectly, that epileptics did not become schizophrenic and therefore, if schizophrenics could be made epileptics they would be cured.[41] Ugo Cerletti (1877-1963) and Bini in approximately 1938 introduced the induction of epileptic fits by the use of electrical current. This method replaced metrazol as the major form of convulsive therapy.[42] The transition from chemical to electrical treatment was a relatively simple methodological change of treatment; however, another physical method of treatment also developed during the 1930s—psychosurgery.

Otto Pötzl, a supporter of Sakel's insulin treatment, described patients with brain lesions as having symptoms similar to schizophrenia. Hoff says that Pötzl:

Found a disturbance of a distinct system in the brain causing such specific signs and symptoms. He described this fiber system of the brain as consisting of thalamocortical and thalamo-commissural connections. He therefore made the attempt in some schizophrenics to change the pathological function of the brain system by causing injury to the thalamus itself. This came close to the starting point of one of the organic treatments of schizophrenia called psychosurgery.[43]

Similarly Pötzl thought that with insulin coma, malfunctioning ganglion cells were destroyed and this destruction made it possible for the remaining cells to work in a normal fashion.[44]   Believing pathological tissue was the cause of mental disturbance, he followed the work of G. Burckhardt who in 1890 published the first modern account of such a procedure and was a contemporary of Egas Moniz (1874-1955). In 1936 Moniz introduced lobotomy and lobectomy for the treatment of functional psychoses basing his conclusions on animal experiments with monkeys and clinical experience with patients. For his work in this area Moniz was awarded a Nobel prize in 1955.[45, 46]

From Moniz's first operation until the late 1950s some 50,000 lobotomies were performed in the United States.[47]   Both closed and open operative techniques were utilized.   Open methods included topectomy, and orbital-medial and orbitoventromedial undercutting.   Closed methods included trans-orbital lobotomy, blind rostral leucotomy, electrocoagulation of the medial ventral quadrant, and stereotaxic thermolesions of the frontal white matter. Recently, ultrasound irradiation of the bimedial and frontal quadrants and stereotaxic implantation of radioactive yttrium Y^{90} in the substantia innominata have been used.[48]   Frontal lobe operations diminished markedly with the introduction of psychotropic drugs in the 1950s.

Prior to the mid-nineteenth century man relieved his anxiety and abnormal mental states with alcohol, cocaine, and opium. Balard (1802-1876) discovered the element bromine in 1826 and Laycock treated epilepsy with it in the 1850s. [49] The drug was first used for sedative and hypnotic purposes in 1864 by Behrend, who treated insomniacs with bromides. Bromides were very popular but were supplanted by the discovery of barbiturates—barbital (1903) and phenobarbital (1912). Today meprobamate, introduced in 1955 [first synthesized in 1952 by Frank Berger (1913-   )] and benzodiazepines (chlordiazepoxide in 1960), have for the most part replaced the bromides and barbiturates for sedative or tranquilizing purposes.[50, 51]

Laborit, a French anesthesiologist, observed that chlorpromazine produced an unusual behavioral effect, i.e., it was sedative but, at the same time, the patient could be easily aroused. This observation led Jean P.L. Delay (1907-   ) and Deniker, in 1952, to try the drug on schizophrenic patients, and indeed they observed a tranquilizing effect.[52]   Similarly S. and Rafat Siddiqui isolated

Rauwolfia serpentina, and Ganneth Sen and Katrick Bose in 1931 used these alkaloids to treat psychoses. Chlorpromazine and Rauwolfia serpentina, the first antipsychotic drugs, and their derivatives had an enormous effect in diminishing hospital admission rates and patient time spent in mental institutions.

Antidepressive drugs and stimulants constitute another relevant contribution. In 1951, iproniazid was used to treat tubercular patients. A euphoric side effect resulted. In 1952, Zeller found it to be a monoamine oxidase inhibitor, a finding later correlated with the biogenic amine theory of depression. By 1957, a commercial monoamine oxidase inhibitor, Marsilid, was introduced for the treatment of depression but because a number of cases of jaundice were attributed to the drug, it was withdrawn from the market. In 1964 another monoamine oxidase inhibitor—tranylcypromine (Parnate)—was also withdrawn from the market, this time due to the occurrence of hypertensive crises. Therefore, this class of drugs has been suspect and its use restricted for years in the United States. However, recently they have again been recommended.[53] The tricyclics, another group of antidepressant drugs, have not had so checkered a history. Imipramine was introduced in 1957 by Kuhn as an antidepressive agent and is still used as the model for all tricyclic medications.[54] The amphetamines are classified as stimulants, not antidepressive drugs, but since the 1930s they have been used to treat depressed patients. In 1949, J.F. Cade introduced lithium for manic excitements and today this drug and derivatives constitute a common method for treating depressed patients.[55]

This century has seen an expansion and elaboration of psychological methods of treatment. Individual therapy is one major method and includes: psychoanalysis (Freud), analytical psychology (Jung), individual psychology (Adler), the holistic approach (Horney, Koffka, Köhler, Werteimer, Goldstein, Angyal), interpersonal relationships (Sullivan), existential psychotherapy (May, Binswanger, Frankl), direct analysis (Rosen), client-centered psychotherapy (Rogers), behavior therapy (Skinner), and so forth. Another type of individual therapy is hypnosis, which started reappearing as a modality in the 1940s. Today psychiatrists are using it alone or in conjunction with other forms of therapy.[56]*

Group therapy began in the United States in 1907 when Joseph Pratt, an internist, gathered tubercular patients together for discussion of their psychological problems. In 1919, L. Cody Marsh worked with groups in mental institutions and from these beginnings this technique spread in several directions. There are those who use the principles learned from individual therapy (Freudian, Jungian, Adlerian, etc.) and apply them to groups, and there are others who modified or innovated different techniques. The latter group includes Samuel Slavson

*Relaxation and training techniques with and without hypnosis and biofeedback electrical apparatus have been used in medical therapeutics since 1910, by Levy, Johan Schultz (autogenic training),[57] and Edmund Jacobson (progressive relaxation).[58, 59]

(children's activity groups), Jacob Moreno (psychodrama), Eric Berne (transactional groups), Joseph Wolpe (behaviorial groups), Frederick Perls (Gestalt groups), Carl Rogers (group-centered psychotherapy), Alexander Lowen (bioenergetic group therapy), and so forth.[60]   Cotherapy, family, conjoint, and milieu are other group forms. The types and variations seem endless, and today patients are even advertising in newspapers and forming their own groups—shades of Alcoholics Anonymous and Recovery, Inc. (Abraham Low).

Despite the diversity of opinions regarding diagnosis, classification, etiology, and treatment of mental illness, there has been progress in this century and history has taught its lessons. The work in genetics is promising. It demonstrates that defective genes and abnormal chromosomes have a relationship to intelligence and behavior. Furthermore, it illustrates that, by diet and drugs, patients are at times treatable if not, in fact, curable. Physical therapies, including controversial psychosurgery, have relieved a great deal of suffering and have helped many individuals to maintain productive, gainful lives outside the walls of mental institutions. All types of psychological therapies can help, but it is indeed unfortunate that psychotherapists have splintered into so many groups. Perhaps, a new group of broadly based psychiatrists can be trained who will attain a balance and correct the massive confusion. Hypnosis is enjoying a revival and biofeedback machines are coming into use. Hospitals, private and public, are better than ever. Although they offer clean and decent surroundings and have larger staff to patient ratios than in former times much can be done to improve the training of the medical and nonmedical staffs.[61]   The social and legal roles of psychiatrists are very confusing. Certain recent trends regarding commitment procedures, privileged communication and informed consent, considered well-intentioned and theoretically humane and right, often on a practical level hamper the psychiatrist's ability to fulfill his obligations to his patients. Only by establishing a firm medical identity can psychiatry properly serve the needs of patients. Although there have been many advances in therapy, psychiatrists still know far too little to enter the entire arena of sociological problems.

TREATMENT PLAN

Adequate examination initiates proper treatment. Examination includes obtaining information regarding complaint or complaints, present illness, current life situation and stresses, biographical and family background, as well as physical and laboratory findings. Organizing and formulating the aforementioned data within the concepts of the comprehensive diagnosis is then followed by a therapeutic plan, thus establishing a logical system for treatment, i.e., examination, diagnosis, and treatment plan.

The treatment plan is often neglected or vaguely defined, and yet its importance cannot be overestimated. In formulating a therapeutic plan the psychiatrist or physician is integrating observations, knowledge, and philosophical orientation. In the words of Thomas Sydenham, the seventeenth century physician:

> It is ruin of our prospects to have departed from our oldest and best guide, Hippocrates, and to have forsaken the original *methodus medendi*. This was built upon the knowledge of immediate and conjunct causes, things of which the evidence is certain. Our modern doctrine is a contrivance of the word-catchers; the art of talking rather than the art of healing.
>
> That I may not seem to speak these things rashly, I must be allowed to make a brief digression; and to prove that those remote and ultimate causes in the determination and exhibition of which the vain speculations of curious and busy men are solely engaged, are altogether incomprehensive and inscrutable; and that the only causes that can be known to us, and the only ones from which we may draw our indications of treatment are those which are proximate, immediate, and conjunct.[62]

Initially, in any treatment, the psychiatrist discusses his findings with the patient. Doctor and patient establish a working relationship with shared therapeutic goals, clearly defined roles, and mutual responsibilities. The physician should make certain that the patient is aware of and comprehends his opinions regarding diagnosis and treatment. Physicians should always be on guard for an agreeing patient who says he understands but does not. Sometimes having the patient repeat the previous explanation in words or writing to the physician may help. Once the physician ascertains that the patient understands both diagnostic opinions and treatment goals and methods treatment may continue. A cooperative, knowledgeable patient will frequently mean the difference between success and failure.[63]

The original plan should be revised periodically with the complete knowledge of the patient, thus allowing flexibility of treatment goals and methods. The initial goal may be relief of painful symptoms, followed by such goals as improvement in the patient's life situation—work, family, friends, and so forth. Therapeutic methods may also change: environmental readjustment, drug therapy, or psychotherapy. The psychiatrist's hope is to maximize his services to the patient in the most expeditious manner.

Compromises in treatment plans may be essential. Generally the least amount of change in the patient's life the better, but sometimes reality dictates exceptions. For example, when a patient is expected to work beyond his ability, he might be wise to change jobs. Similarly, situational changes can be helpful in improving family and marital relationships. Ideally, satisfaction should be derived in as many areas of life as possible and the less a patient is satisfied in any one area the more important it becomes that he derive satisfaction in other areas of life. The simplest and cheapest form of psychiatric treatment is frequently environmental change. Unfortunately this is often not enough and it then becomes necessary to use psychological and physical therapies.

Any method of treatment that affects the mind through bodily influences is referred to as physical treatment. The nomenclature includes drugs, insulin coma, electroconvulsion, prolonged sleep, carbon dioxide, psychosurgery, hydrotherapy, and so forth.

PHYSICAL METHODS OF TREATMENT

Drug Treatment

It is a fact that every day enormous quantities of drugs are used in the United States and the vast majority by far affect the central nervous system. By affecting the brain, and in so doing the mind, these drugs at least temporarily meet one or more needs or desires. Drug takers seek stimulation, happiness, relaxation, rest, sleep, and a means to forget the difficulties and disappointments of everyday life. For these purposes a lavish supply of substances, some legal and some illegal, are available. The exhilaration of alcohol, the relaxation of sedatives and tranquilizers, the pleasant stimulation of coffee and amphetamines, the enchanting visual illusions conjured up on mescaline and LSD, and the peaceful world of hypnotic drug sleep are all very seductive. Once known and used there is no easy way to stop their use or abuse. Whether the patient gets the drug by prescription or from a street pusher, he will find it if he wants it. Besides, many doctors do not resist prescribing drugs, and pharmaceutical companies and street pushers gladly advertise and sell their products for profit. The motives of both buyer and seller are clear enough. Within a permissive, democratic political system the problem of drug control, however, leads to endless complexities.[64]

There are innumerable suggestions regarding the control (a form of treatment) of drug consumption. Public school systems have initiated educational programs for the young. Students are taught about drugs, their effects, legal implications, and available community treatment resources. Detailed curricula have been devised for kindergarten through high school.[65] Federal, state, and local government programs advertise everywhere—radio, television, newspapers, magazines, etc. They too attempt to educate the general public. Politicians promise help for the afflicted and respond with legislative proposals and laws. Psychiatrists propose that physicians prescribe drugs less freely and carelessly, and supervise the manner of their use; that drug manufacturers insure in the most cautious manner that their products reach only legitimate sources; that patients be advised against accumulating drugs and only take them under medical supervision. Psychiatrists also suggest: inculcating the highest of moral values, reorganizing the health care delivery system, promoting health and safety, creating decent jobs and living conditions, improving the quality of life, and so forth.[66] In essence there are many ideas and much talk, but the plain fact is that no viable solution has so far been advanced.

Reliable statistics on the incidence of legal and illegal drug use and abuse are impossible to obtain. A recent study of patients admitted to medical and surgical services in a large city hospital found that 20% of these patients had histories of psychotropic drug use, and this study did not include psychiatric patients.[67] Benzodiazepines are the most frequently prescribed drugs in the United States.[68] It is estimated that over 77,000,000 prescriptions for these drugs were filled in 1972.[69] In the United States, alcohol, the most used and abused drug, is consumed by 71% of the adult population, or 70 to 80 million people. Accordingly, it is estimated that there are from four and one-half million to nine and one-half million alcoholics, and alcoholism accounts for 15% of first admissions to public mental hospitals.[70] It is speculated that there are over 600,000 narcotic addicts[71] and anyone can guess regarding the number of marijuana users.

Despite the abuse of drugs, the professional should not lose his perspective and forget that drugs do have proper and legitimate uses. Physicians obviously should prescribe them sparingly and be aware of the dangers connected with their use. The patient should be carefully told how to use the drug. The written prescription should be legible and the instructions explicitly clear.[72] The physician should know the indications, contraindications, optimum dosage, drug interactions, and side effects. He should be informed regarding diagnosis and treatment for overdose. Although knowledge of basic pharmacology and chemistry is indispensable, the effect of a drug on the individual patient is of utmost importance. Some patients need higher dosages and some lower, to achieve the desired effect. The dose can vary depending on each patient's reaction. Follow-up visits are essential with all drugs. Also, the physician should know the patient's attitude towards taking medication. Some patients follow instructions, others do not. Some take more and some less than prescribed. There are habitual drug takers, and patients who refuse to take medication. These considerations should be foremost in the mind of every thinking physician.

Since there are so many psychotropic drugs, the physician should familiarize himself with at least one in each major group. He should be aware of the indications, contraindications, side effects, interactions, and so forth. He should attempt to follow the literature on the specific drugs he uses and use the lowest possible effective dose, although not necessarily the dosages recommended by pharmaceutical houses. A good rule of thumb is start with a low dosage and increase gradually. If the drug does not work then perhaps another one should be considered before going to higher doses. With psychotropic drugs it is difficult to justify the use of dosages so high that another drug must be prescribed to treat complications of the first. This type of "medication to treat medication" often adds insult to injury and produces serious complications.

Several other points should be kept in mind. First, drugs that have been in use for long periods are preferable to new ones. Before prescribing a new drug short- and long-term complications should be well established. Second, a drug should be used for the shortest period of time; this insures the least amount of difficulty. Likewise no prescription should be given with unlimited refills. If the patient needs the drug for a prolonged time, periodic reviews are necessary. Third, pregnant women, if possible, should not be given psychotropic drugs or Antabuse. Antabuse has toxic effects leading to the acetaldehyde syndrome, and psychotropic drugs frequently pass the placental barrier and affect the fetus.[73]

Several terms need defining. "Drug use" refers to prescribed drugs, properly supervised; "misuse" refers to improper administration of drugs by a physician; "abuse" refers to drug administration by the patient for other than proper medical purposes. "Addiction," "drug dependence," and "drug addiction" are synonymous terms which encompass three phenomena: first, there is tolerance, i.e., a diminished effect from the drug with repeated administration of the same dosage; second, habituation refers to the psychological dependence on the drug; third, physical dependence refers to an altered physiological state that occurs as a result of withdrawal of the drug (abstinence syndrome). Abstinence syndromes occur after prolonged use of narcotics, analgesics, sedatives, hypnotics, minor tranquilizers, alcohol, stimulants, hallucinogens, hashish, marijuana, and other drugs.[74, 75]

With each patient the clinician is confronted with choices regarding drug usage. Does the patient need to be slowed down, speeded up, made happier, or a combination of these? For what duration does the physician anticipate using the drug? Which drug in that general class of drugs should be selected, once a decision regarding desired effect is reached? Are combinations of drugs from several classes necessary? Hopefully, the physician's judgment is correct. In making a choice the doctor uses his experience, his knowledge of the patient, and of the drug.

Drugs inhibiting consciousness are categorized as sedatives, tranquilizers, hypnotics, or anesthetics. Sedatives lower the overall awareness of the patient and should have a calming effect. Tranquilizers (antianxiety drugs) relieve patients of worry, and anxiety, and should not produce undue drowsiness. Hypnotics produce sleep and anesthetics produce coma for surgery. However, not all anesthetic agents can be used as sedatives or hypnotics and conversely not all sedatives and hypnotics are suitable for anesthesia. The effects are usually determined by dosage. The larger the dose the more the patient's alertness is diminished. Higher dosages or drug sensitivity result in incoordination and drowsiness, apathy, and decreased motor responsiveness. Ultimately

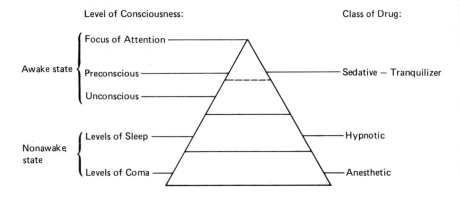

Fig. 12-1.   Relationship of drug effect to level of conscious state.

the patient suffers vasomotor collapse, respiratory depression, and if not reversed, death.   Sedatives, hypnotics, and anesthetics are anticonvulsant, voluntary muscle relaxants and are habituating and addicting.   The triangle shown above (Fig. 12-1) illustrates the approximate relationship of class of drugs to levels of mental alertness.   This applies only when the drug is used appropriately.

The two major classes of sedatives or hypnotics are the barbiturates and non-barbiturates.   The barbiturates are classified as follows: ultrashort thiopental (Pentothal) which is used for intravenous anesthesia; short acting secobarbital (Seconal) and pentobarbital (Nembutal) which have a rapid onset of action, induce sleep, and last approximately three hours; intermediate acting buta-barbital (Butisol) and amobarbital (Amytal) which induce sleep that lasts three to six hours; long acting phenobarbital (Luminal) which has a slow absorption rate, penetrates the brain slowly, lasts over six hours, and does not produce the "high" of the other barbiturates.   Probably, for these reasons phenobarbital is not often used by drug abusers for recreational or nonmedical purposes.   Phenobarbital, used mainly as a daytime sedative, when prescribed in its elixir form (37% alcohol) offers a drug combination that can become habituating.[76, 77]

Acute poisoning and addiction are the consequences of barbiturate misuse and abuse.   Unfortunately, alcohol and many other drugs are synergistic with barbiturates, thereby complicating treatment and increasing the incidence of acutely overdosed patients.   Barbiturates are respiratory depressants producing a decreased rate of breathing, varying levels of coma, cyanotic skin and mucous membranes, diminished or absent reflexes, lowered body temperature and blood pressure, and constricted pupils that may or may not respond to light. Treatment for such patients consists of adequate oxygenation, proper electrolyte balance, activated charcoal, gastric lavage, peritoneal dialysis and hemodialysis, forced diuresis, stimulants (Metrozol, picrotoxin, amphetamines), and other methods.[78,79]

The barbiturate addict is as serious a problem as the narcotic addict. The barbiturate addict behaves as if drunk on alcohol, and can become incoherent and unable to work or participate in friendships, cannot sleep even with increasing dosages of the drug, and is often depressed. Withdrawal is very dangerous and extreme caution must be exercised, while very slowly lowering the dosage. Withdrawal symptoms are anxiety, fear verging on panic, tremors, convulsions, insomnia, anorexia, vomiting, sweating, hyperreflexia, delirium, and craving for the drug. These patients should be hospitalized as soon as possible. The abstinence syndrome begins within 72 hours after drug withdrawal and can be fatal. It is wise to determine the level of addiction. A test dose of 200 mg of pentobarbital is given in an attempt to establish the degree of tolerance. If no physical changes are observed after an hour the level of the habit is probably above 1200 mg of pentobarbital per day. The test can then be re-peated in three or four hours using higher doses of pentobarbital to get some idea of the extent of drug usage. Starting at the test level, systematic lowering of the dose begins. Pentobarbital or phenobarbital are usually given every six hours and the dosage is reduced approximately 10% daily. However, other sedatives, hypnotics, or antianxiety drugs can be just as satisfactory. As an additional safety measure an anticonvulsant such as diphenylhydantoin (Dilantin) is given. Total withdrawal may take two weeks. Outpatient psychotherapy is recommended following discharge.[80]

The nonbarbiturate sedative and hypnotic drugs are used extensively and pre-sent the same problems as barbiturate drugs; namely, overdosage and addiction. In fact the principles of treatment are basically the same.[81] Although some of the newer drugs in this group are called minor tranquilizers not sedatives, they share some common properties. They are all sedative, hypnotic, central muscle relaxants, anticonvulsant, central nervous system depressants, and have drug dependence po-tential. for this reason many workers feel that minor tranquilizers and sedatives should be classified together and should be referred to as antianxiety drugs.[82]

The nonbarbiturate sedative, hypnotic, or antianxiety drugs are classified according to duration of action. The short acting older drugs are chloral hydrate (Noctec) and paraldehyde (Paral). They are helpful in treating elderly patients, those with liver disease, and patients who cannot tolerate barbiturates. Both drugs are metabolized in the liver and 10% of paraldehyde is excreted through the lungs. Paraldehyde has the distinct disadvantage of producing an unpleasant odor as it is exhaled.[83]

Some of the newer short acting sedatives and hypnotics are ethchlorvynol (Placidyl), ethinamate (Valmid), flurazepam (Dalmane), methaqualone (Quaalude, Sopor), and methyprylon (Noludar). Of all these new drugs flurazepam impairs

REM sleep the least and therefore is the most desirable member of this group.[84]

The intermediate acting antianxiety drugs include diazepam (Valium), glutethimide (Doriden), and meprobamate (Equanil, Miltown). Valium, a benzodiazepine is preferred, and Blackwell says:

> Comparing the choice of psychotropic drugs with the comparative criteria for selecting between them, the evidence supports what is happening in everyday practice. In treating minor emotional states with mixtures of anxiety and depression, the benzodiazepines are as effective as any other sedative drug, they have no overdose potential; tolerance, abuse, and abstinence are very rare; and they have remarkably few side effects. They interact with few of the other drugs used in medical practice or daily living except that, like all sedatives, they synergize with alcohol. In addition, their effects are immediate.[85]

> The long acting antianxiety drugs include chlordiazepoxide (Librium), clorazepate (Tranxene) and oxazepam (Serax). Those drugs all have cumulative effects; hence, after withdrawal the abstinence syndrome may be delayed for a week or more.[86]

There are four major criteria in selecting an antianxiety drug: relative efficacy, safety, compatibility with other drugs, and economy. Although difficult to prove, there seems to be a general consensus among investigators that benzodiazepines are the choice antianxiety drugs.[87]

In considering safety, barbiturates produce a high degree of tolerance, drug dependency, and toxicity when taken in an overdose. Meprobamates produce marked tolerance, dependence, and suicidal potential. The benzodiazepines do not depress respiration, hence, they are virtually suicide-proof.

Tolerance does not develop as readily with the benzodiazepines since, unlike barbiturates and meprobamates, they do not induce their own drug metabolizing liver microsomal enzymes and they are longer acting.[88] Because of enzyme-producing activity the meprobamates and barbiturates interact with anticonvulsant and anticoagulant drugs, reducing their efficacy. Benzodiazepines are, on the other hand, compatible with other drugs. As for cost, the barbiturates are about ten times cheaper than either meprobamates or benzodiazepines.[89] There seems little doubt, when applying the aforementioned criteria, that the benzodiazepines are the best antianxiety medication.

Major tranquilizers, neuroleptics, ataractics, antipsychotics, psycholeptics, and psychoinhibitors are synonymous terms.[90] The differences between that group and the antianxiety drugs are significant. Antipsychotic drugs produce quiet, calm, apathy, and sleep, but not profound coma. The patient can be aroused. This is unique and is thought to be caused by decreased dopaminergic transmission in the brain. Under the influence of antipsychotic drugs, the patient often gains enough control to be amenable to psychological therapies (individual, milieu, group) and to live outside of a hospital, capable of work and social relationships. Antipsychotic drugs are responsible to a great extent for ambulatory treatment of psychotic patients, the discharge of patients from mental hospitals, and the return of psychiatrists to biological psychiatry.[91]

Antipsychotic drugs are distinguished by their capacity to ameliorate symptoms of psychoses and the induction of extrapyramidal side effects. There are six major classes of antipsychotic drugs. Each class differs structurally from the other but all have partial molecular similarity.[92]

Major side effects of antipsychotic drugs are classified under central nervous system, autonomic, extrapyramidal, allergic, endocrine, skin, eye, and cardiac actions. These are manifested by such conditions as cataleptic states, decreased convulsive threshold, anticholinergic and antiadrenergic blocking, muscle relaxation, and sedation. There are also some dangerous toxic and sensitivity reactions such as blood dyscrasia, intrahepatic obstructive jaundice and skin reactions (abnormal pigmentations). Some other side effects include Parkinsonism, tartive dyskinesia, akathesia, fainting, palpitations, blurred vision, nasal stuffiness, dry mouth, constipation, weight gain, gynecomastia in males, lactation in females, altered pulse rate, arrhythmias and hypotension. In pregnancy there is a risk of congenital malformation. These side actions are common to all of the classes of antipsychotic drugs in varying degrees. Often the primary basis for selecting a particular drug is the degree to which the drug has a specific side effect. Conversely some drugs have a greater positive action on certain symptoms and are therefore chosen.[93]

The classes of antipsychotic drugs are phenothiazines, butyrophenones (Haldol), thioxanthenes (Taractan, Navane), oxoindoles (Moban), rauwolfia alkaloids (Serpasil), and dibenzoxazepines (Loxitane). The phenothiazines are the most important of all these drugs and are classified according to their side chain as: aliphatics which include chlorpromazine (Thorazine); piperazines (or piperazinyl) which includes fluphenazine (Prolixin), prochlorperazine (Compazine), and trifluoperazine (Stelazine); piperidines which includes thioridazine (Mellaril) and mesoridazine (Serentil). Clinically these groups can be distinguished as follows: the aliphatics produce more sedation, hypotension, dermatitis and convulsions, and less extrapyramidal side effects. Thus they are most useful in patients when sedation is desirable. The piperazine group produces more extrapyramidal effects and less sedation, hypotension, and lens opacities. These drugs are best for patients who need calming, but not motor retardation. The piperidines produce more retinal toxicity, ejaculatory disturbance, and electrocardiographic changes but fewer extrapyramidal symptoms and antiemetic action.[94]

The butyrophenones are low dose drugs with a strong tendency to evoke extrapyramidal symptoms and akathesia. They are alleged to be more effective in treating manic, paranoid, and agitated patients. The thioxanthenes are low dose drugs in which lenticular opacities have occurred and are clinically as effective as the phenothiazines. The oxoindoles and dibenzoxazepines are effective but offer no advantage over the other classes and can be used as an alternative. Rauwolfia alkaloids are rarely used today since they produce severe depression and are not as effective as phenothiazines.[95, 96]

Antipsychotic drugs calm agitation and fear; allay restlessness and excitement; lead to detachment from and often actual loss of delusions, hallucinations, and ideas of reference; improve behavior; and help control thought disorders. Their major use is for patients suffering from schizophrenia, mania, agitated depressed psychoses, Gilles de la Tourette's syndrome, and psychosis with organic brain disease; however, they do have a place in the treatment of neuroses especially those in which anxiety and depression predominate. They are nonaddicting and thus have an advantage over antianxiety drugs. They can be used in relatively low dosages for prolonged periods and at times, work when other drugs fail.[97]

Antidepressants (thymoleptics) are the next major class of drugs and have already been discussed in the chapter on depressive neuroses. Their use is predicated upon the validity of the catecholamine and indolamine hypothesis of affective disorders. They should be used only after acquisition of a thorough knowledge of the biochemistry and neurophysiology of the affective disorders and the pharmacology of the drugs. However, endocrine, electrolyte, and enzyme factors must not be overlooked in the treatment of patients suffering from affective disorders.

Other drugs concern psychiatrists but will be mentioned only briefly because they are not central to the treatment of neuroses. Analgesics may be classified as mild or strong. Strong analgesics raise the threshold of pain, alter psychological response to pain, and suppress anxiety and apprehension. Mild analgesics do all the above but do not influence psychological response to pain. Strong analgesics include opium alkaloids (morphine); semisynthetic modifications of morphine such as hydromorphone (Dilaudid), oxymorphone (Numorphan); and synthetic compounds such as meperidine (Demerol), alphaprodine (Nisentil), anileridine (Leritine), levorphanol (Levo-Dromoran), methadone (Dolophine), methotrimeprazine (Levoprome), and pentazocine (Talwin); and so forth.[98] Mild analgesics include agents chemically related to strong analgesics such as codeine, ethoheptazine (Zactane), and propoxyphene (Darvon); and analgesic-antipyretics, the prototype being acetylsalicylic acid (Aspirin). Others in the mild group include sodium salicylate; acetophenetidin (Phenacetin); mixtures of Aspirin, Phenacetin, Caffeine (APC), mixtures of codeine phosphate with Aspirin, Phenacetin and Caffeine (APC with codeine); mixtures of Darvon with

Aspirin (Darvon with ASA) and Darvon with APC (Darvon Compound); mixtures of oxycodone, APC, and homatropine (Percodan), mixtures of zactane with Aspirin or with APC (Zactirin or Zactirin Compound); and many other substances and mixtures—some more intelligently combined than others.[99]   Since some of these analgesics are classified as narcotics the problems of drug dependency must be considered. Psychiatrists, indeed all physicians, must be concerned with the proper use, abuse, misuse, side effects, and interactions of these drugs.

The hemp plant, cannabis sativa, produces a resin primarily in the leaves and flowering tops that when dried is called marijuana (pot, weed, grass, bhang, ganja, charas, tea, reefers, Mary Jane, muggles). When concentrated and mechanically compressed it is called hashish. The most active substance in the resin is Δ-3-tetrahydrocannabinol (THC) and the concentration of this substance determines the strength or mildness of the effects of the marijuana. Cannabis, whether smoked or taken orally, produces euphoria, giggling, uncontrollable laughter, and mild perceptual distortions; colors are brighter; music better; touch more sensitive; and time seems to pass slowly. These psychic effects usually last two to four hours and are followed by relaxation and sleep. This occurs when the individual has a "good trip"; however, there are "bad trips."[100]

The symptoms of a bad trip vary. The individual may experience excessive anxiety extending to panic; body, spatial, and temporal distortions may become grotesque and frightening; depersonalization, paranoid delusions, and visual hallucinations occur; reddened conjuctiva, an increase in heart rate, a rise in blood pressure, and other somatic complaints are observed; and an individual can, at times, experience a marijuana psychic state without having recently taken the drug (flashback). Because reactions to marijuana vary greatly from individual to individual, and research results conflict, there is controversy regarding both legalization of the drug and its therapeutic use. There are those who claim it is harmless and others who claim it is dangerous. Both sides in this conflict demand proof; claims and counterclaims are made regarding both short-term and long-term use of the drug.[101]

The words of Thomas Maugh may serve as a warning:

> What the evidence does suggest is that the effects of marihuana are cumulative and dose-related, and that prolonged heavy use of marihuana, or less frequent use of the more potent hashish, is associated with at least six different types of potential hazards. The research indicates that cannabis . . . :
>
> ▶   May cause chromosome damage . . .
>
> ▶   May cause disruption of cellular metabolism, including synthesis of DNA, and may interfere with the functioning of the immune system.

▶   May mimic hormones or act on hormonal regulators to produce a variety of effects ranging from impotence and temporary sterility to the development of female-like breasts in men.

▶   Is, with heavy use, severely debilitating to the bronchial tract and lungs.

▶   Causes sharp personality changes that lead to a marked deterioration in what is normally considered good mental health.

▶   And most important, may cause potentially irreversible brain damage.[102]

Marijuana, a psychogenic agent, has, to date, no place in the treatment of mental disorder.

Marijuana is but one of many psychogenic, hallucinogenic, or psychedelic agents.   All may produce hallucinations, delusions, and cognitive, behavioral, and affective disturbances.   The most common are: mescaline which is derived from Lophosphora Williamsii, a cactus plant; lysergic acid diethylamide (LSD) which is related to ergot alkaloids; and phencyclidine (Sernyland, street name: angeldust, PCP, Hog, LBJ, etc.) which was originally investigated as an anesthetic and still sold by pharmaceutical companies for animal use.[103]   In my opinion, these drugs like marijuana, have no place in psychiatry for either human research or as aids in psychotherapy.[104]   Studies should be encouraged, however, to determine the effects of these drugs when they are taken voluntarily by drug users.   Such investigations might help answer controversial questions and can certainly do no harm.[105, 106]

In summary, sedative, hypnotic, analgesic, antianxiety, antipsychotic, and antidepressive drugs are frequently used in treating neurotic patients. Although we know something about the mechanisms of these drugs, their indications and contraindications, we are extremely unclear as to the mechanisms and etiologies of the illnesses which they treat; this is not an ideal situation to say the least.   But the drugs do help and their use is indispensable so the physician is challenged to use them in the most competent manner. First, the physician should be cautious and do no harm to his patient.   Second, his use of drugs should be systematic, logical, and appropriate to the clinical situation.   Several factors must be considered before commencing actual drug treatment: comprehensive diagnosis, knowledge of the natural history of the disease, proper overall choice of treatment as well as choice of drug, dosage, mode of administration, side effects, interactions, and duration of treatment.   In addition the patient should be informed about the drug and the physician must periodically assess the patient's progress and decide when and how to discontinue the drug.   Follow-up treatment must then be determined.   In a word, a rational, thoughtful approach to drug usage is best.[107]

SPECIALIZED DRUG TREATMENT

There are two types of treatment in which regular insulin is injected. Both require hospitalization. The first is called modified insulin treatment and is used for those patients who are anxious or depressed; those experiencing alcohol or narcotic withdrawal; and those with severe anorexia or anorexia nervosa. The technique involves injecting enough insulin to produce a hypoglycemic state. The initial dose consists of five or ten units of insulin. After ascertaining that there is no hypersensitivity the physician may slowly increase the dosage day by day, to 50 units, if necessary. Patients are allowed to experience only mild hypoglycemic symptoms. Sweating is usually the first visible sign, followed by a period of relaxation. Slurred speech or dimming of consciousness call for immediate termination of treatment and a reduction of the dose the next day. Treatments are administered four to six times per week for four to six weeks. Each daily treatment is terminated two or three hours after the injection by having the patient drink a glass of sweetened juice and eat a high carbohydrate meal. In successful cases the patient's appetite and weight increase; his mood elevates and tension decreases; and there is an improvement in overall physical condition.[108]

The second type, called insulin coma treatment, is indicated primarily in the treatment of schizophrenia, but can be used in extremely severe cases of anxiety and obsessive compulsive neuroses. It is sometimes used in combination with electroconvulsive treatment. The techinque is similar to modified insulin but the dosage can go as high as 400-600 units and clinical manifestations are different. The patient goes through various stages: first, a precoma stage in which sweating and relaxation lead to sleep; second, the coma stage, beginning with restlessness, muscle twitching, disoriented speech, and progressing to a quiet, relaxed comatose stage. This is thought to be the therapeutic stage. If the patient sinks deeper into coma, he reaches a stage where he no longer responds to stimuli, pupils are miotic, corneal and tendon reflexes disappear, and respiratory difficulties appear. Death may occur if there is no medical intervention. Treatments are terminated by intravenous glucose. When the patient awakens, in 10 to 15 minutes, oral sugar preparations and high protein foods are taken. Termination can be facilitated by intravenous or intramuscular glucogen. Depending on the patient's response, a series of 25 to 60 comas is administered at the rate of 5 treatments per week. Major complications are convulsions, prolonged comas, and cardiovascular collapse. Major contraindications are heart, renal, liver, and respiratory disease; pregnancy; insulin sensitivity; and diabetes mellitus. Insulin coma and modified insulin treatments are rarely used today because a team of specially trained individuals is necessary to administer the treatment; and an area of a ward must be isolated so that these patients are continually and carefully observed. Because of these difficulties and the high cost factor, insulin treatment has largely been replaced by electro-convulsive treatment and the newer drugs.[109]

Continuous sleep therapy is another form of treatment which requires trained personnel and supervision. It too has been largely replaced by tranquilizers, electroconvulsive treatment, and antidepressive drugs. It is used for manic excitements, severe intractable anxiety states, and in certain psychosomatic disorders. The technique consists of administering 100 to 300 mg of amobarbital (Amytal) every two to three hours until the patient goes to sleep followed by enough drugs to maintain sleep from 16 to 20 hours a day. The treatment lasts approximately two weeks with the deepest levels of sleep occurring within the first three days. The drug is gradually withdrawn until, at termination, the patient sleeps only at night. Chloral hydrate or chlorpromazine (Thorazine), may be used to facilitate the barbiturate. Complications are those of an over-dose of barbiturates—pneumonitis, atelectasis, shock, cardiac arrhythmias, venous thrombosis, and infection are the most serious. There can be no doubt that sleep and rest are beneficial to the nervous system and the mind. Were it not for the difficulty in administration this treatment might meet with more acceptance in the United States. In the Soviet Union, where sleep is viewed from the Pavlovian viewpoint as a protective inhibition this type of therapy is extensively utilized.[110]

Narcosynthesis, narcoanalysis, and narcotherapy are synonymous terms describing a method which employs drugs—hypnotics, stimulants, and hallu-cinogens—to produce a state of mind in which the patient's conscious control and inhibitions diminish. The patient becomes more communicative and suggest-ible. He expresses thoughts and feelings that are unknown to his conscious mind or that he will not or cannot express under normal conditions. By in-fluencing the patient to talk, feel, abreact, and seek insights, the drug supposedly facilitates the therapeutic process.[111]

Narcotherapy is useful for diagnostic and therapeutic purposes. It can aid in differentiating an organic from a functional illness. For instance, intravenous stimulants or hypnotics can increase the confusion, negativism, and mutism of a patient with an organic brain syndrome; whereas, they can for varying periods of time clear these symptoms in a depressed, hysterical, or catatonic patient. Conversely, in a patient with masked or suspected depression or schizophrenia, an intravenous stimulant or hypnotic can evoke overt depressive or psychotic symptomatology. Narcotherapeutic methods are employed as a treatment in conversion and dissociative (amnesia, fugues) neuroses; as a quick way to explore patients with emotional problems due to traumatic onset; as a means of helping patients who suffer from excessive anxiety or guilt to talk; and as an adjunct to psychotherapy. The drugs that are used during narcotherapy do not function as "truth serum." In fact, fantasies and thoughts may be stimulated or, in cases of criminals, they may be deliberately fabricated.[112]

Since hallucinogens are not recommended, the choice between hypnotics or stimulants depends upon the diagnostic and therapeutic problems. In many cases, however, the choice of drug may make little difference. Both hypnotic and stimulant may be employed in sequence, with the hypnotic usually given first. Stimulants have the advantage of increasing the patient's awareness; hence, the effects may be more easily remembered than with hypnotics. The disadvantage of stimulants is that they may release overwhelming anxiety, thoughts, and affects that can result in extremely disturbed behavior. Stimulants are to be avoided in anxious, overtly psychotic, and organic brain damaged patients. Hypnotics have the advantage of relaxing the patient, thus permitting him to relate certain thoughts and feelings that are normally hidden or difficult to express. The disadvantage is that these patients often forget what was discussed and this can be an especially disturbing experience for paranoid patients. A major disadvantage to the repeated use of both hypnotics and stimulants is that the patient may enjoy the euphoria and relaxation and repeatedly return for those effects rather than understanding or working through his problems.[113]

The technique with both the hypnotic and stimulant drugs is basically the same. Amobarbital (Amytal) or thiopental (Pentothal) are the most common drugs employed in the hypnotic group. A 2.5% solution (25 mg/cc) is injected intravenously at the rate of 2 cc per minute until the patient becomes drowsy, speech begins to slur, or eyelid tone decreases. Then the patient is encouraged to speak and, when drowsiness lifts, more drug is injected to a maximum of 500 mg. Methamphetamine (Methedrine) and methylphenidate (Ritalin) are the most common drugs used in the stimulant group. Doses of 25-40 mg are slowly injected intravenously over a five minute period and within five to ten minutes physiological and psychological effects of the drug begin to appear. Although those effects may initially be uncomfortable they abate within 10 or 15 minutes and the patient talks and the diagnostic or therapeutic exploration begins.[114]

A different type of drug therapy (orthomolecular or megavitamin), is based on the theory that mental health is dependent on the molecular structure of the brain and other organs of the body as well as on the optimum concentration of certain substances in the organism. The substances deemed important are vitamins and according to Linus Pauling, who in 1954 coined the term "orthomolecular psychiatry," vitamins such as niacin, pyridoxine, ascorbic acid, and cyanocobalamin are useful in the treatment of schizophrenia. The treatment consists of massive dosages of one or more of these vitamins.[115] The importance of vitamins for mental health cannot be denied and many physicians and psychiatrists recommend daily multivitamins for those patients who are undernourished or lack proper nutrition. But most psychiatrists do not find evidence to support the contention that massive dosages are helpful in treating schizophrenia or any other mental illness.[116-118]

Some other specialized treatments are employed. Intravenous acetylcholine (up to 600 mg) is a form of convulsive treatment for schizophrenics. When used in nonconvulsive dosages (up to 200 mg) claims are made for its therapeutic value in anxiety neurosis.[119] Atropine and scopolamine injected intramuscularly are used for treating neuroses and psychoses. Carbon dioxide in a mixture of 30% CO_2 + 70% O_2 is inhaled for the treatment of anxiety and other neurotic conditions.[120]   Lastly, inhalation of the anesthetic flurothyl (Indoklon) produces a convulsion and has the same indications and effectiveness as electroconvulsive therapy. None of the aforementioned therapies has met with much acceptance among psychiatrists. Generally their side effects are too undesirable or they have no advantage over other modes of treatment.

ELECTRICAL TREATMENT

Electricity has multiple uses in medicine. Diagnostic procedures such as the electrocardiogram and the electroencephalogram depend on the interpretation of graphs of certain types of activity that emanate from the heart and brain. Therapeutic uses for electricity are numerous and diverse. They include such methods as electroconvulsive, nonconvulsive electrostimulation, electrosleep, biofeedback, electrical stimulation of nerves, electrical aversion techniques, and surgical electrocoagulation treatments. Hence, electricity is used diagnostically and therapeutically; and in the treatment of neuroses as well as other mental and physical conditions.

Electroconvulsive treatment is synonymous with electroshock, electroplexy, electrical treatment, ECT, or EST. The psychiatrist's preference for any of these terms seems to be a matter of esthetics. Some psychiatrists feel that the words "convulsive" or "shock" have frightening connotations to the patient and prefer the other terms. Regardless of what term is used the indications, contraindications, side effects, and method of administration are the same.

Convulsive therapy has its best results in the treatment of affective disorders. In suicidal depression it can be life saving. Usually six to nine treatments administered over a two to three week period will yield results and change the patient's depressive mood. It is also used in the treatment of patients who suffer from schizophrenia, anxiety neurosis, and in the hysterical patient with chronic bodily pain.[121]

The treatment consists of placing electrodes on the temporal areas of the head. Bilateral stimulation involves placing electrodes on both temples, and unilateral stimulation involves placing one electrode on the nondominant side. Electrical stimulation is delivered by different types of machines with varying pulse width, frequencies, and enough intensity to cause a grand mal convulsion.[122] Prior to electrical stimulation the patient is given succinylcholine (Anectine, Sucostrin), to decrease the impact of the convulsion; and an ultrashort acting barbiturate, to lower the patient's apprehension. These drugs are given intra-venously, preferably by the drip method. After the convulsion, the patient remains in bed until enough consciousness returns to allow him to arise safely.[123]

The overall death rate from the treatment is 0.08% and major complications are fractures, bruises, dislocations, respiratory and cardiovascular arrest, coronaries, confusion, amnesia, and electroencephalogram changes.[124] The most trouble-some psychiatric complications are memory loss for recent events, disorienta-tion, and confusion.[125] These complications usually clear up within a week or ten days. However, at times the patients complain of memory loss for long periods following the cessation of treatment. Whether the memory failures are due to psychological or physical factors is not known.

Patients who receive unilateral treatment have fewer short-term memory problems than those who receive bilateral treatment. The frequency of memory loss over periods of six to nine months, however, is the same with both types of treatment and there is no proof of permanent long-term loss. Squire con-cludes the following:

> Nevertheless, subjects who had received bilateral ECT frequently reported that their memory was not as good as before treatment. The marked memory impairment initially associated with bilateral ECT might cause some individuals to become more alert to subsequent memory failures and then to under-estimate their memory abilities. Alternatively, it is difficult to rule out the possibility that occasional failures of recall persist after ECT that are not detected by conventional memory tests.[126]

The nonsuicidal death and sickness rates in depressed patients offer some interesting comparisons. The untreated depressed patient is malnourished, suffers from intercurrent infections, and has a higher incidence of cardiovascular disease and death than either treated patients or the general population. Depressed patients treated with ECT have a more rapid treatment response, a greater percentage of recovery, and a lower mortality rate than those treated by anti-depressive drugs. Myocardial infarctions are more frequent in inadequately treated depressed patients than those adequately treated by either ECT or antidepressive drugs. These findings apply mainly to males of any age and older people of both sexes, and emphasize not only the superiority but also the necessity of ECT over all other forms of treatment for the severely depressed patient.[127]

Some psychiatrists believe that the convulsion is not responsible for the therapeutic effect of ECT; therefore, machines have been developed to induce clonic movements and autonomic effects without the convulsion. There are two such types of treatment: subconvulsive (E Snc) and high-frequency stimulative electrotherapy (Sedac). The technique is to anesthetize the patient as for ECT; then electrically stimulate the head, legs, or lumbar region until the anesthetic wears off. Both psychoses and varying types of disabling neuroses are treated in this manner. Reported results of this therapy vary from no significant effect[128] to highly effective.[129]

Electrosleep therapy is used for anxiety and depressive symptoms, sleep disturbances, psychophysiological disorders, and some neuroses. The equipment for electrosleep consists of an electrical apparatus with two cathodes and two anodes. In central electrical stimulation, the cathodes are placed above the eyes and the anodes over the mastoids; in peripheral stimulation, one supraorbital electrode is an anode, the other a cathode, and both mastoid electrodes are dummies. There are daily sessions that last one to two hours during which the patient receives small modulated electric impulses. The patient should relax and experience some light sleep; however, sleep is not induced in all subjects and for this reason the name is considered a misnomer. Electrosleep, like continuous drug sleep treatment is popular in the Soviet Union but is used infrequently in the United States. Claims vary as to its therapeutic efficacy.[130-133]

Biofeedback training consists of continually monitoring a patient by electro-encephalograph, myelograph, cardiograph, voltmeter, or other apparatus that can measure temperature (thermister), blood pressure, pulse, and so forth. The patient is trained to recognize, by visual or auditory signals, when a desired effect is attained. The purpose of biofeedback is to teach the patient conscious control over body functions—voluntary, involuntary, and rhythmical. By immediate feedback transmitted from machine to patient, he is able to associate an otherwise imperceptible physiological change with a specific thought, feeling, fantasy, or image.[134]

For voluntary functions the electromyelograph is employed. Electrodes on the skin record muscle tension. The patient wears earphones and listens for sounds that vary in proportion to the tension, or observes colored lights that indicate various levels of tension, i.e., red, maximum tension; amber, medium tension; green, maximum relaxation. Through this method the patient becomes newly conscious of muscle tensions. Herein lies the therapeutic value of bio-feedback. For example, patients suffering from tension headaches receive feedback training with electrodes attached to the frontalis muscle. Twenty minute training sessions occur twice a week and as the cues are recognized the patient becomes conscious of previously unrecognized muscle tensions. The patient, with practice, eventually becomes aware of muscle tensions without the aid of the machine. Then no further training is necessary. Furthermore, by learning to relax one muscle or group of muscles the patient is encouraged to seek more generalized body relaxation. Techniques such as progressive relaxation, autogenic training, yoga, hypnosis, and behavior therapy are often used in conjunction with biofeedback training.[135]

Variations of the above biofeedback technique are used to treat or study certain rhythmical body activities. The electroencephalograph as well as the electromyelograph are used for treatment of insomnia. After frontalis relaxation is achieved (alpha rhythms—8-13 cps) until these change to theta (4-7 cps), the patient is taught to prolong theta; hence, sleep. For study of twilight stages of consciousness a three-phase procedure is used: EMG to monitor muscle relaxation; thermister to monitor increase in body temperature; and EEG feedback which assists the patient to enhance theta waves. Thus, explorations are made of the domain between wakefulness and sleep—the hypnagogic state.[136] There is no experimental evidence that alpha waves are of therapeutic value, but EEG feedback has helped some epileptics to detect seizure prodromata and thereby abort the seizure.[137]

Conditioning experiments show that the involuntary or autonomic nervous system can be trained: increasing or decreasing salivation, gastric secretions, peristaltic movements, heart rate, blood pressure, uterine contractions, etc. Now feedback machines can be used to attain the same results. Although results with humans are not comparable to those attained in animal experiments, there has been some progress. Patients with essential hypertension can temporarily lower their blood pressure while in the laboratory, but little is accomplished if they do not change harmful dietary, smoking, or stressful life patterns. Biofeedback training has more success, however, with cardiac arrhythmias. These patients are trained to accelerate or decrease heart rate. Patients with paroxysmal auricular tachycardia or premature ventricular contractions can be taught to maintain their heart rate within a normal range; migraine sufferers can abort their headaches by directing blood from the head to their hand: asthmatics are taught diaphragmatic breathing; and so forth.[138] Biofeedback is now enjoying immense popularity, but with the exception of its ability to control heart rate, its real therapeutic value for autonomic disturbances is not firmly established. It can, however, be of value as an adjunct to psychotherapy in the treatment of tension states as well as anxiety, phobic, depressive, and neurasthenic neuroses, and as a means of decreasing drug usage.[139-141]

Pain is the most common patient complaint. Pain is not a simple phenomena in which a particular sensation is directly proportional to the degree of tissue damage. Rather, it is a highly complex phenomenon in which the patient's psychological state is intimately connected to the pain response whether it is based upon a demonstrable or nondemonstrable lesion. Pain has many causes and the comprehensive concepts of etiology, diagnosis, and treatment are extremely relevant.[142]

Patients complain of three types of pain. Pricking pain (fast) is sharp, localized, acute, disappears with removal of stimulus, and has no chronic emotional sequelae. Burning pain (slow) takes about 0.5 to 1 second until experienced, is not distinctly localized, remains a few seconds after removal of stimulus, and momentarily produces a mental change in the patient. Aching pain comes from the viscera and deep somatic structures, can be accompanied by burning, and is difficult to localize since it is perceived in distant areas of the body rather than in the actual location of the stimulus (referred).[143] This last type of pain can lead to mental problems. All types of pain, however, can become chronic and when it does, treatment becomes very difficult.

Chronic pain is treated by innumerable methods which include: subarachnoid saline infusion, drugs, psychotherapy, nerve blocks, surgery, cold applications, acupuncture, operant conditioning, electrical stimulation, biofeedback, and Zen, among others. The patient's reaction to, and threshold of pain are of prime importance. Conservative treatment is preferred, irrespective of primary etiology. The physician will at times be pressured to resort to drastic treatments to relieve the patient's chronic pain and he should, if possible, resist these pressures. However, when unavoidable, such treatments as invasive central nervous system neurosurgery should be withheld until more moderate neurosurgical treatments have been tried. Two types of electrical stimulation are used—peripheral and central. Peripheral stimulation requires implantation of an electrode in the vicinity of the painful area; central nervous system stimulation requires implantation of electrodes on the dorsal surface of the spinal cord via laminectomy. In both methods the patient voluntarily activates the electrodes with a signal transmitter. Supposedly the electrical stimulation amplifies the inhibitory mechanisms for pain.[144]

The various diagnostic and therapeutic uses of electricity are, in conjunction with drugs and surgery, leading the psychiatrist to return to the clinic, laboratory, and hospital. Psychiatrists are working on medical and surgical services and in pain clinics. The physiology of sleep and of the nervous system and the mechanisms of pain and electroconvulsive treatment are again the concern of the physician-psychiatrist. The ancient force of magnetism is drawing psychiatrists and psychologists back to the material body and its functions and lessening their recent concentration on metaphysical speculation and psychotherapy.

PSYCHOSURGERY

Psychosurgery, perhaps more than any other form of psychiatric treatment, has in recent years caused a great deal of controversy both inside and outside the profession. Lawyers, physicians, psychologists, behavioral scientists, judges, and laymen are all involved. Phil Zakowski, a lawyer, expounded as follows:

PUBLIC OUTCRY occasioned by questionable uses of psychosurgery has underscored the need for regulation of this controversial technique. Its irreversibility, unpredictable side effects, and the lack of precise knowledge about the brain areas affected have lent strength to demands for stricter governmental controls.   Although the procedure itself is strictly medical, its social, moral, and ethical implications are such that its supervision cannot remain solely within the realm of medicine.   The term "psychosurgery" generally denotes brain surgery done primarily for behavior control rather than for removal of pathologic tissue . . . .[145]

Yet the National Commission for the Protection of Human Subjects of Biomedical and Behavioral Research, released a report in October 1976 that approved of psychosurgery in carefully defined circumstances.   That report was based on the findings of scientists who were appointed by the commission to study psychosurgery.   These individuals reviewed world literature on this subject for the last five years, and personally evaluated the psychological and neurological status of patients who had psychosurgery between 1965 and 1975.   Although the scientists did not approve of the old prefrontal lobotomy they did approve of newer procedures such as cingulotomy.   The prestigious magazine "Science" quotes an interview with the commission's chairman J. Kenneth Ryan, of Harvard Medical School, in which he stated:

We looked at the data and saw they did not support our prejudices. I, for one, did not expect to come out in favor of psychosurgery. But we saw that some very sick people had been helped by it, and that it did not destroy their intelligence or rob them of feelings. Their marriages were intact. They were able to work. The operation shouldn't be banned.[146]

The commission's principal recommendations were that psychosurgery be performed only at hospitals that have review boards; the board must certify that the surgeon is competent; the patient must be evaluated carefully before and after surgery and be operated on for the right reasons; that there be informed consent; and children, prisoners, or involuntarily confined mental patients must be taken before a court to determine whether the operation is in the patient's best interest.[147]   In effect, the commission regards psychosurgery as another medical procedure and insists only on quality practice.   The question, however, of what constitutes "informed consent" could be the one provision in the recommendations to cause considerable difficulty since this is a complex legal issue.[148]

Procedures include standard lobotomy, transorbital lobotomy, cingulectomy, topectomy, gyrectomy, bimedial leucotomy, and others.   These methods vary in the amount of brain tissue that is isolated from the rest of the brain.   It varies from 160 square centimeters of frontal cortex in standard lobotomy to 8 square centimeters in stereotactic tractotomy.   The older methods that destroyed the most tissue—standard lobotomy, transorbital lobotomy, gyrectomy, and topectomy—are only of historical interest and need not be discussed.   The newer methods attempt to cut the connection between the medial and frontal cortices and the limbic system and are named according to the exact location and surgical method. The details are more the concern of the neurosurgeon than the psychiatrist. For example, stereotactic subcaudal tractotomy uses radioactive yttrium, Y90, stereotactically placed by orbital undercuttings in the substantia inaminata; and cingulectomy cuts a specific bundle of nerve fibers connecting the frontal lobes with the limbic system. Stereotactic subcaudal tractotomy has an operative mortality rate of less than 1%, postoperative epilepsy rate of 1-2.2%, behavioral and psychological disturbances of 3% and 7%, respectively, and around 90% of the patients show no undesirable side effects. In comparison to the older lobotomies these are remarkable statistics.[149, 150]

Psychosurgery is advised for those chronic mental patients who have been unsuccessfully treated by other methods. They should be considered intractable cases. Best results are obtained with the affective disorders but patient with obsessive compulsive and anxiety neuroses and/or schizophrenia may benefit. It is also recommended for drug addiction, ulcerative colitis, hypochondriasis, and behavior disorders among others. Amygdalotomy and other psychosurgical methods are recommended for treatment of aggressive behavior, be it of a criminal or noncriminal nature, and for sexual deviation—again controversial. Is it punishment and "behavior control" or is it a medical treatment, that relieves pain and discomfort for these patients? These are difficult questions to answer. Each case should be considered carefully not only by the attending therapist but also by several colleagues.[151, 152]

Studies need to be done on these patients who are "successfully" treated by psychosurgery; those where indications for treatment are agreed upon by psychiatrists and where no deleterious side effects occur—epilepsy, hemorrhage, behavioral, and psychological disturbances. Evaluations of the total effect upon the patient are necessary, above and beyond the removal of the chronic disease and its symptoms. For instance, the effects of the operation are that the patient feels less anxious and worries less. Does this also mean that he experiences a reduction in depth of feeling, initiative, and creative thinking? Likewise, some patients feel less restrained and freer to do and to say things. Does this also mean they use less thought and deliberation in directing their behavior? Intelligence supposedly is not impaired. What kind of intelligence? Brain damaged individuals tend to be more concrete, less abstract, and attend more to immediate situations, often not realizing or is it ignoring remote consequences? Do these patients have more difficulty with complex situations and are their short- and long-term judgments impaired? Only when these questions are answered can the physician properly evaluate the pros and cons of psychosurgery for the individual patient and place it in perspective as a medical treatment. The legal, social, moral, and ethical issues then boil down to a medical judgment and this is no different than what it has always been.

PSYCHOTHERAPY

The term psychotherapy is defined in a variety of ways. In the narrow sense it refers to "a systematized professional technique whereby mental symptoms can be ameliorated or disordered behavior brought under control by means of an ongoing structured relationship between a trained physician and a patient."[153] Broadly, "Psychotherapy is the name given to all those methods of treatment that affect both psyche and body by measures which proceed via the psyche."[154] Somewhere between these two definitions is the one that is followed here. Psychotherapy refers to an art, not a science. There are many techniques of psychotherapy—some structured, some unstructured; some systematized, some unsystematized; some requiring and some not requiring an ongoing relationship. Yet, people do influence people and all human interactions are not called psychotherapy. A definition of psychotherapy should include the influencing of mind or body via consciousness, the necessity of professionally trained personnel to administer the treatment, and the description of the methods. Psychotherapists work with one or more patients for the following purposes: to alleviate or remove the cause or causes of symptoms originating from primary or secondary mental illness; to improve adaptive behavior; to promote positive changes in growth and development; and to explore knowledge of self and interpersonal relationships.

Psychotherapeutic methods vary considerably: individual therapy—one therapist, one patient; conjoint (triangular, triadic, couples)—one therapist and a couple, usually married; family—one therapist plus parents and children; cotherapy—more than one therapist with one or more patients; sex—single or dual therapists with patient partners; group—one or more therapists with two or more patients. There is also bibliotherapy in which the patient assimilates psychological, sociological, and aesthetic values from books; and other types that are self-explanatory such as occupational, art, music, poetry, dance, psychodrama, milieu therapy, among others. Autogenic training, progressive relaxation, behavior modification, and hypnosis are also forms of psychotherapy. There are also variations in the number of visits. Short (brief) term limits patient visits to approximately 10-25 and long term (intensive) has an unlimited and regular number of visits.

Within each of the above approaches there are variations dependent upon the therapist's ability and variations dependent upon the school of thought to which the therapist adheres. There are followers of Freud, Jung, Adler, Grinker, Sullivan, Horney, Erikson, Perls, Moreno, Slavson, Maslow, Skinner, Wolpe, Binswanger, to name just some of the better known persons. It should be clear that in psychotherapy there are many variations of theoretical and clinical approaches.

Jung wrote the following:

Since the mind is common to mankind it may seem to the layman that there can be only one psychology, and he may therefore suppose the divergences between the schools to be either subjective quibbling, or else a commonplace disguise for the efforts of mediocrities who seek to exalt themselves upon a throne . . . . There are, in fact, many methods, standpoints, views and convictions which are all at war with one another—the main reason for this being that, since they fail to be mutually comprehensible, none of them can grant the validity of any other. The many-sidedness and variety of psychological opinions in our time is nothing less than astonishing, . . .

When we find the most diverse remedies prescribed in a text-book of pathology for a given disease, we may confidently assume that none of these remedies is particularly efficacious. So, when many different ways of approaching the psyche are recommended, we may rest assured that none of them leads with absolute certainty to the goal, least of all those advocated in a fanatical way.[155]

The principal methods of psychotherapy are individual, behavioral, group, and hypnosis.

INDIVIDUAL PSYCHOTHERAPY

There are many levels of understanding and claims are made that one form of therapy is more suited than another to attain insight. For instance, supportive (suppressive) is said to be more superficial, uses ego-strengthening methods such as reassurance, ventilation, suggestion, discussion, reeducation, etc., and is little concerned with "analyzing" the patient. On the other hand, expressive (deep) therapy provides insight into conscious and unconscious conflicts and achieves changes in the personality structure. Further, it is said that the goal of supportive is adaption to existing conditions, while the goal of expressive is internal change so that the patient can change the conditions of his existence.[156–158] This separation is simply not true. Insights are not limited to one form of therapy or another. Sometimes the most profound insights can come as a sudden flash, or as the result of some seemingly insignificant experience or word. Therefore, all psychotherapy, regardless of methodology, may broaden and deepen the patient's insights; and a division such as suppressive versus expressive is artificial and misleading.[159]

There are five aspects of psychotherapy that are of particular importance: the doctor–patient relationship; the ability of the patient to talk to the therapist and unburden himself of guilt, conflict, anxiety, shame, etc.; the value of education, reeducation, and suggestion; the increase of understanding by explanation; and the resultant change or transformation that occurs within the patient's total being. With each patient these aspects have varying degrees of importance; hence, there is tremendous variety in the management of each individual.

The patient's relationship with the doctor begins at the time an appointment is made. The manner in which it is done has relevance. Does a cold and efficient, or warm and friendly secretary make the appointment? Does the doctor make the appointment? With this, the first contact, the patient's feelings and thoughts regarding the therapist begin to develop. From this point, through the comprehensive evaluation, diagnosis, treatment plan, and continuing therapy, both patient and doctor form opinions and feelings toward each other. An effective relationship ideally is based upon mutual respect, confidence, and trust. The physician should be knowledgeable, available, affable, flexible, and both patient and physician should participate in the therapeutic process with a feeling of openness and frankness. Expectations and limitations should be defined and false promises should not be explicitly or implicitly implied by the therapist. Faith in both the therapist and the procedure is a great ally to successful treatment and should be recognized as having healing power. Patients become attached to and dependent upon the therapist and this must be understood by both the patient and the physician in order to prevent endless therapy. A time must come when optimum benefit has been attained and when treatment is ended. Too long or too short a period of time can be detrimental. The difficulties of differences—likes, dislikes, morals, ethics, religion, race, prejudices, etc.—should be evaluated. Negatives hinder treatment and need to be resolved or at least recognized and understood. The doctor-patient relationship is basic for without an effective one there will be no therapy.

The value of communication has been recognized since time began. To share one's thoughts, feelings, and activities—to sense and touch another person—removes individuals from feelings of isolation and loneliness. In therapy the value of talking, confessing, ventilating, and abreacting affords the patient not only relief and the feeling of communion with another human being, but also the opportunity to reveal his inner secrets. Revealing secrets—be they conscious or unconscious thoughts or feelings in which shame and guilt play a predominant role—can free the patient to see and understand himself and his behavior as never before. These shared insights open pathways for change. These insights may be based upon past or present fantasies or real experiences— it makes no difference, for the fact remains that unexpressed conscious and unconscious thoughts, feelings, fantasies, and behavior are forces and influences that inhibit and inhibited the patient's growth, development, and functioning. Prior to being shared with another, they were a source of pain and suffering. The therapist's attitudes toward these patient revelations is of extreme importance as he must help to relieve not to reinforce the guilt and shame. The therapist by interpreting the transference of past feelings and attitudes and relating this to the current life situation may add a further dimension of insight.[160]

The value of education and reeducation will increase and expand the abilities of the mind and relieve uncertainties and doubts. Ignorance can foster fear which knowledge can dissolve. There are many areas about which patients can become informed and when the therapist tells him that he does not have cancer and/or is not insane, the patient can be relieved of anxiety, self-recrimination, and worry. To be informed of the scope of a normal range is especially reassuring. Likewise, suggestions made by the therapist and followed by the patient may lead to success and this in turn can remove symptoms or improve function and change the patient's attitudes and orientation. Suggestion may provide temporary or permanent relief of symptoms and improvement of overall functioning. Besides, interpretation or explanation may be a suggestion in disguise—there is no scientific way to prove otherwise. Perhaps the most potent form of treatment—both for physical and mental illness—is suggestion. The effectiveness of suggestion depends upon who gives it, how it is given, and to whom it is given.[161]

Explanations need not be formalized or ritualized but can be based on common sense and rational thought. Rational thought is a complex process that involves reasoning, judgment, and intellectual ideals. Reasoning is a form of logic that is related to the data from which a conclusion is drawn. Tart writes:

> Note that a *logic* is a self-contained, arbitrary system. Two and two do not make four in any "real" sense; they make four because they have been *defined* that way. That a particular logic is highly useful in dealing with the physical world should not blind us to the fact that it is basically an arbitrary, self-contained, assumptive system. Thus when I define the Evaluation and Decision-Making subsystem as processing information in accordance with a logic, I do not intend to give it an ultimate validity, but just to note that there is an assumptive system, heavily influenced by culture and personal history, which processes data . . . . We should also note, as honest self-observation will reveal, that much of what passes as rationality . . . is in fact rationalization. We want something so we make up "good" reasons for it.[162]

Since logic involves a system which in turn involves values or judgments, the question arises as to what to base these judgments upon? Information reaches the brain via sensations and is interpreted there. But the imagery is not the same as the stimulus that produced that imagery, e.g., a "real" pencil is not the same as the "idea" pencil. Our ideas such as morality, causality, abstract thought, and so forth are removed from the stimulus. The more abstract and the further removed from the actual sense data, the more universal are the conclusions. The more explanations are based on the particular and sense perceptions, the less abstract and less universal are the conclusions.[163] Hence for therapists, universals should be avoided as much as possible since that form of abstraction removes the patient and physician too far from the sense perceptions and it presupposes a universal image of man. This type of thinking forces the patient and doctor into a closed philosophical system and should be avoided. On the other hand a rational common sense explanation that is not too abstract and close to the patient material is preferable. Yet intellectual explanation or knowing by itself is not enough. The patient must "feel" the explanation as well as intellectually know it. In this sense, there is "knowing" and "knowing."

Although the goals of therapy vary from more satisfactory adjustments to home, family, and social relationships, or symptom removal, among others, the highest goal a psychiatrist seeks is to help a patient make responsible choices and to attain personal freedom. The patient can change not into what the psychiatrist, the patient's family, or society thinks he ought to be but change into what he can be and wants to be—a personal choice. For this, the patient must remove inner obstacles to his thought, feeling, desires, and will. In attaining personal freedom the patient will then experience harmony between his action and the goal, and accept the responsibility for the consequences of his action. He has in effect attained a level of personal freedom within certain predetermined organic limits to make conscious choices and to act according to these choices.[164, 165] This does not imply that the needs of others are not considered; they are. But it is the patient who chooses the degree to which others can influence him. When this occurs, however, it may create a variety of new conflicts, for he now views himself and the world differently. This may promote changes in life-style or values, uproot families, or shift occupations. No therapist can predict when such far-reaching changes will occur and the hope is that these changes are beneficial and not destructive to the patient or to others. The hope is that with personal freedom, a patient will devote his energies toward constructive activities with himself, his family, friends, and society. It is indeed, however, the rare patient who seeks or reaches this level of attainment; hence, for the most part the therapist's work is directed towards the other goals of treatment.

PSYCHOANALYSIS

Psychoanalysis is a method of psychotherapy designed to explore the unconscious mind. The method employs the technique of free association, i.e., the analysand (patient) lies on a couch and is encouraged to utter spontaneously any thought or feeling that comes to his mind; and the interpretation of dreams, unconscious resistances, and transferences. The manifest dream is thought to represent unconscious wishes, fantasies, and desires in disguised form. The analyst's work is to remove the censorship (resistance) in the conscious mind and in this manner to arrive at the meaning of the dream (latent content). Applying the same principles to manifest conscious activity such as slips of tongue, forgetfulness, and everyday activities among others, the analyst interprets the resistances and arrives at the meanings. Resistances can be manifested by mechanisms of defense (repression, identification, overcompensation, substitution, sublimation, etc.) that represent a failure in the ego to integrate impulses with one another or with the environmental situation. Transference is the repetition of early life patterns displaced by the analysand towards the analyst. Transference neurosis is a regressed state in which the patient re-experiences with the analyst the most intense emotional involvements prior to age 6. The resolution of the transference neurosis is the goal of therapy. Analyzing or demonstrating the true nature of the resistances, transferences, and the transference neurosis is the basic method of psychoanalytic therapy. The aim is to include into the conscious personality those portions of the mind which were previously excluded; thereby enabling the analysand to experience growth and maturation, to remove the cause of the symptoms and in so doing remove the symptoms, and to promote conscious control and flexibility in dealing with the changing conditions of the patient's current life.[166]

Classical psychoanalysis can be used for the treatment of personality disorders and neuroses. The major difficulties with classical analysis are its expense, the time consumed (3-5 times per week for several years), and the limited number of suitable patients for this form of treatment. Generally, psychotic patients cannot be analyzed by the classical method, and those with certain types of defenses who do not form transferences are also unanalyzable. Besides the patient should be below the ages of 40-45, of at least average intelligence, and strongly motivated. Other disadvantages are: the increase in introspection and egocentricity may cause difficulties in the patient's social life; the limited number of qualified analysts creates a relative unavailability for those who seek this type of treatment; and proof is lacking that the therapeutic outcome is better than other treatment modalities.[167]

BEHAVIOR THERAPY

The term refers to a group of dissimilar methods of treatment that are all based on learning or conditioning theory. The goal of treatment is to abolish old patterns of maladaptive behavior or to establish new appropriate ones. Symptom removal is primary and cause is either secondary or not considered since the symptom is regarded as an inadvertent conditioned or poorly learned response; in effect then, to behavior therapists the symptom is the disease. Obviously, this approach is the antithesis of classical psychoanalysis and since both methods do have successes it should again impress therapists that in psychiatry there is room for everything but dogma. To dismiss any notion that the behavior therapist is some sort of mechanical robot, it should be remembered that he is a person, talks with his patients, and offers encouragement, advice, and reassurance.[168]

The indications for behavior therapy are broad. Claims are made for its use in the treatment of various types of mental illness and in certain educational, social, and other nonpsychiatric settings.[169]   These claims by enthusiastic users of the methods, however, have not as yet been satisfactorily substantiated and caution in its use is recommended.[170]   The enthusiasts claim that behavior therapy can help about 10% of all adult psychiatric patients; that it is the best approach for phobias including social anxieties and obsessive compulsive rituals; that it is helpful in impotence, frigidity, and exhibitionism; that it may be useful in obsessive thinking, social skill problems, stammering, hair pulling, self-mutilation, compulsive gambling, obesity, anorexia, and so on.[171]   This list, while incomplete, should be enough to stimulate an interest in some of the principal applications of behavior therapy.

The behavior therapist, like all other therapists, starts treatment by carefully evaluating the patient. The evaluation concentrates on the exact circumstances that provoke the appearance of symptoms in the patient. Once this is determined, a treatment plan is formulated in which one of the innumerable methods of behavior therapy is selected.   Any method requires the cooperation of the patient and may need the help of the family, residential treatment center, or a hospital.   The treatments can vary from 1 to 30 sessions, and last from one-half hour to two hours per session.[172]

Desensitization (reciprocal inhibition) is the most common form of treatment and is used mainly for phobias, anxiety, psychosomatic disorders, and sexual dysfunctions or perversions.   Two methods of desensitization are employed: the in vivo method in which the patient is placed in the real life situation and the fantasy method in which the patient imagines the situation that provokes symptoms. Both the in vivo and fantasy methods may employ muscle relaxation technics.   One type of desensitization involves the arrangement of a series or hierarchy of symptom-provoking situations in which the patient is gradually exposed, either in fantasy or in vivo, to the symptom-provocative circumstances. Another method, called implosion or flooding, suddenly places the patient in the symptom-provoking situations.   In both types the therapist hopes to extinguish the maladaptive response in the patient and exposure to provocative circumstances is the common denominator.[173]

Paradoxical intention or self-regulation is a variation of desensitization. In this type of treatment the patient is encouraged to keep the symptom, embellish, or even practice it.   The therapist attempts to abolish the symptom by encouraging its existence, hence the name paradoxical intention. Varieties of this technic are called negative practice, directive therapy, direct analysis, symptom prescription approach, and symptom simulation. Whatever the name, this form of behavior therapy has been used to treat a variety of mental illnesses.[174]

Modeling or imitation therapy presents a live situation in which the patient observes the behavior of others. It can be produced by live people, a movie, puppet theatre, etc. The basis for this treatment is that the patient will model his behavior after the examples selected by the therapist.

Operant conditioning or positive reinforcement attempts to modify behavior by altering the consequences of behavior. This method rewards satisfactory behavior, thereby encouraging new patterns of behavior and eliminating undesirable responses. Its main use has been in the treatment of autistic children, hospitalized adults, and in childhood behavior problems. In contrast, aversion or negative reinforcement therapy is that in which behavior is not rewarded but punished. Unpleasant, painful electric shocks are used in treating enuretics and sexual perverts. Alcoholics are treated with Antabuse, a drug that interferes with the enzymatic breakdown of alcohol and causes acute acetaldehyde intoxication—flushing, headaches, nausea, vomiting, palpitations, tachycardia, dyspnea, hyperventilation, and hypotension. For details of these and other methods of behavior therapy the student is referred elsewhere.[175]

The shortcomings of behavior therapy are many. At times it does not work and if the symptom is removed it may be replaced by another. When symptoms are removed with behavior therapy such disturbances as divorce, broken homes, depression, or aggressive behavior may result. For these reasons combinations of behavior therapy with other forms of psychotherapy are advised. With symptom removal, the patient may need help toward developing an integrated personality with appropriate adaptive patterns of behavior. A cooperative rather than a competitive attitude among the various types of psychiatric therapies is encouraged.[176, 177]

GROUP THERAPY

The term group therapy refers to yet another type of psychotherapy in which there are marked divergences of approaches. Theoretical and practical considerations are so diverse that there is no one satisfactory method of classification. In fact, not all groups are organized for the purpose of treating the mentally ill. T groups enable individuals to evaluate their behavior and its effect on others; hence, T groups are used in schools, industry, and government. Encounter, sensitivity, and variations such as primal scream, Gestalt (existentialist), body movement, aquanude therapy, love massage, among others are concerned with the expression of feelings. Transactional analysis groups, in contrast to the expressive or didactic groups, are concerned with the covert meanings of interpersonal communication. Traditional groups, on the other hand, follow one of the established schools of individual psychotherapy and apply its theoretical principles to the group. Each group borrows rather freely from other groups and there are no "pure" groups.[178]

Group psychotherapy is conducted by a professionally trained individual. There are usually no more than ten participants in a group and the group meets from one to five times per week in sessions that usually last 1½ hours. Groups may be of the same or mixed sex; leaders, depending on orientation, may behave in an active, passive, authoritarian or democratic manner and follow a structured or unstructured approach; participants' ages vary from 20–50, and they suffer from various types of mental illness. In each group the leader selects patients on the basis of compatibility and the type of illness from which they suffer. Hence there are groups of schizophrenics, neurotics, homosexuals, personality disorders, or various combinations.[179]

The patients and leader help one another. Open discussion, self-disclosure, and give and take relationships are encouraged. Members of the group help each other seek solutions to individual problems. Belonging and participating helps to relieve feelings of isolation, shyness, and inhibition, removes symptoms, and stimulates adaptive behavior. The patient's role is that of an individual equal to all others in the group. His concerns and problems are recognized and evaluated. Acceptable behavior and attitudes that increase self-esteem, self-respect, and a more realistic evaluation of social relationships are encouraged. At times, peer pressures are more effective than the "dictates" of the authoritarian leader. This, plus an economy of cost to the patient and time to the therapist are the major advantages. For some patients, groups are without a doubt the treatment of choice and not a secondary or "cheap" form of treatment.[180]

The major disadvantages of group therapy are: a patient may be placed in an unduly stressful situation or may receive too much criticism and disapproval and therefore drop out of treatment and lose self-esteem and respect; the members of the group may reveal secret or privileged information about another member; all persons are not suitable for this type of treatment; and some patients need more personal attention to enable them to make meaningful connections. Combinations of group and individual therapies may overcome the latter difficulty. Further disadvantages of group therapy are the need to clarify what constitutes proper training for a group leader and what types of activity are appropriate and inappropriate for group participation. Experimental groups continue to appear and some limits must be set in terms of professional activity and type of setting. Male and females swimming in the nude may be fun, but is this modality professional or therapeutic?[181]

Family and marital therapies are forms of group therapy. They, however, assume a direct relationship between the total family constellation and its influence on each individual member's growth, development, and psychic state. This paradigm lends itself to the supposition that the family member who comes for psychiatric treatment may not be the most disturbed one in the family. Indeed, the patient who develops the symptoms may reflect a dysfunction within the family constellation. Some other member or members of the family may be more disturbed and may be the actual reason the patient develops his difficulties. By examining the family as a group it is possible to evaluate the patient in a way that is not permitted by individual methods. Family therapy, like all other forms of psychotherapy, confronts the therapist with particularly difficult situations. For example, a child is brought for treatment for either a symptom or behavioral disturbance and the therapist determines that the "real" pathology is not in the child but in the marriage or in one of the parents. Alternatives are to treat the child individually or to treat the parents (one or both); to advise separation of the child from the family, or divorce; to maintain the status quo that will perpetuate the pathology of the child; or to treat the whole family. The basic assumption that the environmental circumstances caused the disturbance in the child must be questioned. This assumption is difficult to prove. Yet a great deal of psychotherapy makes this assumption and it is the basis for many important decisions. Family therapy is still in its early stages of development and caution by the therapist must be a principal concern.[182-184]

HYPNOSIS

Hypnosis is a specialized technique in which the patient enters a hypnagogic or trancelike state of consciousness. With a patient in the hypnotic state, the therapist can, by suggestion, remove symptoms or probe for repressed memories, situations, or emotions (hypnoanalysis). In the posthypnotic state suggestions made during the trance can be followed by the patient and can influence the patient's behavior and symptoms. Hypnosis is used for treatment of amnesias, fugues, conversion reactions, psychosomatic disorders, anxiety states, phobias, anesthesia, intractable hiccupping, severe malnutrition from neurotic vomiting, anorexia nervosa, and so forth. There are those who believe that hypnosis like narcoanalysis, although recommended for many conditions, has in fact a very limited usage and nothing can be done for the patient with hypnosis that cannot be done with other forms of psychotherapy.[185, 186] Others claim that hypnosis does have unique features with broad applications and usages.[187]

The mechanism of hypnosis is not known. Some consider it the result of suggestion, role playing, or a type of self-protective behavior characterized by motor inhibition. Psychoanalysts consider hypnosis a regressive phenomenon, and Pavlovians view it as a partial cortical inhibition.[188] Posthypnotic amnesia is considered one of the most important phenomena of hypnosis. Speculations regarding why the patient fails to recall the events in the trance vary from poor memory, implicit or explicit suggestions not to remember, problems of memory storage, to decay of memory traces, etc. Others claim that posthypnotic amnesia is an active dynamic process in which information is kept at a level out of the patient's awareness.[189] To date these are all theories but with further investigation they can have relevance to the mechanism of memory as well as to the meaning and mechanisms of varying levels of states of consciousness.

Hypnosis requires a relatively brief period of time and can be used in conjunction with other forms of physical and psychological therapies. A 30–60 minute session can remove symptoms, and repeated sessions (hypnoanalysis) can explore areas of thought and feeling in a shorter time than other forms of psychotherapy. The symptoms, however, may return or be replaced by others. The most dangerous risk is that at times patients become psychotic, depressed, or suicidal.[190] Even with careful pretreatment evaluations, the therapist is not assured that the proximate or ultimate results will be to his and the patient's satisfaction. The advantages and disadvantages should be evaluated with each patient.

An excellent summary of all psychiatric treatments was written by Raskin as follows:

It is a truism that almost any therapeutic move works once with some patients—and nothing works well with all or should be ventured by all practitioners. It is understandable, nonetheless, that we are tempted by the proclamation of The Theory or The Strategy of personality and therapy. Theories and strategies are simpler than patients and psychiatrists. Only recently has it become professionally respectable to call oneself either theoretically or technically an "eclectic."

It is not surprising that experienced and successful clinicians often act alike with patients, despite the language and constructs they use when initiating their juniors into the fraternity. There are even relatively few niceties of theories that clearly separate the therapies into opposing camps—the theory may not count for much.[191]

REFERENCES

REFERENCES

1. Ludwig, A.M., The proper domain of psychiatry. *Psychiatric Dig.* 37(1):15–24 (1976).
2. Ibid., p. 23.
3. Szasz, T.S., Psychiatry, psychotherapy, and psychology. *Arch. Gen. Psychiatry* 1:455–463 (1959).

4. Offenkrantz, W. and Tobin, A., Psychoanalytic psychotherapy. *Arch. Gen. Psychiatry* 30:593-606 (1974).

5. Robinson, L.R., Basic concepts in family therapy: A differential comparison with individual treatment. *Amer. J. Psychiatry* 132(10):1045-1048 (1975).

6. Cabral, R.J., Best, J., and Paton, A., Patients' and observers' assessments of process and outcome in group therapy: A follow-up study. *Amer. J. Psychiatry* 132(10): 1052-1054 (1975).

7. Harbin, H., Some advantages and disadvantages of conjoint family therapy by the same therapist. *Dis. Nerv. Syst.* 36(1):20-23 (1975).

8. Marks, I.M., The current status of behavioral psychotherapy: Theory and practice. *Amer. J. Psychiatry* 133(3):253-261 (1976).

9. Kopolow, L.E. and Cohen, G.D., Milieu therapy: Towards a definition of reimbursement. *Amer. J. Psychiatry* 133(9):1060-1063 (1976).

10. Blanchard, E.B., et. al., Clinical applications of biofeedback training: A review of evidence. *Arch. Gen. Psychiatry* 30:573-589 (1974).

11. Cartwright, R.D. and Weiss, M.R., The effects of electrosleep on insomnia revisited. *J. Nerv. Ment. Dis.* 161(2):134-137 (1975).

12. Fleck, S., A general systems approach to severe family pathology. *Amer. J. Psychiatry* 133(6):669-673 (1976).

13. Seigler, M. and Osmond, H., *Models of Madness, Models of Medicine.* New York: Macmillan, 1974.

14. Brown, B.S., The life of psychiatry. *Amer. J. Psychiatry* 133(5):489-495 (1976).

15. Ibid., p. 495.

16. Marmor, J., Presidential address: Psychiatry 1976—The continuing revolution. *Amer. J. Psychiatry* 133(7):743-744 (1976).

17. Engelhardt, Jr., H.T., Explanatory models in medicine: Facts, theories, and values. *Tex. Rep. Biol. Med.* 32(1):225-239 (1974).

18. Marmor, J., op. cit., pp. 742-743.

19. Davis, D.R., *An Introduction to Psychopathology,* 3rd ed. London: Oxford Univ. Press, 1972, p. 1.

20. Jaspers, K., *General Psychopathology* (transl. by Hoenig, J. and Hamilton, N.W.). Chicago: Univ. of Chicago Press, 1963, pp. 1-2.

21. King, L.S., Empiricism, rationalism, and diabetes. *J. Amer. Med. Assoc.* 187(7):521-526 (1964).

22. Batchelor, I.R.C., *Henderson and Gillespie's Textbook of Psychiatry,* 10th ed. London: Oxford Univ. Press, 1969, pp. 3-15.

23. Brown, B.S., op. cit., p. 491.

24. Lieberman, M.A. and Gardner, J., Institutional alternatives to psychotherapy: A study of growth center users. *Arch. Gen. Psychiatry* 33(2):157-162 (1976).

25. Brown, B.S., op. cit., pp. 493-495.

26. Marmor, J., op. cit., pp. 740-745.

27. Thompson, J.S. and Thompson, M.W., *Genetics in Medicine.* Philadelphia: Saunders, 1967, pp. 255-265.

28. Garrison, F.H., *An Introduction to the History of Medicine,* 4th ed. reprinted. Philadelphia: Saunders, 1929, p. 516.

29. Thompson, J.S. and Thompson, M.W., op. cit., p. 260.

30. Engelhardt, Jr., H.T., The patient as a person: An empty phrase? *Tex. Med.* 71(9): 57-63 (1975).

31. Hsia, D.Y., *Inborn Errors of Metabolism,* 2nd ed. Chicago: Year Book Pub. Co., 1966, p. 134.

32. Ibid., pp. 134–143.
33. Durell, J., "Introduction," in *Biological Psychiatry* (Mendels, J., Ed.). New York: Wiley, 1973, p. 7.
34. Roth, M., Kay, D.W.K., and Kiloh, L.G., "The results of biological (physical) treatment in psychiatry and their bearing on the classification of disease," in *Biological Treatment of Mental Illness* (Rinkel, M., Ed.). New York: Farrar, Straus, and Geroux, 1966, p. 72.
35. Hoff, H., "The invention of insulin shock treatment of schizophrenia, a milestone in the development of psychiatry," in *Biological Treatment of Mental Illness* (Rinkel, M., Ed.). New York: Farrar, Straus, and Geroux, 1966, pp. 47–49.
36. Beeson, P.B. and McDermott, W., *Cecil-Loeb Textbook of Medicine*, vol. 2. Philadelphia: Saunders, 1971, p. 1442.
37. Garrison, F.H., op. cit., p. 706.
38. Hoff, H., "History of the organic treatment of schizophrenia," in *Insulin Treatment in Psychiatry*, (Rinkel, M. and Himwich, H., Eds.). New York: Philosophical Library, 1959, pp. 8–9.
39. Gottlieb, J.S., "Introductory greetings," in *Insulin Treatment in Psychiatry* (Rinkel, M. and Himwich, H., Eds.). New York: Philosophical Library, 1959, p. xxvii.
40. Noyes, A.P., *Modern Clinical Psychiatry*, 2nd ed. Philadelphia: Saunders, 1944, p. 475.
41. Hoff, H., "History of the organic treatment of schizophrenia," op. cit., pp. 11–12.
42. Rossi, M., "History of psychiatry," in *Handbook of Psychiatry*, 3rd ed. (Solomon, P. and Patch, B.V., Eds.). Los Altos, Calif.: Lange Medical Publications, 1974, p. 167.
43. Hoff, H., "History of the organic treatment of schizophrenia," op. cit., p. 9.
44. Ibid., p. 11.
45. Rossi, M., op. cit., p. 167.
46. Detre, T.P. and Jarecki, H.G., *Modern Psychiatric Treatment*. Philadelphia: Lippincott, 1971, p. 663.
47. Zakowski, P., Psychosurgery. *J. Legal Med.* 26, April (1976).
48. Detre, T.P. and Jarecki, H.G., op. cit., p. 663.
49. Burch, E.A., Bromide intoxication–1976 literature review and case report. *Curr. Concepts Psychiatry* 2(4):13 (1976).
50. Aagaard, G.N. and Elliott, H.W., Clinical pharmacology: Drug therapy of anxiety. *Postgrad. Med.* 54(1):159–160 (1973).
51. Rossi, M., op. cit., p. 167.
52. Ibid.
53. Johnson, W.C., A neglected modality in psychiatric treatment–the monoamine oxidase inhibitors. *Dis. Nerv. Syst.* 36:521–525 (1975).
54. Batchelor, I.R.C., op. cit., p. 336.
55. Rossi, M., op. cit., p. 167.
56. Freedman, A.M., Kaplan, H.I., and Sadock, B.J., *Modern Synopsis of Comprehensive Psychiatry/II*, 2nd ed. Baltimore: Williams & Wilkins, 1976, pp. 905–908.
57. Jaspers, K., op. cit., pp. 380, 802, 836.
58. Jacobson, E., *Direct Electrical Measurement of Mental Activities in Action-Potentials*, vol. 1. Chicago: Laboratory for Clinical Physiology, reprints from 1927–1946.
59. Jacobson, E., *Progressive Relaxation*, 2nd. ed. Chicago: Univ. of Chicago Press, 1938.
60. Freedman, A.M., Kaplan, H.I., and Sadock, B.J., *Modern Synopsis of Comprehensive Psychiatry*, 1st ed. Baltimore: Williams & Wilkins, 1972, pp. 518–521.

61. Seitz, P.F.D., et al., *The Manpower Problem in Mental Hospitals.* New York: International Universities Press, 1976.

62. Sydenham, T., "Medical observations concerning the history and cure of acute diseases." [3rd ed., 1676], in *The Works of Thomas Sydenham*, translated by R.G. Latham, Vol. 1, The Sydenham Society, 1848, pp.11-12. All of this taken from: King, L., (Ed.), *A History of Medicine*, Baltimore, Penquin Books, 1977, pp.122-123.

63. Enelow, A.J. and Swisher, S., *Interviewing and Patient Care.* New York: Oxford University Press, 1972, pp. 168-170.

64. Kaplan, S.A., Drug abuse and drug addiction: Why the numbers game? *Psychiatric Annals* 4(12):7-10(1974).

65. Redmond, J.F., *Education About Drugs: Kindergarten Through High School Program.* Chicago: Board of Education, 1971.

66. Farnsworth, D.L., Toward a theory of drug control. *Psychiatric Annals* 3(4):73-93 (1973).

67. Greenblatt, D.J., Shader, R.I., and Koch-Wesser, J., Psychotropic drug use in the Boston area: A report from the Boston collaborative drug surveillance program. *Arch. Gen. Psychiatry* 32:518-521 (1975).

68. Cohen, S. (Ed.), Valium: Its use and abuse. *Drug Abuse and Alcoholism Newsletter:* 5(4): May 1976).

69. Greenblatt, D.J., et al., op. cit., pp. 520-521.

70. Rowe, C.J., *An Outline of Psychiatry.* Dubuque, Iowa: William C. Brown Co., 1975, p. 137.

71. Ibid., p. 152.

72. Mazzullo, J.M., Methods of improving patient compliance. *Drug Therapy:* 6:148-155 (March 1976).

73. Detre, T.P. and Jarecki, H.G., op. cit., pp. 306, 464, 465.

74. Rowe, C.J., op. cit., pp. 151-152.

75. Maugh, II, T.H., Marihuana: The grass may no longer be greener. *Science* 185:683-685 (1974).

76. Goth, A., *Medical Pharmacology: Principles and Concepts*, 4th ed. St. Louis: Mosby, 1968, pp. 260-261.

77. AMA Committee on Alcoholism and Drug Dependence: Barbiturates and Barbiturate-Like Drugs: Considerations in Their Medical Use. *J. Amer. Med. Assoc.* 230(10): 1440-1441 (1974).

78. Goth, A., op. cit., pp. 268-270.

79. Greenblatt, D.J. and Shader, R.I., "Psychotropic drug overdose," in *Manual of Psychiatric Therapeutics: Practical Psychiatry and Psychopharmacology* (Shader, R.I., Ed.). Boston: Little, Brown, 1975, pp. 237-260.

80. Shader, R.I., Caine, E.D., and Meyer, R.E., "Treatment of dependence on barbiturates and sedative-hypnotics," in *Manual of Psychiatric Therapeutics: Practical Psychiatry and Psychopharmacology* (Shader, R.I., Ed.). Boston: Little, Brown, 1975, pp. 195-202.

81. Shader, R.I. (Ed.), Ibid., pp. 195-202, 237-262.

82. Freedman, A.M., Kaplan, H.I., and Sadock, B.J., *Modern Synopsis of Comprehensive Psychiatry/II*, op. cit., pp. 976-977.

83. Greenblatt, D.J., and Shader, R.I., "Treatment of the alcohol withdrawal syndrome," in *Manual of Psychiatric Therapeutics: Practical Psychiatry and Psychopharmacology* (Shader, R.I., Ed.). Boston: Little, Brown, 1975, p. 218.

84. Greenblatt, D.J. and Shader, R.I., "Psychotropic drugs in the general hospital," in *Manual of Psychiatric Therapeutics: Practical Psychiatry and Psychopharmacology* (Shader, R.I., Ed.). Boston: Little, Brown, 1975, p. 7.

85. Blackwell, B., Psychotropic drugs in use today: The role of diazepam in medical practice. *J. Amer. Med. Assoc.* **225**(13):1640 (1973).
86. Hollister, L.E., Uses of psychotherapeutic drugs. *Ann. Int. Med.* **79**(1):90 (1973).
87. Greenblatt, D.J. and Shader, R.I., *Benzodiazepines in Clinical Practice.* New York: Raven Press, 1974, pp. 78–79.
88. Hollister, L.E., op. cit., p. 90.
89. Blackwell, B., Rational drug use in the management of anxiety. *Rational Drug Therapy* **9**(6):5 (1975).
90. Hollister, L.E., Clinical use of psychotherapeutic drugs: Current status. *Clin. Pharmacol. Ther.* **10**(2):171 (1969).
91. Hollister, L.E., Uses of psychotherapeutic drugs. op. cit., p. 95.
92. Appleton, W.S., Third psychoactive drug usage guide. *Dis. Nerv. Syst.* **37**(1):39–44 (1976).
93. Detre, T.P. and Jarecki, H.G., op. cit., pp. 534–591.
94. Appleton, W.S., op. cit., pp. 39–44.
95. Ibid., pp. 43–44.
96. Hollister, L.E., Clinical use of psychotherapeutic drugs: Current status, op. cit., p. 186.
97. Hollister, L.E., Uses of psychotherapeutic drugs, op. cit., pp. 96–97.
98. AMA Council on Drugs: AMA Drug Evaluations, 1st ed. Chicago: American Medical Association, 1971, pp. 169–176.
99. Ibid., pp. 177–188.
100. Freedman, A.M., Kaplan, H.I., and Sadock, B.J., *Modern Synopsis of Comprehensive Textbook of Psychiatry/II,* op. cit., pp. 209, 665.
101. Ibid., pp. 665–668, 1313–1314.
102. Maugh, T.H., op. cit., p. 683.
103. Cohen, S., Angel dust: The pervasive psychedelic. *Drug Abuse and Alcoholism Newsletter* **5**(7): (Sept. 1976).
104. Ulett, G.A., *A Synopsis of Contemporary Psychiatry,* 5th ed. St. Louis: Mosby, 1972, p. 304.
105. Grant, I., Mohns, L., Miller, M., and Reiton, R., A neuropsychological study of polydrug users. *Arch. Gen. Psychiatry* **33**(8):973–978 (1976).
106. Grant, I. and Lewis, L.J., Neuropsychological and EEG Disturbances in Polydrug Users. *Amer. J. Psychiatry* **133**(9):1039–1042 (1976).
107. Blackwell, B., "Rational drug use in psychiatry," in *Rational Psychopharmacotherapy and the Right to Treatment* (Ayd, F.J., Ed.). Baltimore: Ayd Medical Communications Ltd., 1975, pp. 187–199.
108. Curran, D., Partridge, M., and Storey, P., *Psychological Medicine: An Introduction to Psychiatry.* Edinburgh and London: Churchill, Livingstone, 1972, pp. 390–391.
109. Freedman, A.M., Kaplan, H.I., and Sadock, B.J., *Modern Synopsis of Comprehensive Textbook of Psychiatry/II,* op. cit., pp. 993–995.
110. Detre, T.P. and Jarecki, H.G., op. cit., pp. 665–666.
111. Freedman, A.M., Kaplan, H.I., and Sadock, B.J., *Modern Synopsis of Comprehensive Textbook of Psychiatry/II,* op. cit., pp. 988–989.
112. Batchelor, I.R.C., op. cit., pp. 338–339.
113. Detre, T.P. and Jarecki, H.G., op. cit., pp. 660–662.
114. Ibid., pp. 656–659.
115. Pauling, L., On the orthomolecular environment of the mind: Orthomolecular theory. *Amer. J. Psychiatry* **131**(11):1251–1257 (1974).
116. Wyatt, R.J., Comment. *Amer. J. Psychiatry* **131**(11):1258–1262 (1974).

117. Klein, D.F., Comment. *Amer. J. Psychiatry* **131**(11):1263-1265 (1974).
118. Lipton, M., Comment. *Amer. J. Psychiatry* **131**(11):1266-1267 (1974).
119. Freedman, A.M., Kaplan, H.I., and Sadock, B.J., *Modern Synopsis of Comprehensive Textbook of Psychiatry/II,* op. cit., p. 1000.
120. Ibid., pp. 1000-1001.
121. Arnot, R.E., Observations on the effects of electric convulsive treatment in man— psychological. *Dis. Nerv. Syst.* **36**(9):499 (1975).
122. Blachly, P.H., New developments in electroconvulsive therapy. *Dis. Nerv. Syst.* **37**(6):357-358 (1976).
123. Ulett, G.A., op. cit., pp. 282-287.
124. Ibid., pp. 285-286.
125. Arnot, R.E., op. cit., pp. 500-501.
126. Squire, L.R. and Chace, P.M., Memory functions six to nine months after electroconvulsive therapy. *Arch. Gen. Psychiatry* **32**(12):1564 (1975).
127. Avery, D. and Winokur, G., Mortality in depressed patients treated with electroconvulsive therapy and antidepressants. *Arch. Gen. Psychiatry* **33**(9):1029-1037 (1976).
128. Ulett, G.A., op. cit., p. 288.
129. Friedman, E., Andrus, P., Sedac electrotherapy III—A ten year study of therapeutic efficiency and indications. *Dis. Nerv. Syst.* **37**(8):451-455 (1976).
130. Scallet, A., Cloninger, C.B., and Othmer, E., The management of chronic hysteria: A review and double-blind trial of electrosleep and other relaxation methods. *Dis. Nerv. Syst.* **37**(6):347-353 (1976).
131. Chumakova, L.T. and Kirillova, Z.A., "Electrosleep as an effective outpatient treatment for nervous and psychological disorders," in *Innovative Medical-Psychiatric Therapies* (Suinn, R.M. and Weigel, R.G., Eds.). Baltimore: University Park Press, 1976, pp. 291-297.
132. Ulett, G.A., op. cit., pp. 288-289.
133. Cartwright, R.D. and Weiss, M.F., The effects of electrosleep on insomnia revisited. *J. Nerv. Ment. Dis.* **161**(2):134-137 (1975).
134. Diamond, S., Kemler, N., Kohli, D., Schwartz, G., and Whitmore, G. (Consultants), Biofeedback: Therapy with electronic aids. *Patient Care:* August 1 (1975).
135. Stovya, J. and Budzynski, T. (Investigators), Application of muscle and EEG feedback for anxiety, stress disorders, and exploration of conscious states. (Prepared by Luce, G.) Mental Health Prog. Rep. 6, DHEW Pub. HSM 73-9139, 1973, pp. 109-117.
136. Ibid., pp. 117-121.
137. Diamond, S., et al., op. cit., pp. 2-4.
138. Marti-Ibañez, F. (Ed.), Biofeedback training. *Medical News Magazine* **16**(1):65-67 (1972).
139. Diamond, S., et al., op. cit., pp. 4-16.
140. Leitenberg, H., Agras, W.S., Allen, R., Butz, R., and Edwards, J., Feedback and therapist praise during treatment of phobia. *J. Consult. Clin. Psychol.* **43**(3):396-404 (1975).
141. Townsend, R.E., House, J.F., and Addario, D., A comparison of biofeedback-mediated relaxation and group therapy in the treatment of chronic anxiety. *Amer. J. Psychiatry* **132**(6):598-601 (1975).
142. Pos, R., Psychological assessment of factors affecting pain. *Canadian Medical Association Journal* **111**:1213-1215 (1974).
143. Nakahama, H., Pain mechanisms in the central nervous system. *Int. Anesthesiol. Clin.* **13**(1):109-110 (1975).

144. O'Neal, J.T., Managing chronic pain. *American Family Physician* 10(6):75-84 (1974).
145. Zakowski, P., op. cit., p. 26.
146. Culliton, B.J., Psychosurgery: National commission issues surprisingly favorable report. *Science* 194(4262):299 (1976).
147. Ibid., p. 301.
148. Slovenko, R., Commentary on psychosurgery: A perspective on informed consent. *Reflections* XL(3):46-53 (1976).
149. Shevitz, S.A., Psychosurgery: Some current observations. *Amer. J. Psychiatry* 133(3):266-267 (1976).
150. Knight, G., "The orbital cortex as an objective in the surgical treatment of mental illness: The results of 450 cases of open operation and the development of the stereotactic approach," in *Innovative Medical-Psychiatric Therapies* (Suinn, R.M. and Weigel, R.G., Eds.).   Baltimore: University Park Press, 1976, pp. 195-221.
151. Shevitz, S.A., op. cit., pp. 268-269.
152. Mark, V.H. and Neville, R., Brain surgery in aggressive epileptics: Social and ethical implications. *J. Amer. Med. Assoc.* 226(7):765-772 (1973).
153. Kleeman, S.T. and Solomon, P., "Psychotherapy," in *Handbook of Psychiatry*, 3rd ed. (Solomon, P. and Patch, B.V., Eds.).   Los Altos, Calif.:   Lange Medical Publications, 1974, p. 341.
154. Jaspers, K., op. cit., p. 834.
155. Jung, C.G., *Modern Man in Search of a Soul.*   New York: Harcourt, Brace and Co., 1934, p. 33.
156. Wolberg, L.R., *The Technique of Psychotherapy,* 2nd ed.   New York: Grune & Stratton, 1967, pp. 71-91.
157. Urasano, R.J. and Dressler, D.M., Brief vs. long term psychotherapy: A treatment decision. *J. Nerv. Ment. Dis.* 159(3):164-171 (1974).
158. Offenkrantz, W. and Tobin, A., Psychoanalytic psychotherapy. *Arch. Gen. Psychiatry* 30:593-606 (1974).
159. Bromberg, W., *Man Above Humanity: A History of Psychotherapy.*   Philadelphia: Lippincott, 1954, pp. 274-275.
160. Freedman, A., Kaplan, H.I., and Sadock, B.J., *Modern Synopsis of Comprehensive Textbook of Psychiatry/II,* op. cit., pp. 885-886.
161. Wolberg, L.R., op. cit., pp. 80-83.
162. Tart, C.T., *States of Consciousness.*   New York: Dutton, 1975, p. 114.
163. Gruender, H., *Psychology Without a Soul: A Criticism,* 2nd ed.   St. Louis: Herder, 1917, pp. 149-159.
164. Ingle, D.J., The nature of personal freedom. *Zygon* 6(1):39-47 (1971).
165. Ingle, D.J., Boundaries of human freedom. *Persp. Biol. Med.* 16(1):51-68 (1972).
166. Offenkrantz, W. and Tobin, A., op. cit., pp. 593-594.
167. Harty, M. and Harwitz, L.R., Therapeutic outcome as rated by patients, therapists, and judges. *Arch. Gen. Psychiatry* 33(8):957-961 (1976).
168. Staples, F.R., Sloane, R.B., Whipple, K., Cristol, A., and Yorkston, N.J., Differences between behavior therapists and psychotherapists. *Arch. Gen. Psychiatry* 32(12): 1517-1522 (1975).
169. Marks, I.M., The current status of behavioral psychotherapy: Theory and practice. *Amer. J. Psychiatry* 133(3):254 (1976).
170. Shapiro, A.K., The behavior therapies: Therapeutic breakthrough or latest fad? *Amer. J. Psychiatry* 133(2):154-159 (1976).
171. Marks, I.M., op. cit., p. 254.
172. Ibid., pp. 255-257.

173. Ibid., pp. 255-258.
174. Raskin, D.E. and Klein, Z.E., Losing a symptom through keeping it: A review of paradoxical treatment techniques and rationale. *Arch. Gen. Psychiatry* 33(5):548-555 (1976).
175. Wolpe, J., *The Practice of Behavior Therapy*, 2nd ed.   New York: Pergamon, 1973.
176. Seagraves, R.T. and Smith, R.C., Concurrent psychotherapy and behavior therapy: Treatment of psychoneurotic outpatients. *Arch. Gen. Psychiatry* 33(6):756-763 (1976).
177. Braff, D.L., Raskin, M., and Geisinger, D., Management of interpersonal issues in systematic desensitization. *Amer. J. Psychiatry* 133(7):791-794 (1976).
178. Everett, H. and Solomon, P., "Special psychotherapies," in *Handbook of Psychiatry*, 3rd ed. (Solomon, P. and Patch, B.V., Eds.).   Los Altos, Calif.: Lange Medical Publications, 1974, pp. 379-384.
179. Ibid., pp. 384-386.
180. Ibid., pp. 386-387.
181. Fidler, J.W., Group therapy: Future prospects. *Psychiatric Ann.* 2(4):51-62 (1972).
182. Fleck, S., A general systems approach to severe family pathology. *Amer. J. Psychiatry* 133(6):669-673 (1976).
183. Robinson, L.R., Basic concepts in family therapy: A differential comparison with individual treatment. *Amer. J. Psychiatry* 132(10):1045-1048 (1975).
184. Sander, F.M., "Misleading" concepts in family therapy. *Amer. J. Psychiatry* 133(3): 344 (1976).
185. Polatin, P., *A Guide to Treatment in Psychiatry.*   Philadelphia: Lippincott, 1967, pp. 46-47.
186. Freedman, A.M., Kaplan, H.I., and Sadock, B.J., *Modern Synopsis of Comprehensive Textbook of Psychiatry/II*, op. cit., p. 905.
187. Peterfly, G., The present status of hypnosis. *Can. Med. Ass. J.* 109:397-407 (1973).
188. Ibid., pp. 400-401.
189. Nace, E.P., Orne, M.T., and Hammer, A.G., Posthypnotic amnesia as an active psychic process. *Arch. Gen. Psychiatry* 31(8):257-260 (1974).
190. Peterfly, G., op. cit., p. 403.
191. Raskin, D.E. and Klein, Z.E., op. cit., p. 554.

NAME INDEX

Abimelech, 5
Abraham, Karl, 5, 177, 188
Ackerknecht, Erwin H., 2, 10, 11, 19, 20
Ackerman, S.H., 92, 93
Ackner, Brian, 221
Addams, Jane, 207
Adler, Alfred, 28, 53, 274, 297
Akhtar, Salman, 149, 155
Akiskal, Hagop S., 189
Alexander, Franz, 251
Alexander the Great, 9
Allen, M., 22
Angyal, Andras, 274
Apollo, 7
Aquinas, Saint Thomas, 12, 13
Aretaeus, 112
Aristophanes, 21
Aristotle, 6, 7, 13, 59
Asklepios, 7
Augustine, Saint, 12

Babinski, Joseph 113
Bailey, Percival, 13
Baillarger, Jules, 21, 175
Balard, Antoine Jerome, 273
Beck, Aaron, 172, 179
Beard, George Miller, 22, 83, 205, 206, 207, 215, 241, 243
Bechterev, Vladimir, 30
Behrend, 273
Berger, Frank, 273
Bernard, Claude, 83, 84, 85
Berne, Eric, 53, 275
Bernheim, Hippolyte-Marie, 27, 113, 209
Berze, J., 22
Bini, L., 272
Binswanger, Ludwig, 274, 297
Black, Richard G., 255

Blackwell, Barry, 282
Bleuler, Eugen, 23, 24, 115, 242, 243
Boerhaave, Hermann, 1
Bose, Katrick, 274
Boswell, James, 241
Braid, James, 27
Breuer, Joseph, 28, 111
Briquet, Paul, 108
Broca, Pierre Paul, 17, 18
Brown, Bertram S., 265
Brown, Felix, 242, 243
Burckhardt, G., 273
Burns, B. H., 246
Burton, Robert, 173, 174, 240

Cade, J.F., 274
Cannon, Walter B., 85, 87
Carter, Robert, 112, 113
Celani, David, 117
Celsus, Aurelius Cornelius, 112, 133
Cerletti, Ugo, 272
Charcot, Jean-Martin, 26, 27, 30, 113
Cheyne, George, 174, 241
Chiarugi, Vincenzo, 18
Chrzanowski, Gerard, 49
Cooke, Alistair, 243, 244, 245
Coronis, 7
Coué, Emile, 113
Cowan, John, 252
Cullen, William, 1, 2, 17, 18, 205, 241
Curran, Desmond, 73, 154

DaCosta, Jacob, 83, 210, 214
Darwin, Charles, 25, 84, 224, 270
Davis, D. Russell, 268
Dejerine, Jules, 208, 209
Delay, Jean P. L., 273
Democritus, 6

315

Deniker, P., 273
Descartes, René, 15
Dewey, John, 84, 110
Diethelm, Oscar, 49
Dix, Dorothea Lynde, 270
Dornblüth, Otto, 154
Dreyssig, Guilielmus Fridericus, 174
Dugas, L., 22, 223
Dunham, J.W., 74
Durell, Jack, 271

Eddy, Mary Baker, 26, 27, 113
Elliotson, John, 26
Engel, George, 75, 76, 122, 123
Engelhardt, H. Tristram, Jr., 48, 64, 66
Epicurus, 6
Erikson, Erik Homburger, 28, 297
Esdaile, James, 26
Esquirol, Jean E.-D., 19, 21, 152, 154, 175, 222
Ewald, G., 177
Eysenck, Hans J., 71
Ezekiel, 5

Falret, Jean-Pierre, 21, 152, 175, 241
Federn, Paul, 209
Fenichel, Otto, 250
Ferenczi, Sandor, 249
Feuchtersleben, Baron Ernst von, 22
Flemming, C.F., 22
Fölling, A., 271
Foulds, G.A., 182
Frankl, Viktor E., 274
Freud, Sigmund, 24, 27, 28, 29, 45, 74, 83, 93, 94, 111, 113, 134, 135, 138, 153, 154, 177, 188, 209, 210, 214, 242, 243, 249, 274, 297
Fromm, Erich, 53

Galen, 10, 11, 12, 112, 173, 240
Gall, Franz Joseph, 17
Galton, Sir Francis, 270
Garrison, Fielding H., 8
Gauckler, E., 208
Georget, Etienne Jean, 241, 243
Gillespie, R.D., 242, 243
Goldberger, Joseph, 272
Goldstein, Kurt, 93, 96, 274
Griesinger, Wilhelm, 19, 20, 21, 112, 152, 154
Grinker, Roy Richard, Sr., vii, 38, 297
Guislain, Joseph, 22

Hagen, Thomas, 187
Hall, G. Stanley, 134

Hart, Bernard, 177
Hecker, Ewald, 21, 176, 209
Heinroth, Johann C., 19, 22
Heraclitus, 5, 6
Herrick, C. Judson, 212
Hippocrates, 8, 9, 10, 21, 112, 173, 239, 240, 243, 276
Hoche, Alfred, 24
Hoff, Hans, 272
Hollister, Leo, 102
Homer, 5
Horney, Karen, 28, 53, 274, 297

Imhotep, 4
Ingle, Dwight, 60

Jackson, Hughlings, 25, 224
Jacobson, Edmund, 274
James, William, 20, 84
Janet, Pierre, 24, 25, 26, 74, 83, 111, 113, 120, 134, 153, 154, 209, 223, 243
Jaspers, Karl, 20, 111, 120, 268
Jauregg, Julius Wagner Von, 271
Jehovah, 5
Jelliffe, Smith Ely, 175, 176, 210
Jones, H. Gwynne, 159, 160
Jung, Carl, 24, 28, 274, 297, 298

Kahlbaum, Karl Ludwig, 21, 44, 175, 176
Kant, Immanuel, 17, 44, 175
Kendall, R.E., 63, 180
Kenyon, F.E., 245, 253, 257
Kety, Seymour, 51
Kierkegaard, Søren A., 83, 93
King, Lester, 61
Kläsi, Jacob, 272
Kleist, K., 177
Koffka, Kurt, 274
Köhler, Wolfgang, 274
Kraepelin, Emil, 21, 22, 23, 24, 44, 45, 134, 176, 179, 209, 242, 243
Krafft-Ebing, Richard Von, 21, 152, 154
Kretschmer, Ernst, 71, 115, 177, 213
Krishaber, Maurice, 223
Kuhn, R., 274

Laborit, Henri-Marie, 273
Lader, Malcolm H., 90, 91
Lang, P.J., 136
Lange, Karl C., 84, 179
Laughlin, Henry P., 211
Laycock, Thomas, 273
Lazarus, Richard S., 80
Levy, 274
Lewis, Aubrey J., 134, 153, 154, 174

Liébeault, Ambroise-Auguste, 27, 113
Lindegård, B., 71
Lindsley, D.R., 31
Linnaeus (von Linné, Carl), 1
Linné, Carl von (Linnaeus), 1
Littré, Emile, 16, 18
Ljungberg, L., 114
Locke, John, 15, 16
Lockridge, Ross, Jr., 187
Loewy, H., 223
Lombroso, Cesare, 22
Low, Abraham, 275
Lowen, Alexander, 275
Lucretius, 6
Ludwig, Arnold, 109

McKinney, W.T., 189
McReynolds, P., 93
Macfayden, Heather W., 181
Makhlouf-Norris, Fawzeya, 158, 159, 160
Mandeville, Bernard, 241
Mapother, E., 223
Margetts, Edward L., 19
Marks, Isaac, 90, 99, 123, 142, 150, 165, 227
Marmor, Judd, 266
Marsh, L. Cody, 274
Maslow, Abraham, 297
Maugh, Thomas, 285
May, Rollo, 93, 274
Mayer-Gross, W., 223, 224
Mead, George Herbert, 110
Mechanic, David, 248
Meduna, Ladislas J. Von, 272
Melville, Herman, 187
Mendels, Joseph 185
Menninger, Karl, 18, 23, 49
Menninger, William, 45
Mesmer, Franz Anton, 26, 27, 113
Meyer, Adolf, 20, 22, 24, 25, 176, 177,
    209, 243
Mitchell, S. Weir, 22, 113, 207, 217, 272
Molière, (Poquelin, Jean Baptiste), 241
Moniz, Egas, 273
Moore, J.W., 271
Morel, Benedict Augustin, 20, 21, 22, 44,
    152, 154
Moreno, Jacob, 275, 297
Murray, L.G., 92

Nakahama, Hiroshi, 236
Nathan, P.W., 237

Nebuchadnezzar, 5
Nichols, Madeline A., 246
Noguchi, Hideyo, 271
Norris, Hugh, 159, 160

Oberndorf, C.P., 49
Oesterreich, K., 223
Oppenheim, Hermann, 83

Paracelsus, 13, 14, 26, 27
Pauling, Linus, 289
Pavlov, Ivan Petrovich, 29, 30, 53
Perls, Frederick, 275, 297
Pick, A., 223
Pilowsky, I., 245
Pinel, Philippe, 18, 19, 21, 175
Pitres, A., 134
Plato, 5, 6, 7, 10, 59, 64, 112
Platter, Felix, 14, 173
Pluto, 7
Pötzl, Otto, 272, 273
Pope, Alexander, 15
Poquelin, Jean Baptiste (Molière), 241
Poyen, Charles, 26
Pratt, Joseph, 274
Pythagoras, 5, 6

Quimby, Phineas P., 26

Rado, Sandor, 177
Raecke, J., 242
Raggi, A., 134
Raskin, D.E., 307
Rees, W. Linford, 71
Régis, E., 134
Reil, Johann Christian, 222
Ribot, Théodule A., 25, 223
Rickman, John, 177
Riese, Walther, 18
Rittelmeyer, Louis F., Jr., 252
Roberts, W.W., 226
Robin, G., 16, 18
Rogers, Carl, 93, 274, 275
Rosen, John, 274
Rudge, P., 237
Rush, Benjamin, 18
Russell, Bertrand, 59, 133
Ryan, J. Kenneth, 295

Sakel, Manfred, 272
Salzman, Leon, 138, 161

Sarah, 5
Sartre, Jean-Paul, 228, 229
Saul, 5
Sauvages, François Boissier de, 1
Schilder, Paul, 223, 243
Schneider, Kurt, 153, 154
Schultz, Johannes Heinrich, 274
Sedman, G., 225
Selye, Hans, 87, 88, 95, 98
Sen, Ganneth, 274
Sheldon, William, 74, 213
Sherrington, Sir Charles, 84
Shindell, S., 40, 41
Siddiqui, Rafat, 273
Siddiqui, S., 273
Sigaud, Claude, 71
Skinner, Burrhus F., 31, 94, 212, 274, 297
Slater, Eliot, 114
Slavson, Samuel R., 274, 297
Smollius, G., 241
Socrates, 59, 134
Soranus, 10, 11, 112
Spencer, Herbert, 25
Spinoza, Baruch S., 134
Spitz, René, 188
Spurzheim, Johann C., 17
Squire, L.R., 291
Stahl, Georg Ernst, 16, 17, 174
Stekel, Wilhelm, 209
Stillé, Alfred, 83
Stransky, E., 177
Sullivan, Harry Stack, 28, 53, 274, 297
Sydenham, Thomas, 14, 241, 276

Taine, Hippolyte Adolphe, 223
Tanner, J.M., 71
Tart, Charles T., 38, 300
Tempkin, Owsei, 31
Thalbitzer, Sophus, 177
Tuke, William, 18

Vaughn, M., 157
Veith, Ilza, 9
Videbeck, Thomas, 157
Viola, Giacento, 71

Walker, L., 99
Walshe, Francis, 121
Watson, John B., 30
Watson, Robert, 15
Wernicke, Carl, 20
Wertheimer, Max, 274
Westphal, Carl, 133, 134, 152, 154
White, William A., 210
Willis, Thomas, 14, 173
Wittels, Fritz, 115
Wolpe, Joseph, 94, 136, 275, 297
Wollenberg, Robert, 242
Wordsworth, William, 229
Wundt, Wilhelm, 20, 30, 44

Yahweh, 4

Zakowski, Phil, 294
Zeller, A., 22
Zeller, E.A., 274
Zeus, 7
Zilboorg, Gregory, 26
Zubin, Joseph, 178

SUBJECT INDEX

Abreacting, 299
Abstinence syndrome, 279, 281, 282
Acetaldehyde syndrome, 279
Acetylcholine, 87, 290
Acetylsalicylic acid, 284-285
Acrophobia, 135
ACTH, See Adrenocorticotropic hormone
Acupuncture, 294
Acute anxiety, 97
Acute obsessional neurosis, 156
Acute organic brain syndrome, 72
Adapin. See Doxepin HCL
Adaptation versus disease, 63-64
Addiction, 279, 280
    barbiturate, 281
    and psychosurgery, 296
Addison's disease, 100
Adolescence, 73. See also Etiology of individual disorders
Adrenal glands, 87
Adrenocorticoids, 88, 89
Adrenocorticotropic hormone, 88
Advice, in therapy, 101
Adynamia, 1
Affect. See also Feelings: Emotion
    definition, 79
    and instincts, 25
    regression, 25
    self-reported, 80
Affective diseases. See also names of individual diseases
    and electroconvulsive treatment, 290
    and psychosurgery, 296
Affective disorders, 47, 180. See also names of individual disorders

Affective psychoses, 257. See also names of individual psychoses
Affective responses, 81
Age of Enlightenment, 15-16
Aggression, 86
    and anxiety, 94
    and depression, 177
    and neurasthenia, 214
    and phobias, 138
    and psychosurgery, 296
Aggressive obsessions, 157
Agitated depressed psychoses, 284
Agitation, 284
Agoraphobia
    and anxiety neurosis, 99
    and depersonalization, 227
    diagnosis, 140-142
    incidence, 133
    and other illnesses, 137
    prognosis, 145
    treatment, 146
Ailurophobia, 135
Air swallowing, 192
Akinesias, 108
Alarm reaction, 188. See also Panic
Alcohol, 273, 277. See also Alcoholism
    abstinence syndrome, 279
    abuse, 278
    and amnesia, 125
    and anxiety, 100
    and barbiturates, 280
    withdrawal, 287
Alcoholics Anonymous, 275

Alcoholism
    aversion therapy, 304
    and disease concepts, 62
    psychological symptoms, 72
    as symptom, 19
Aldosterone, 88
Alkaloids, 187. *See also* names of individual
        drugs
Alkalosis, 92
Alteration of consciousness. *See*
        Consciousness
Altered state of consciousness. *See*
        Consciousness
Amenorrhea, 73, 118
American disease. *See* Neurasthenia
American Psychiatric Association, 266. *See
        also* DSM I, DSM II, DSM III
Amino acids, 87
Amitriptyline HCL, 196, 197
    for anxiety, 102, 103
Amnesia, 125
    and hypnosis, 366
    in hysteria, 108, 113, 119, 125
    and narcotherapy, 288
Amobarbital, 280, 288, 289
Amphetamines, 100, 196, 217, 274, 277
Amygdaloid, 86, 132
Amygdalotomy, 296
Amytal. *See* Amobarbital
Anaclitic depression, 188
Anafranil, 167
Analgesia, 116
Analgesic-antipyretics, 284
Analgesics, 279, 284-285. *See also* names
        of individual drugs
    mild, 284-285
    synthetic compounds, 284
Anal personality, 161-162
Anal-sadistic stage, 153
Analysand, 301, 302
Anancasm, 149. *See also* Compulsion;
        Obsession
Anaphylactic reactions, 87
Androgyny, 71-72
Anemia, 187
Anesthesias
    and hypnosis, 306
    in hysteria, 108, 118, 124
Anesthetic effects, 279
Angel dust. *See* phencyclidine
Anger, 87, 157
Animal magnetism. *See* Mesmerism
Anorexia, 287, 303

Anorexia nervosa, 118-119
    and depression, 192
    and hypnosis, 306
    and modified insulin treatment, 287
    and obsessive compulsive neurosis, 156
Anosmia, 108, 118
Antabuse, 279, 304
Antianxiety drugs, 279, 281, 282-283. *See
        also* Minor tranquilizers; Sedatives;
        names of individual drugs
Anticholinergic side effects, 197
Anticipation, 81
Anticoagulant drugs, 260, 282
Anticonvulsant drugs, 281, 282
Antidepressant drugs, 196-199, 217, 260,
        274, 284. *See also* names of indi-
        vidual drugs
Antihistamine side effects, 197
Antihypertensive drugs, 216
Antipsychotic drugs, 274, 282-284. *See
        also* names of individual drugs
Anxiety, 41, 81-82. *See also* Anxiety
        neurosis
    and antipsychotic drugs, 284
    in barbiturate addiction, 281
    barbiturates for, 101, 103
    and benzodiazepines, 282
    and body type, 71
    biological basis, 85-90
    and carbon dioxide, 290
    and continuous sleep therapy, 288
    and depersonalization, 227
    and desensitization, 303
    and electrosleep therapy, 292
    expressing, 298, 300
    versus fear, 81-82, 131
    and hypnosis, 306
    and hypochondriasis, 235, 251, 257
    and hysteria, 121-122, 123
    insight in, 133
    and instincts, 28
    and insulin coma treatment, 287
    and modified insulin treatment, 287
    and narcotherapy, 288, 289
    in neuroses, 49-50
    in obsessive compulsive neurosis, 149,
        156, 157
    in phobias, 99, 137, 140, 141, 142, 143
    psychodynamic theory, 75
    similar symptoms, 72

Anxiety (continued)
  and sleep therapy, 288
  and somatization, 123
  and stress, 81, 89
  and tranquilizers, 279
  in unitary theory of diseases, 65-66
Anxiety hysteria, 134
Anxiety neurosis, 79-106. *See also* Anxiety
  and behavior therapy, 103
  classification, 28, 29, 37
  course and prognosis, 100
  and depression, 98-100, 187, 193
  development, 66
  diagnosis, 41, 96-100
  drugs, 101-103
  electroconvulsive treatment for, 290
  etiology, 90-96
  history, 83-85
  and intravenous acetylcholine, 290
  and neurasthenia, 215, 216
  and personality, 91, 92, 98
  and phobias, 99, 137
  and phobic neurosis, 143
  psychological theories, 93-95
  and psychosurgery, 103, 296
  and psychotherapy, 103
  and somatics, 92
  and stress, 82, 87-88, 89, 95-96, 99
Anxiety reaction, 82. *See also* Anxiety
    neurosis
Anxiety state, 82, 97. *See also* Anxiety
    neurosis
Anxiety trait, 82, 97, 101. *See also* Anxiety
    neurosis
Aphasia, 18, 20
Aphonia, 127
Aquanude therapy, 304
Aquaphobia, 135
Archetypes, 6
Arousal, 86, 183
Art therapy, 297
Asexuality, 86
Asklepieia, 7
Aspirin, 284-285
Associative reflex theory, 30
Assyrians, 4
Asthenic type, 71, 92, 213
Asthma, 89, 122
Ataractics. *See* Antipsychotic drugs
Atarax. *See* Hydroxyzine

Ataxias, 108
Atherogenesis, 88
Athletic type, 71
Atomistic explanation, 6
Atropine, 290
Atypical somatoform disorder, 113
Authenticity, 111
Autistic children, 304
Autogenic training, 292, 297
Autohypnosis, 120
Automatized behavior, 248-249
Autonomic nervous system, 73, 122, 123
    conditioning, 293
Aventyl. *See* Nortriptyline HCL
Aversion therapy, 304
Avitaminosis, 187
Avoidance
  active, 132
  in obsessive compulsive neurosis, 158
  passive, 132
  response, 133
Axons, 86

Babylonians, 4
Barbiturates, 102, 103, 272, 273
  addiction, 281
  for anxiety, 101, 103
  classes, 280
  misuse, 280-281
  overdose, 282
  for panic, 101
Beard's syndrome. *See* Neurasthenia
Behavior
  and anxiety, 81
  control, 296
  and genetics, 68, 275
  problems, 304
Behavioral groups, 275
Behavioral model, 53-54
Behavior disorders, 73, 296. *See also* names
    of individual disorder
Behaviorism
  beliefs, 30-31, 74
  and psychodynamics, 75
  theories of anxiety, 94-95
  theories of depression, 188
  theories of fatigue, 212
  theories of obsessive compulsive neuro-
    sis, 162
Behavior therapist, 269

Behavior therapy, 31, 265, 274, 297, 302–
304
  and anxiety, 103
  basis, 302
  and biofeedback, 292
  and classical analysis, 303
  dangers, 32
  and depersonalization, 232
  and hypochondria, 259–260
  indications, 303
  methods, 303–304
  and obsessive compulsive neurosis, 167
  and phobias, 145, 146
  shortcomings, 304
Being, 6
Benedryl. See Diphenyldramine
Benzodiazepines, 102, 103, 273, 278, 282
  for anxiety, 101, 103, 282
  for depression, 198, 282
  for panic, 101
  for obsessive compulsive neurosis, 167
  and safety, 282
Beta adrenergic blocking agent, 101, 103
Bibliotherapy, 297
Bimedial leucotomy, 295
Bioenergetic group therapy, 275
Biofeedback, 265, 274, 275
  anxiety as, 95
  anxiety therapy, 103
  for pain, 294
  self-regulating, 88
  training, 292–293
Biogenic amine hypothesis, 183–185, 284
Biological disadvantage, 64
Biological psychiatry, 271, 283
Biosocial adaptation, 188–189
Bipolar depression personality. See
        Personality
Bipolar disease, 182
Blindness, 108, 116, 118
Blood lactate level, 90, 92
Bloodletting, 269
Bodily complaints, 122–123
Bodily dysfunctions, 44
Bodily preoccupation, 98
Body defenses, 88
Body functions, conscious control, 292
Body movement groups, 304
Body size, 71. See also Somatics
Body structure changes, 72

Body weight, 19, 71. See also Somatics
Borderline states, 41, 42
Brain
  anatomy, 86
  lesions, 72, 152
  physiology, 86
  structural changes, 72
  surgery. See Psychosurgery
Brain-damaged persons, 296
Brain stem, 86, 87
Brain to mind relationship, 17, 18
Breath, 5
Brief term therapy, 297
Briquet's disorder, 107–108, 113, 114
Bromazepam, 167
Bromine, 273
Butabarbital, 103, 280
Butisol, 280
Butyrophenone, 283, 284

Cachexias, 192
Caffeine, 100
Cancer, 187, 192
Cannon-Bard theory, 85, 87
Carbon dioxide, 290
Cardiac arrhythmias, 293
Cardiac neurosis, 83
Cardiac symptoms, 100
Cardiazol shock treatment, 272
Cardiovascular disorder, 215
Cardiovascular system, 88
Carotid sinus syndrome, 100
Catalepsy, 193
Catatonia, 21, 24, 288
Catecholamine hypothesis. See Biogenic
        amine hypothesis
Catecholamines, 87, 88, 184–185
Catharsis, 28
Causes of mental illness. See Etiology of
        mental illness
Cell body, 86
Central nervous system (CNS), 86–88. See
        also Brain; individual parts of the
        brain
  and depression, 183, 184–185, 192
  drugs affecting, 277
  and fatigue, 212
Central nervous system depressants, 216
Central nervous system stimulants, 196
Cerebellar disturbances, 100

Cerebellum, 86
Cerebral arteriosclerosis, 38, 72
Cerebral cortex, 73, 86, 88
Cerebral localization, 14, 17-18
Cerebrocortical functioning, 14
Cerebrotonia, 71
Change, 5
Characteristics. *See* Personality; Traits
Chemical disturbances, 121
Chemical treatment. *See* individual
    treatments
Child-guidance clinics, 39
Children's activity groups, 275
Children's disorders, 73
Chloral hydrate, 281, 288
Chlordiazepoxide, 92, 103, 282
Chlorimipramine, 167
Chlorpromazine, 283, 288
Choking, 192
Christian Science, 26-27, 113
Chromosomes, 68, 69-70
Chronic anxiety neurosis. *See* Anxiety
    neurosis; Anxiety state
Chronic factitious illness, 114
Chronic mental patients, 296
Chronic obsessional neurosis, 156
Chronic pain syndrome (CPS), 255-256
Cingulectomy, 295
Classical psychoanalysis, 302
Classification of mental illness, 37-58
    by affective life or ideas and will, 22
    by Bleuler, 23-24
    by botanical principles, 1
    contemporary, 31-32
    by Cullen, 1-2
    DSM *(Diagnostic and Statistical Manual
        of Mental Disorders)*
        I, 45, 46, 47, 83, 113, 135, 154,
            179-180, 223
        II, 38, 46-47, 49-50, 83, 113, 135,
            154, 180, 182, 211, 223, 239
        III, 47, 113, 135, 154, 180, 182,
            211, 223, 251
    by Esquirol, 19
    by Freud, 28, 29
    by Heinroth, 19
    by Hippocrates, 9
    international, 37
    by Kant, 17
    by Kraepelin, 22-23, 44-45

Classification of mental illness (continued)
    by Meyer, 24-25
    by Morel, 20-21
    multifactorial, 37
    national, 37
    by New York Academy of Medicine, 45
    nineteenth century, 18
    by Paracelsus, 13-14
    by Pinel, 18
    by Platter, 14
    psychological, 16
    reliability, 43-44
    by Soranus, 10-11
    by Sydenham, 14
    by Wernicke, 20
    by Willis, 14
    in World War II, 45
    validity, 44
Class I phobias, 136, 139-142
Class II phobias, 136, 142-143
Claustrophobia, 135
Client-centered psychotherapy, 274
Climacteric, 73. *See also* Menopause
Clinical psychiatrists, 40
Clorazepate, 282
Closed operative techniques, 273
Cocaine, 273
Codeine, 284
Coffee, 277
Cognition, 93
Cognito ergo sum, 15
Cold applications, 294
Colitis, 100
Collective unconsciousness, 25
Comata, 1
Commitment procedures, 275
Communication
    in hysteria, 117
    between patient and therapist, 298, 299-
        300, 305
    among schools of psychiatry, 269
Community, return of patient to, 270
Community mental health centers, 270
Community period of treatment, 270
Community therapy, 265
Compazine. *See* Prochlorperazine
Comprehensive theory of disease, 67-68
Compulsion, 149
Compulsion neurosis. *See* Obsessive com-
    pulsive neurosis

Compulsive personality, 213
Computer, 41
Conditioned reflex, 29–30
Conditioning, 93. *See also* Behaviorism, Operant Conditioning
Conditioning theory, 302
Conditioning therapy. *See* Behavior therapy
Confession, 299
Conflict
    and anxiety, 81
    and anxiety neurosis, 82
    expression, 298
    and fatigue, 211
    in hysteria, 114–115
    insights into, 298
    in psychodynamic theory, 75
Conflict theory, 84
Confusion
    with electroconvulsive treatment, 291
    hospitalization for, 267
Congestive heart failure, 192
Conjoint therapy, 265, 275, 297
Consciousness
    alterations of, 220, 225
    altered states of, 108, 116, 119
    in psychotherapy, 126, 297
    requirements for, 110
    and self, 109–112
    split. *See* Dissociation
Consciousness inhibiting drugs, 279
Constitutional factors in etiology, 67, 68–70. *See also* etiology portion of specific neurosis
Constitutional syndrome. *See* Obsessive compulsive neurosis
Construct theory, 158
    and obsessive compulsive neurosis, 158–161
Continuous sleep therapy (narcosis). *See* Narcotherapy
Control, 138, 141
Controlling compulsion, 150
Conversion reaction, 288, 306
Conversion type, hysterical neurosis, 108, 109, 117
    and anxiety, 123
    as defense mechanism, 123
    etiology, 116
    and psychoses, 124–125

Convulsions
    with electroconvulsive treatment, 290, 291
    as side effects of drugs, 281, 283
Convulsive therapy. *See* names of individual types of therapies
Coping, 81
Cornell Medical Index, 238
Corticoid hormones. *See* Adrenocorticoids
Corticosterone, 88
Cortisol, 88
Cortisone, 88
Cosmetic procedures, 254
Co-therapy, 275
Craniology, 17
Cranioscopy, 17
Creative process, 192
Criminal anthropology, 22
Criminal degenerate, 22
Criminality
    and body type, 71
    and heredity, 69, 70
Criminals, 295, 296
Crowds, fear of. *See* Agoraphobia
Cultural factors, 67, 74
Cure, 266
Current life situation, 67
Cushing's syndrome, 89
Cyclic pattern, 163
Cycloid personality. *See* Personality
Cyclothymia, 21, 175
Cyclothymic personality. *See* Personality
Cynophobia, 135

Da Costa's syndrome. *See* Functional cardiac disorder
Dalmane. *See* Flurazepam
Dance therapy, 297
Dancing mania. *See* Vitus chorea
Darvon, 284–285
Darwin's theory of emotion, 84
Day centers, 270
Daydreaming, 120
Deaffectualization, 222
Deafness, 108, 116, 118
Deconditioning, 167
Deep therapy. *See* Expressive therapy
Defense hysteria, 113
Defense mechanisms, 28, 111, 302
Deities, 3

Déjà vu, 120, 222
Delirious patients, 267
Deliriums, 120
Delusional conviction, 163
Delusional systems, 133
Delusions, 157-158, 221, 222
  in unitary theory of disease, 66
Dementia, 9, 66
Dementia praecox, 21, 24
Demonology, 4, 13
Demons, 3, 4
Dendrites, 86
Dependency
  in anxiety neurotic, 91, 97
  in phobics, 141
  on therapist, 299
Dependency needs, 214
Depersonalization. See also Depersonaliza-
    tion neurosis
  in agoraphobia, 140
  in hysteria, 109, 111, 113
  and neurasthenia, 215
  and obsessive compulsive neurosis, 156
  in phobias, 143, 144
  term origination, 22
Depersonalization neurosis, 220-234. See
    also Depersonalization
  classification, 223
  course and prognosis, 231
  diagnosis, 228-230
  differential diagnosis, 230-231
  etiology, 223-228
  history, 222-223
  Koro, 230
  treatment, 232
Depersonification, 222
Depletion theory, 183-185
Depression. See also Depressive neurosis;
    Melancholia
  and agoraphobia, 140
  and antipsychotic drugs, 284
  and anxiety, 98
  and anxiety personality, 91-92
  in barbiturate addicts, 281
  and benzodiazepines, 282
  and body type, 71, 72
  and depersonalization, 227, 231
  and drug therapy, 32
  and electroconvulsive treatment, 290,
    291

Depression (continued)
  and electrosleep therapy, 292
  and endocrine glands, 89
  and hypochondriasis, 235, 243, 256-
    257, 258
  and hysteria, 115, 121, 122
  and integration, 119
  as melancholia, 173-176
  in all mental disorders, 22
  and modified insulin treatment, 287
  and narcotherapy, 222
  and neurasthenia, 215, 216
  and obsessive compulsive neurosis, 99,
    152-153, 156, 157-158, 164, 165
  and obsessive phobias, 142
  personality, 91-92
  and somatization, 124
  and spontaneous remission, 269
Depressive neurosis, 171-203. See also
    Depression
  affects, 171
  and antidepressants, 284
  and anxiety neurosis, 98, 99
  classification, 179-182
  course and prognosis, 194-195, 199
  diagnosis, 41, 185, 190-192
  differential diagnosis, 192-194
  etiology, 182-190
  genetic findings, 181
  history, 173-179
  personality in, 98, 186
  and phobias, 137
  physiological changes in, 183-186
  psychoanalytic formulations, 177
  and stress, 99
  treatment, 195-199
Derealization, 222, 223, 226
Dermatologists, 254
Dermatitis artifacta, 118
Desensitization, 303
  and phobias, 145, 146
  and obsessive compulsive neurosis, 167
Desipramine HCL, 196
Desomatization, 222
Desoxyn. See Methamphetamine
Deviant behavior, 62
Deviant personality types. See Personality
Devils, 3
Dexedrine. See Dextroamphetamine
Dextroamphetamine, 196, 232

Diagnosis. *See also* names of individual
    neurosis
  components, 43
  and computers, 41
  criteria for, 32
  definition, 37
  factors, 38
  importance of, 31
  multiaxial, 54-55
  and narcotherapy, 288
  problems, 41
  in psychotherapy, 299
  validity, 44
Diagnostic and Statistical Manual. *See*
    Classification of mental illness;
    DSM I, II, III
Diagnostic models, 51-55
Diazepam, 103, 282
Dibenzoxazepines, 283, 284
Didactic groups, 305
Diencephalic lesions, 100
Diet, 5
Differential diagnosis. *See* names of individ-
    ual conditions
Diffuse phobia, 135
Dilantin, 281
Dilaudid, 284
Dimensional model, 52-53
Diphenylbutylpiperidine, 260
Diphenyldramine, 103
Diphenylhydantoin, 281
Diphenylmethane antihistamines, 101,
    103
Direct analysis, 274, 304
Directive therapy, 304
Disease concepts, 62-68
  Aristotelian, 64, 65
  comprehensive (multiaxial), 67-68
  Hippocratic, 64
  natural disease entity, 66, 68
  Platonic, 64
  psychiatric, 65-68
  unitary, 65-66, 98, 172
Disorientation, 29
Dissociation
  and anorexia nervosa, 118
  and autohypnosis, 120
  and hypnosis, 120, 125
  and hysteria, 111, 122
  Ribot's theories, 25

Dissociation (continued)
  and sleep, 120
  and other states, 120
Dissociative disorders, 113. *See also* names
    of individual disorders
Dissociative type of hysteria, 108-109,
    117
Dissolution, 224
Diuretics, 216
Divination, 4
DNA molecules, 68
Doctor-patient relationship, 250-253, 259,
    298, 299
Dopamine, 32, 87, 184-185
Doriden. *See* Glutethimide
Double personality. *See* Personality
Down's syndrome, 68, 69
Doxepin HCL, 102, 103, 196, 197
Dreams
  ancient Greek interpretation, 7
  Babylonian interpretation, 4
  Freud's interpretation, 28
  Hebrew interpretation, 5
  in phobias, 141
  in psychoanalysis, 301
Dreamy state, 116
Drug. *See also* Addiction; Drug therapy;
    names of individual drugs
  abuse, 277, 278, 279
  combinations, 279, 280
  control, 277
  intoxication, 72, 222, 224, 231
  overdose, 278
  poisoning, 280-281
  statistics, 278
  tolerance, 279
  use, 277, 278, 279
  withdrawal, 100
Drug therapy, 265, 270, 277-290. *See also*
    names of individual disorders
  primitive, 3
  recent advances, 31-32
  specialized, 287-290
DSM I, II, III. *See* Classification of mental
    illness
Duality, 6
Duodenal ulcer, 156
Dynamic school, 23-27, 42-43, 91, 167
Dynamics, 25
Dyskinesias, 108

Dysmorphophobia, 253, 254, 260
Dysthymia, 175-176

Early man. *See* Primitive man
Economic factors, 67
ECT. *See* Electroconvulsive treatment
Ectomorph, 71, 213
Education, 101, 174, 299, 300
EEG, 73, 290, 292, 293
Effort syndrome, 83
Ego, 28, 93, 302
Egocentricity, 114, 118
Ego psychology, 28
Ego-strengthening methods, 298
Egyptians, 4
Einheitpsychose, 22
Elavil. *See* Amitriptyline HCL
Elderly patients, 260, 281
Electrical treatment, 290-294. *See also* names of individual treatments
Electroconvulsive treatment, 232, 260, 267, 290-292, 294
    bilateral stimulation, 290, 291
    complications, 291
    death rate, 291
    for depression, 199
    for obsessive compulsive neurosis, 167
    unilateral stimulation, 290, 291
Electroencephalogram. *See* EEG
Electrolyte disturbance, 183
Electrolyte system, 73
Electromyelograph, 293
Electroplexy. *See* Electroconvulsive treatment
Electroshock. *See* Electroconvulsive treatment
Electrosleep, 265, 292
Electrotherapy, 272, 292
Emotion
    adaptive, 80-81
    anxiety, 81-82
    biological basis, 85-90
    classification, 80-81
    components, 79-80
    in depersonalization, 220, 227
    fear, 81-82
    history, 83-85
    normal and abnormal, 80-81
Emotional lability, 98
Empirical psychology, 16

Empiricism, 15-16
Encephalitis, 73, 152
Encounter group, 304
Endep. *See* Amitriptyline HCL
Endocrine disorders, 187
Endocrine glands, 89
Endocrine system, 73, 87
Endomorph, 71
Energy, 204-205
English malady, 174, 241
Enjoyment, 87
Enteritis, 100
Enuretics, 304
Environment and heredity, 69
Enzymes, 88, 271
Epilepsy
    in ancient Greece, 7, 8
    and anxiety, 100
    and biofeedback, 293
    classifications, 9, 13
    and depersonalization, 231
    and EEG, 73
    and hysteria, 125
    and integration, 119
    and phobias, 143
    and relatives, 73
    and schizophrenia, 272
    treatment, 273
Epinephrine, 87, 92, 154
Equanil. *See* meprobamate
Ergasia, 24
Ergasiology. *See* Psychobiology
Eskalith. *See* Lithium carbonate
Essence, 6
Essential hypertension. *See* hypertension
EST. *See* Electroconvulsive treatment
Estrogen, 73
Ethchlorvynol, 281
Ether abrication, 232
Ethics
    difficulties, 270
    Hebrew, 5
    psychiatric, 267
    and psychosurgery, 295, 297
    in therapy, 299
Ethinamate, 281
Ethoheptazine, 284
Etiology of mental illness, 59-78. *See also* names of individual disorders
    ancient Greek theories, 7

Etiology of mental illness (continued)
    Babylonian theories, 4
    constitutional factors, 68–70
    contemporary theories, 31–32
    Cullen's theories, 17
    current life situations and, 75–76
    disease concepts, 62–68
    Egyptian theories, 4
    Freud's theories, 27–29
    Griesinger's theories, 19–20
    Hebrew theories, 5
    Hippocratic theories, 8–9
    medical, 14–15
    Mesopotamian theories, 4
    Middle Ages concepts, 13
    multiple causes, 61
    organic versus functionalists, 16–17, 18
    Paracelsus' theory, 13
    Pavlov's theory, 30
    philosophical, 15
    physical factors in, 71–73
    psychological factors in, 74–75
    primitive theories of, 3
    and scientific method, 60, 61
    Soranus' theory, 10–11
    Stahl's theory, 16
    theological explanation, 14–15
    Willis's theory, 14
Eugenics, 270
Euphoria, 87
Eurymorphic. *See* Pyknic
Euthanasia, 270
Exhaustion, 22, 92, 98
Exhibitionism, 303
Existential psychotherapy, 274, 304
Existentialist, 269
Exophthalmos, 100
Exorcism, 13, 112
Explanation in therapy, 43, 101, 300–301
Expressive groups, 305
Expressive therapy, 298
Extrapyramidal effects, 283, 284
Extraversion-introversion, 238
Eysenck Personality Inventory, 137, 238

Factitious Disorders, 47, 113–114
Faculties, 6
Fainting, 42, 100, 141, 283
Faith in therapy, 299
Faith healers, 126

Family relationships in treatment, 276
Family therapy, 103, 260, 265, 275, 297, 305–306
Fantasy, 120, 145, 299, 302
Fantasy method, 303
Fatigue. *See also* Neurasthenia
    in anxiety, 98
    and central nervous system, 212
    and conflict, 211
    definition, 205
    and depersonalization, 222, 224
    and physical illness, 213–214
    and repetition, 152
Fear, 81–82
    and anxiety, 81–82, 131
    and barbiturates, 281
    behaviorist theory, 94
    in conflict theory, 84
    and Darwin's theory of emotion, 84
    environmentally conditioned response, 131, 132
    excessive, 132
    insight in, 133
    as instinct, 131
    in James-Lange theory, 84
    in obsessive compulsive neurosis, 149, 157
    in phobic neurosis, 132, 143
    and primitive man, 3
Fear Survey Schedule III, 136
Federal Drug Administration, 198
Feeling, 79, 80, 221–222
Fetishes, 3
Fever, 72, 271–272
Fight or flight, 85, 87
Fits, 116. *See also* Seizures and convulsions
Flooding, 145, 146
Fluphenazine, 103, 283
Flurazepam, 198, 281–282
Flurothyl, 290
Folie à double form, 21, 175
Folie circulaire, 21, 175
Folie de doute, 157
Food intolerance, 192
Foresight, 133
Free association, 301
Freedom, 301
Free-floating anxiety, 94
Fright response, 131, 132
Frigidity, 141, 303

Frustration, 82, 115, 250-251
Fugue
    in hypnosis, 306
    in hysteria, 108, 113, 119, 125
    and narcotherapy, 288
Functional cardiac disorder, 83
Functional changes, 72
Functional disturbance, 16, 18
Functional psychoses, 271, 273. *See also*
    names of individual psychoses
Functionalism, 84

Gambling, 303
Gamma-aminobutyric acid (GABA), 87
Ganser syndrome, 114, 119, 125
Gastrointestinal complaints, 192
Gastrointestinal system, 88
Gate-control theory, 237
General adaptation system, 88, 98, 188
General paresis, 271-272
General psychiatrist, 269
Genes, 68, 69
Genetics, 69, 270-271, 275
Genotype, 69
Gestalt groups, 275, 304
Gestalts, 74
Gilles de la Tourette's syndrome, 284
Glossalgia, 192
Glove and stocking anesthesia, 124
Glucocorticoids, 88
Gluconeogenesis, 88
Glutethimide, 282
Goals of psychiatry, 267
God, 4-5
Gods, 3, 4
Gout, 1
Government controls, 270
Grand mal, 290
Greco-Roman culture, 10
Greece, ancient, 5-9
Group-centered therapy, 275
Group therapy, 265, 274-275, 304-306
    for anxiety, 103
    disadvantages, 305
    types, 304-305
Guilt, 191, 250, 298
Gyrectomy, 295

Haldol. *See* Butyrophenone
Halfway houses, 270

Hallucinations, 119
Hallucinogens, 279, 285-286, 288-289
Hashish, 279, 285
Headaches, 89, 193
Health care delivery system, 277
Health, 48-49, 277
Heart disease, 187
Hebephrenia, 21, 24
Hebrews, 4-5
Hematologic system, 88
Hemophilia, 69
Hepatitis, 187
Hereditary diseases, 270-271
Heredity, 67, 68-70, 270-271
Hibernation, 183
High-frequency stimulative electrotherapy,
    292. *See also* Electrotherapy
Hippocratic writings, 8
Histamine, 87
History, 1-36
Hog. *See* Phencyclidine
Homeostasis, 83-84, 85, 88
Homeric age, 5
Homicidal obsession, 157
Homosexuality 11, 62, 72, 214
Hospitalization, 267-268, 270, 274, 304
    for agoraphobia, 146
    for barbiturate withdrawal, 281
    for behavior therapy, 303
    for homicidal patient, 267
    for hypochondriasis, 260
    for insulin treatment, 287-288
    for panic, 101
Hospital period of treatment, 270
Hospitals, 7, 275, 278, 295
Humane reforms, 269-270
Humanists, 17
Humoural theory, 8-9, 173, 241
Huntington's chorea, 68, 69
Hydromorphone, 284
Hydrophobia, 133
Hydrotherapy, 17
Hydroxyzine, 103
Hygienic laws, 5
Hyperinsulinism, 89, 100
Hyperparathyroidism, 72
Hypersexuality, 86
Hypertension, 89, 122, 293
Hyperthyroidism, 89, 99-100

Hyperventilation, 141, 193
Hypnagogic states, 152, 222, 224
Hypnoanalysis, 306, 307
Hypnosis, 274, 275, 297, 306–307
    and anxiety, 103
    and biofeedback, 292
    and Charcot, 26, 27
    and Christian Science, 26–27
    conditions used for, 306
    and dermatitis artifacta, 118
    and dissociation, 120
    and hysteria, 26, 27, 28, 113
    Pavlovian view, 306
    in phobias, 145
    psychoanalytic view, 306
    risk, 307
    for surgery, 26
Hypnotic drugs, 101, 197–198, 277, 280,
        288–289
Hypnotist, 269
Hypocalcemia, 92
Hypochondria. See also Hypochondriacal
        neurosis
    diagnosis, 41
    and depression, 187
    and hysteria, 121, 122, 241
    and neurasthenia, 215
    and obsessive compulsive neurosis, 156,
        165
    patient's goal, 252
    and psychosurgery, 296
    and somatization, 123
Hypochondriacal neurosis, 235–264. See
        also Hypochondria
    classification, 243–246
    course and prognosis, 258
    and depersonalization, 230
    diagnosis, 251–255
    differential diagnosis, 255–258
    doctor-patient relationship, 250–253,
        259
    etiology, 246–251
    history, 239–243
    monosymptomatic hypochondriasis, 253,
        260
    personality, 246–247
    treatment, 254–255, 258–261
Hypoglycemia, 100, 287
Hypomanic personality. See Personality
Hypothalamus, 73, 86–88, 183

Hysteria. See also Hysterical neurosis
    and anxiety, 99, 121–122
    and bodily complaints, 122–123
    and body type, 71
    and Briquet's syndrome, 107–108
    classification, 1, 9, 25–26
    and depression, 122
    differential diagnosis, 121–124
    etiology, 27
    and electroconvulsive treatment, 290
    and hypnotism, 26, 27, 28
    and hypochondria, 257
    insight in, 133
    interpersonal communication, 117
    and malingering, 120
    and narcotherapy, 288
    and neurasthenia, 216
    and stress, 117
    and suggestion, 26
    terminology, 112, 113–114
Hysterical Neurosis, 107–130.   See also
        Hysteria
    course and prognosis, 125
    and depersonalization, 231
    diagnosis, 117–121
    etiology, 114–117
    history, 112–113
    personality, 114–115
    treatment, 125–127
Hysterical personality.   See Personality

Id, 28, 93
Idealism, 6
Ideas, 6
Identification, 302
Illness phobias, 142
Imavate. See Imipramine HCL
Imipramine HCL, 102, 103, 196, 197, 274
Imipramine pamoate, 196
Imitation therapy, 304
Immaturity, 97, 114
Immortality, 4, 6
Implosion. See Flooding
Impotence, 303
Inderal. See Propranolol
Individual psychotherapy, 265, 274, 297,
        298–301
    for anxiety, 103
    goals, 301
    types, 298

Individual unconscious, 25
Indoklon, 290
Indolamine hypothesis. *See* Biogenic amine
    hypothesis
Indolealkylamines, 184–185
Industrialization, 207
Informed consent, 275, 295
Insanity, 11, 14, 21–22
Insecure personality. *See* Personality
Insight, 115, 143, 298, 300
Insight psychotherapy, 145
Instability, 97, 114
Instinctive reactions, 116
Instinct theory, 28
Insulin, 146, 167, 232, 267
    treatments using, 287–288
Insulin coma treatment, 272, 287–
    288
Intelligence
    as classification, 44
    and genetics, 275
    and heredity, 70
    and hysteria, 116
    and insight, 133
    Mesopotamian theories, 4
    and psychosurgery, 296
Intensive therapy, 297
Interviewing, 40
Intoxications, 72
Intramuscular glucogen, 287
Intravenous acetylcholine, 290
Introspection, 302
Introspective psychological models of treat-
    ment, 265
Introspective school. *See* Dynamic school
Introversion, 91, 137
In vivo method, 303
Involutional melancholia, 176, 180, 194
Iproniazid, 196
Irrational soul, 6
Irritability, 98
Isocarboxazid, 196, 198

James-Lange theory, 84
Janimine. *See* Imipramine HCL

Kidney disease, 187
Klinefelter's syndrome, 69, 70
Koro, syndrome and folk illness. *See*
    Depersonalization neurosis

Labeling, 2–3
La belle indifférence, 108–109, 118, 121
Lactate, 92–93
Lactate theory, 90
Lactic acid, 214
LBJ. *See* Phencyclidine
L-dopa, 187
Learning, 73, 93, 138
Learning theory, 95, 162, 302
Legal considerations, 39, 40, 275, 294–295
Leucotomy, 146, 232, 260, 273
Libido, 28, 75
Librium. *See* Chlordiazepoxide
Limbic system, 86
Lithane. *See* Lithium carbonate
Lithium carbonate, 196, 198, 199, 274
Liver disease, 192
Lobectomy, 273
Lobotomy, 273
Local diseases, 1, 2
Long term therapy, 297
Loss, 188
Love, 250–251
Love massage, 304
Loxitane, 283, 284
LSD (lysergic acid diethylamide), 100, 277,
    286
Luminol, 280
Lying, 115
Lypemania, 22

Magic, 3, 4
Magnetism, 26, 269, 294
Major tranquilizers.   *See* Antipsychotic
    drugs
Malabsorptive disease, 192
Malignancies, 187, 192
Malingering, 123, 257
Mania, 1, 2.   *See also* Manic-depressive
    disease
    and antipsychotic drugs, 284
    and continuous sleep therapy, 288
    and differential diagnosis of anxiety,
        99
    history, 9, 11, 13, 14, 21
    hospitalization for, 267
Manic-depressive disease, 179, 194. *See also*
    Depression; Mania
    and body type, 71
    classification, 180

Manic-depressive disease (continued)
  clinical descriptions, 21
  and genetic factor, 68
  history, 175
  physiological changes in, 183–186
  and repetition, 152
Marijuana, 278, 279, 285–286
Marital groups, 305–306
Marital relationships, 276
Marplan, 196. *See also* Isocarboxazid
Masturbation, 19
Maturity, 91
Mechanical restraints, 270
Mediating factors, 95
Medical model, 51
Medical schools, in ancient Greece, 7–8
Medical specialists, in Egypt, 4
Medicine, ancient, 4, 7–9
Medicine men, 3
Megavitamin therapy, 289
Melancholia, 173–176. *See also* Depression
  Cullen's classification, 1
  definitions, 21–22
  Hippocrates' classification, 9
  and hypochondriasis, 239–240, 242
  in nineteenth century, 21
  Paracelsus' classification, 13, 14
  Soranus' definition, 11
Mellaril. *See* Thioridazine
Memory, 25, 220, 291
Menopause, 73, 89
Menstruation, 73
Mental deficiency, 270–271
Mental health professionals, 265
Mental hospitals, 39. *See also* Hospitals
Mental institutions, 270, 275
Mental retardation, 44, 271
Meprobamates, 101, 102, 103, 273, 282
Mescaline, 100, 277, 286
Mesmerism, 26, 113
Mesomorph, 71
Mesopotamians, 4
Mesoridazine, 283
Metabolic disease, 192
Metabolism, 73
Metaphysics, 294
Metapsychosis, 5–6
Methamphetamine, 196, 289
Methaqualone, 281
Methedrine. *See* Methamphetamine

Methylphenidate, 196, 198, 289
Methyprylon, 281
Metrazol shock treatment. *See* Cardiazol
  shock treatment
Middle Ages, 12–15
Migraine headaches, 122, 156
Milieu therapy, 260, 265, 275, 297
Military classification, 39
Miltown. *See* meprobamates
Mind-body relationship, 110
Mineralocorticoids, 88
Minnesota Multiphasic Personality Inventory (MMPI), 41
Minor tranquilizers, 281
Moban. *See* Oxoindoles
Model of mind, 28
Modeling therapy, 304
Modified insulin treatment, 287
Monoamine oxidase inhibitors, 196, 198
Monomania, 22
Mononucleosis, 187
Monosymptomatic hypochondriasis. *See* Hypochondriacal neurosis
Monosymptomatic phobia, 135
Mood, 79, 157, 190–191
Mood changes, 137, 172, 194
Moral insanity, 18
Morality, 267, 270, 277, 299
  and psychosurgery, 294, 297
Moral neurosis. *See* Moral insanity
Moral treatment, 18
Morbid pathological jealousy. *See* Obsessivedelusional jealousy
Morphine, 284
Mortal soul. *See* Irrational soul
Motor symptoms, 118
Mourning, 191–192
Movement, 5
Moving madness, 11
Mucous membrane diseases, 122
Multiaxial theory of disease. *See* Comprehensive theory of disease
Multiple personality. *See* Personality
Multiple sclerosis, 72, 187
Multivariate analytic techniques, 180
Mumia, 26
Munchausen syndrome, 114, 120
Muscle relaxation techniques, 303
Muscular exhaustion of the heart, 83
Musculoskeletal system symptoms, 192
Music therapy, 297

Myelograph, 292
Myocardial infarction, 267
Mysophobia, 135
Mysticism, 3, 4
Mythology, 3, 7

Narcissism, 118
Narcoanalysis. *See* Narcotherapy
Narcolepsy, 193. *See also* Sleep paralysis
Narcosynthesis. *See* Narcotherapy
Narcotherapy, 232, 272, 288–289
Narcotic addicts, 278
Narcotics, 279
Narcotic withdrawal, 287
Nardil. *See* Phenelzine dihydrogen sulfate
National Commission for the Protection of Human Subjects of Biomedical and Behavioral Research, 295
National Institute of Mental Health, 265
Natural disease entity theory. *See* Disease concepts
Nausea, 89
Navane. *See* Thioxanthenes
Negative practice, 304
Negative reinforcement therapy, 304
Nembutal, 280
Neoplatonism, 10
Nerve blocks, 294
Nerve cell. *See* Neuron
Nerve impulses, 86–87
Nervous exhaustion. *See* Neurasthenia
Nervous functions, 25
Nervousness, 205, 206
Neurasthenia, 204–219
    course and prognosis, 216–217
    and depression, 179, 187, 193–194
    diagnosis, 215
    differential diagnosis, 215–216
    etiology, 211–215
    and Freud, 28, 29, 83, 209
    history, 22, 83, 205–210
    and hypochondria, 243
    and somatization, 123
Neurochemistry, 266
Neurocirculatory asthenia, 83
Neuroleptics. *See* Antipsychotic drugs
Neurons, 86
Neurophysiology, 266. *See also* Brain

Neuroses. *See also* Psychoneuroses; names of individual neuroses
    behavioral theory, 74
    and body type, 72
    and classical analysis, 302
    classification, 1–2, 38, 46, 49–50
    diagnosis, 49–50
    as diseases of sensation and motion, 2
    and electrosleep therapy, 292
    and Freud, 28, 29, 83
    and heredity, 70
    psychodynamic, 75
    types, 45–47
Neurotic depression, 179, 182
Neurotransmitters, 86–87, 184–185
Nialamide, 196
Niamid. *See* Nialamide
Night centers, 270
Nightmares, 3, 97, 120
Night terrors, 120
Noctec, 281, 288
Noludar, 281
Nomenclature. *See* Classification of mental illness
Nonbarbiturate sedatives, 280, 281–282
Norepinephrine, 32, 87, 184–185
Normality, 48–49
Norpramin. *See* Desipramine HCL
Nortriptyline HCL, 196
Nosology. *See* Classification of mental illness
Nosophobia, 164–165
Nous (mind), 5
Numorphan, 284

Obesity, 303
Obsession, 149, 163, 164. *See also* Obsessive compulsive neurosis
    and agoraphobia, 140
    and heredity, 70
    and hypochondria, 238
    and neurasthenia, 215
Obsessional personality. *See* Obsessive compulsive personality under Personality
Obsessional-ruminative state. *See* Obsessive compulsive neurosis
Obsessional state. *See* Obsessive compulsive neurosis

Obsessive compulsive neurosis, 149–170.
  See also Obsession
  and anxiety, 99, 157
  and behavior therapy, 303
  and body type, 71
  course and prognosis, 155–156, 166
  and depersonalization, 230
  and depression, 99, 152–153, 157–158,
    164
  diagnosis, 162–164
  differential diagnosis, 164–166
  etiology, 152–162
  and insulin coma treatment, 287
  and neurasthenia, 216
  and phobias, 137, 138, 142, 143–144,
    156, 164–165
  and psychosurgery, 296
  treatment, 166–167
Obsessive compulsive personality. *See*
  Personality
Obsessive-delusional jealousy, 163
Obsessive doubt, 149
Obsessive fear, 150
Obsessive image, 150
Obsessive impulse, 150
Obsessive phobias, 142
Obsessive rumination, 150, 163
Occupational therapy, 297
Occupations of hysterics, 115
Open operative techniques, 273
Operant conditioning, 304
  for agoraphobia, 146
  for pain, 294
Operationalism, 38–39
Operative myxedema, 192
Opium, 273
Opium alkaloids, 284
Organic brain disease
  as classification, 44
  and depression, 187
  and hypochondria, 255
  and hysteria, 121
  insight in, 133
  and narcotherapy, 288, 289
  and obsessive compulsive neurosis, 156,
    165
  and repetition, 152
Organic dementia, 125
Organic disability, 124
Organic disease, 99–100, 216

Organicists, 17
Organic neuroses, 16–17, 18
Organic pathology, 72–73
Organ neurosis, 98
Organology, 17
Orthomolecular therapy. *See* Megavitamin
  therapy
Osseous system, 88
Outpatients, 32, 39
Overcompensation, 302
Oxazepam, 103, 282
Oxoindoles, 283, 284
Oxymorphone, 284

Pain, 236–238, 260, 266, 293–294
  anxiety and, 94
  fear and, 94
  and hypochondria, 247
  and psychosurgery, 296
  treatment, 294
  types, 293–294
Pain clinics, 260–261, 294
Pain threshold, 237–238
Palebral fissure, 100
Palpitations of the heart, 83, 89
Panhypopituitarism, 192
Panic, 98, 267
  and agoraphobia, 140
  treatment, 101
Paradigms, 6
Paradoxical intention, 303–304
Paral. *See* Paraldehyde
Paraldehyde, 281
Paralysis, 108, 116, 118, 124
Paranoia
  and butyrophenones, 284
  and dementia praecox, 24
  and hospitalization, 267
  and hypochondria, 257
  and hysteria, 115
  and narcotherapy, 289
Paranoid personality, 114
Parasympathetic nervous system, 87
Parental attitudes, 74
Paresis, 31
Paresthesias, 118
Parkinson's disease, 87, 100
Parnate. *See* Tranylcypromine
Paroxysmal auricular tachycardia, 193
Paroxysmic accidents, 13

Passion, 79
Passive aggressive trait, 114
Pattern theory, 237
PCP. *See* Phencyclidine
Peer review, 270
Pentobarbital, 280
Pentothal, 280, 289
Peptic ulcer, 100, 122, 192
Pellagra, 31, 272
Perception, 220
Perceptual cognitive aberrations, 222
Perphenazine, 103
Personal construct theory. *See* Construct
    theory
Personality
    anancastic type, 149
    and anxiety neurotics, 91-92
    and bipolar depression, 91-92
    cycloid type, 186
    cyclothymic, 186
    definition, 70
    and depersonalization, 226
    and depression, 186
    deviant types, 44
    double personality. *See* multiple
        personality
    in etiology, 67
    and heredity, 70
    and hypochondriasis, 246-247
    Hypomanic type, 180
    and hysterical neurosis, 114-116
    hysterical type, 114-116
    insecure type, 213
    integration, 155
    multiple personality, 108, 113, 119
    and neurasthenia, 213
    and obsessive compulsive neurosis, 155,
        156, 161
    obsessive compulsive type, 149, 155-156,
        161, 186, 246-247
    and phobias, 137, 141
    postencephalitic type, 73
    rigid type. *See* obsessive compulsive
        type
    schizoid type, 114
    sensitive type, 213
    and somatics, 71-72
    and therapy, 298
    and unipolar depression, 91-92
Personality disorders, 18

Personality theories, Mesopotamian, 4
Personal unconscious, 25
Pertofrane. *See* Desipramine HCL
Pharmacotherapy. *See* Drug therapy
Phencyclidine, 286
Phenelzine dihydrogen sulfate, 196, 198
Phenobarbital, 102, 103, 280
Phenothiazines, 101, 102, 103, 167, 232
    283, 284
Phenotype, 69
Phenylketonuria, 68, 270-271
Pheochromocytoma, 72, 89, 100
Philosophy, 15
Phobias. *See also* Phobic neurosis
    and behavior therapy, 138, 303
    and depersonalization, 227
    and hypnosis, 306
    and hypochondria, 235, 257
    and obsessive compulsive neurosis, 156,
        164-165
Phobic neurosis, 131-148. *See also* Phobias
    course and prognosis, 144-145
    diagnosis, 139-143
    differential diagnosis, 143-144
    etiology, 137-138
    treatment, 145-146
Phobic-ruminative state. *See* Obsessive
    compulsive neurosis
Phrenitis, 9, 11, 13
Phrenology, 17
Physical factors in etiology, 67, 71-73, 116
Physical illness, 67, 82
Physical methods of treatment, 265, 267,
    275, 277-297. *See also* names of
    individual treatment
Physician-priests, 3, 7
Physiognomy, 17
Physiological disturbance, 121
Pimozide. *See* diphenylbutylpiperidine
Piperazines, 283
Piperazinyl, 283
Piperidines, 283
Pituitary adrenocortical system, 87-88
Pituitary gland, 73, 86
Placidyl. *See* ethchlorvynol
Plants. *See* Drug therapy
Plastic surgery, 254
Pleasure, 87
Poetry therapy, 297
Political factors, 67

Politicians, 270, 277
Porphyria, 72
Positive reinforcement, 158, 304
Postconcussional syndrome, 100, 122, 123
Postencephalitic personality. *See* Personality
Postepileptic automatism, 125
Posthypnotic amnesia, 306-307
Posthypnotic state, 306
Postpartum, 89, 187
Posttraumatic syndromes, 214-215
Power of suggestion, 27
Prayer, 3
Prediction, 43
Pregnancy, 279
Premenstrual, 89
Presamine. *See* Imipramine HCL
Prescription, 278, 279
Priests, 3, 4
Primal scream, 304
Primary affective disorders, 182, 192-194
Primitive man, 3
Prison, 39, 40
Privileged communication, 275
Prochlorperazine, 103, 283
Progressive relaxation, 292, 297
Prolixin. *See* Fluphenazine
Propanediols, 101, 103
Propranolol, 92, 103
Propoxyphene, 284-285
Prototypes, 6
Protriptyline HCL, 196, 197
Pseudo-dementia, 114, 119
Pseudologic, 115
Pseudo-psychosis, 114
Pseudo-stupidity, 119
Psuche, 5
Psychalgia, 113
Psychasthenia, 25, 83, 134, 209. *See also* obsessive compulsive neurosis
Psychedelic drugs. *See* Hallucinogens
Psychiatric therapy. *See* names of individual therapies
Psychiatric training, 269
Psychiatrist, 32, 275
Psychic energy, 204-205
Psychoanalysis, 274, 301-302
    disadvantages, 302
    techniques, 301

Psychoanalysis (continued)
    theories, 27-28
        of anxiety, 93-94
        of depersonalization, 228
        of hypochondria, 249-251
        of neurasthenia, 214
        of obsessive compulsive neurosis, 161-162
Psychoanalyst, 269
Psychobiology, 24
Psychodrama, 275, 297
Psychodynamics, 42-43, 74-75, 187-188
Psychogenic depression. *See* Reactive depression
Psychogenic drugs. *See* Hallucinogens
Psychoinhibitors. *See* Antipsychotic drugs
Psycholeptics. *See* Antipsychotic drugs
Psychological etiology, 16
Psychological factors in etiology, 67, 74-75
Psychological methods, 265, 267, 274-275
Psychological model, 53, 265
Psychological testing, 40
Psychologist, 265
Psychoneurosis, 27, 29, 45, 46
Psychopathology, 268
Psychopaths, 73, 141
Psychopharmacologist, 269
Psychophysiological disorders. *See* Psychosomatic disorders
Psychophysiologic asthenic reaction. *See* Neurasthenia
Psychoses, 22, 253, 284, 288-289. *See also* names of individual psychoses
Psychosomatic disorders, 19, 22
    and desensitization, 303
    and hypnosis, 306
    and hypochondria, 258
    and sleep therapy, 288
Psychosurgery, 272, 275, 294-297
    for anxiety, 103
    for depression, 199
    for obsessive compulsive neurosis, 167
Psychotherapy, 265, 267, 294, 297-307. *See also* names of individual therapies
    for anxiety, 101, 103
    as art, 297
    for depression, 196, 199
    for depersonalization, 232
    for hypochondria, 259
    for hysteria, 127

Psychotherapy (continued)
   for neurasthenia, 217
   for obsessive compulsive neurosis, 167
   for pain, 294
   for panic, 101
   for phobias, 145, 146
   and primitive man, 3
   and psychopathology, 268
Psychotic depression, 179-180, 182
Psychotropic drugs, 273, 278-279. *See also*
   names of individual drugs
Puberty, 89
Public places, fear of. *See* Agoraphobia
Purifactions, 7
Pyknic type, 71
Pyramids, 4
Pyrexias, 1
Pyrophobia, 135

Quaalude. *See* methaqualone

Rabies, 133
Rage, 86
Raphe nuclei, 87
Rationalism, 15, 17
Rational soul. *See* Soul
Rauwolfia, 183, 187, 274, 283, 284
Reaction type, 24
Reactive depression, 179
Reality, 5
Reassurance, 298, 303
Reciprocal inhibition. *See* Desensitization
Recovery, Inc., 275
Reeducation, 101, 298, 299, 300
Reflexology, 30
Regressive phenomena, 116
Rehabilitation centers, 270
Reinforcement, 167
Relaxation techniques, 103, 167, 274
Religion, 4, 19, 74, 151-152
REM sleep, 183, 193, 213, 281-282
Renaissance, 12-15
Repetitive phenomena, 149, 151-152, 153-
   154
Repression, 93, 94, 302, 306-307
Research, 39, 40
Residential treatment center, 303
Resistance, 98, 302
Respiratory systems, 193
Response, 29-30

Response prevention, 167
Rest cure, 22, 217, 272
Resurrection of the body, 4
Reticular activating system, 86
Rheumatism, 1
Rheumatoid arthritis, 122, 187
Rigid personality. *See* Personality
Ritalin. *See* methylphenidate
Rituals, religious, 151-152
Role playing, 306
Roles in treatment, 276
Rome, 10-12

St. Vitus dance. *See* Vitus chorea
Salt metabolism, 88
Sacred disease. *See* Epilepsy
Salmonella, 214
Sanctuaries, 7
Satanism, 112
Scarification, 14
Schizoaffective disorder, 180, 194
Schizoid personality. *See* Personality
Schizophrenia, 23-24, 271, 273
   and anorexia nervosa, 119
   and antipsychotic drugs, 284
   and body type, 71, 72
   and depersonalization, 227-228, 231
   and depression, 180, 187, 194
   and drug therapy, 32
   and electroconvulsive therapy, 290
   and etiology, 113
   genetic factor, 68
   and hypochondria, 243, 257
   and hysteria, 124-125
   and insulin coma treatment, 287
   and integration, 119
   and intravenous acetylcholine, 290
   and megavitamin therapy, 289
   and obsessive compulsive neurosis, 156,
      157, 165
   and phobic neurosis, 144
   and psychosurgery, 296
   and repetition, 152
   treatment, 272, 273
School phobia, 142-143
Scientific method, 60, 61, 269
Scopolamine, 290
Scythian disease, 9
Secobarbital, 280
Seconal, 280

Secondary affective disorders, 182, 192–194
Secondary gains, 125, 216, 267
Secondary reactions, 267
Second wind, 205
Sedative side effects, 197
Sedatives, 267, 277, 279–280, 281
Seers, 3
Seizures, 7
Self, 25, 110
Self-concept, 109–110, 160–161
Self-deception, 115
Self-preservation, 133
Semicircular canal disturbances, 100
Senility, 72, 100, 152
Sensation and motion diseases, 2
Sense identity, 220
Senses, 4
Sensitive personality. See Personality
Sensitivity group, 304
Sensory deprivation, 224
Separation loss, 187–188
Serax. See Oxazepam
Serentil. See Mesoridazine
Sernyland. See Phencyclidine
Serotonin, 87, 184–185
Serpasil. See Rauwolfia
Sex
    and neurasthenia, 214
    and neuroses, 29
    and obsessive compulsive neurosis, 153
    and phobias, 138
    and hysteria, 111, 112, 116
Sex chromosomes, 68, 69
Sex drive, 73
Sex hormones, 89
Sex-linked inheritance, 69
Sex therapy, 297
Sexual deviation, 296
Sexual dysfunctions, 303
Sexual excitement, 87
Sexual frigidity, 97
Sexual perversions, 86, 303, 304
Shamans. See Medicine men
Shame, 298
Short term therapy, 297
Side effects, 197, 198
Simple schizophrenia, 24
Sinequan. See Doxepin HCL
Skin diseases, 122
SK-Pramine. See Imipramine HCL

Sleep, 87, 294
    and anxiety, 92
    in depression, 183
    and dissociation, 120
    Pavlovian view, 288
Sleep disturbances
    in anxiety, 97
    and biofeedback, 293
    and depersonalization, 224
    and electrosleep therapy, 292
    in neurasthenia, 215
    in phobias, 141
Sleep paralysis, 120
Sleep talking, 120
Sleep therapy. See Continuous sleep therapy
Sleep-wakefulness cycle, 224
Sleepwalking, 120
Social anxiety, 303
Social factors, 67
Social relations, 115
Social stress, 95
Social worker, 265
Sociological models, 265
Sodium amytal, 199
Sodium lactate, 90
Soldier's heart, 83
Somatics, 19, 67, 70, 71–72, 92
Somatization disorder. See Briquet's disorder
Somatization, 113, 122, 123–124, and names of individual neuroses and psychoses
Somatoform neuroses, 47, 113
Somatotonia, 71
Somnambulism, 108, 119
Sopor. See methaqualone
Sorcerers, 3
Soul, concept of
    ancient, 5, 6–7, 10
    debates, 265
    Middle Ages, 12–13
    Renaissance, 13–15
Spasm, 1
Specificity theory, 236–237
Speech disturbances, 73
Spinal cord, 86
Spirits, 3
Split consciousness. See Dissociation
Spontaneous remission. See names of individual disorders

Spontaneous symptomatic recovery, 128
Stability, 91
Standard lobotomy, 295
Starvation, 118-119
State of established tension. *See* state of resistance
State of exhaustion, 98, 189
State of resistance, 98, 189
State hospitals, 270
Statistics, 180-181
Stelazine. *See* trifluoperazine
Stereotactic subcaudal tractotomy, 296
Stimulants, 274, 279, 288-289. *See also* names of individual drugs
Stimulus, 29-30
Street pusher, 277
Stress
    and adrenal glands, 87-88
    and anxiety neurosis, 81, 82, 87-88, 89, 95-96, 99
    definition, 95
    and depersonalization, 228
    and depression, 99, 188
    in etiology, 67, 75-76
    general adaptation syndrome, 88
    and hysteria, 117
    and neurasthenia, 214
    and obsessive compulsive neurosis, 162
    and phobias, 141
    and physical illness, 75-76
    responses, 88, 89
Stupors, 120
Subacute anxiety. *See* Anxiety trait
Subacute obsessional neurosis, 156
Subarachnoid saline infusion, 294
Subconscious, 25, 111-112
Subconvulsive treatment, 291-292
Sublimation, 302
Substitution, 302
Suffocation of the intellect, 13, 14
Suggestibility, 109, 114, 118
Suggestion, 101, 298, 299, 300, 306-307
Suicidal obsessions, 157
Suicidal patient, 267
Suicide, 195
    and anorexia nervosa, 119
    and depression, 194-195, 199
    and drugs, 282
    and hypnosis, 307
    and hypochondria, 258

Suicide (continued)
    and obsessive compulsive neurosis, 157
    statistics, 195
Sulfonamides, 187
Sumerians, 4
Superego, 28, 93
Superficiality, 114
Supernaturalism, 3, 13
Superstition, 151
Supportive measures, 101
Supportive psychotherapy, 145, 167, 298
Suppressive therapy. *See* Supportive psychotherapy
Surgery, 3, 187, 265, 267, 294. *See also* Psychosurgery
Swallowing, 192
Sweating, 89
Swindlers, 115
Symbolism, 138, 164
Symbols, 81
Sympathetic nervous system, 87
Symptom prescription approach, 304
Symptoms, 155. *See also* names of individual disorders
Symptom simulation, 304
Synapses, 86, 184
Synergistic, 102, 279, 280
Syphilis, 271
Systematic desensitization, 145
Systematics. *See* Classification of mental illness
Systemic diseases, 100

Taboos, 3
Tachycardia, 100
Taractan. *See* Thioxanthenes
Taste, 118
Taxonomy. *See* Classification of mental illness
Teeth grinding, 192
Temperament, 70
Terminology. *See* Classification of mental illness
Testosterone, 73
Tetany, 141
Textbooks, early, 19, 19-20
T groups, 304
Thalamus, 73
Theologians, 14-15
Theory of ideas or forms, 6

Therapeutic goals, 276
Therapy. *See also* names of individual
    therapies
  Babylonian, 4
  behavior, 31
  contemporary, 31-32
  Egyptian, 4
  eighteenth century, 17
  Greek, 7-9
  Hebrew, 5
  humanist, 18
  hypnotism, 26-27
  mesmerism, 26-27
  Mesopotamian, 4
  Paracelsus and, 14
  primitive, 3
  psychoanalysis, 27-28
  psychobiology, 24
  religious, 19
Thiopental, 280, 289
Thioridazine, 283
Thioxanthenes, 283, 284
Third party payment, 270
Thorazine. *See* chlorpromazine
Thymoleptics. *See* Antidepressant drugs
Thyroid, 198
Thyroid enlargement, 100
Thyroid releasing hormone, 198
Thyroid stimulating hormones, 198
Thyrotoxicosis, 72, 122
Tics, 73, 97
Time, 222
Tofranil. *See* Imipramine HCL
Tofranil-PM. *See* Imipramine pamoate
Topectomy, 273, 295
Total person concept, 25, 266, 299
Totems, 3
Tradition, 74
Training techniques, 274
Traits, 2, 69, 155. *See also* Personality
Trance
  hypnotic, 306, 307
  hysterical, 119, 125
Tranquilizers, 146, 197, 267, 277, 279, 281.
    See also names of individual drugs
Transactional analysis groups, 275, 304-305
Transference, 300, 302
Transference neurosis, 302
Transformation, 299
Transmigration of the soul, 5-6

Transorbital lobotomy, 295
Tranxene. *See* clorazepate
Tranylcypromine, 196, 198
Trauma, 158, 288
Traumatic injuries, 72
Treatment, 265-307. *See also* names of indi-
    vidual treatment
  physical methods, 265, 267, 271-274,
    275, 277-297
  psychological methods, 265, 267, 274-
    275, 297-307
Treatment plan, 275-277, 299
Trepanation, 3, 269
Tricyclic antidepressant drugs, 102-103,
    146, 167, 196-198, 274. *See also*
    names of individual drugs
Trifluoperazine, 103, 283
Triiodothyronine, 198
Trilafon. *See* perphenazine
Trophic changes, 118
Truth serum, 288
Tryptamine, 184
Twilight state, 116, 125
Twins
  and EEG, 73
  studies, 70, 91, 114, 137, 186
  types, 68-69
Tybamate, 103
Typological model, 51-52
Tyrosine, 87

Ulcerative colitis, 122, 296
Ulcers, 89
Unconscious mind, 25, 28, 301, 302
Unipolar affective disease, 182
Unipolar depression, 91-92
Unitary theory of disease, 64, 65-66, 98,
    172
Unreality, 221
Urticarial reactions, 87
Uterus, 112

Valium. *See* Diazepam
Valmid. *See* ethinamate
Values, 66, 80, 267, 300, 301
Vasodilators, 232
Vasomotor neuroses, 83
Venn diagrams, 55
Ventilating, 298, 299
Vesania, 1

Visceral symptoms, 118
Viscerotonia, 71
Vistaril. *See* Hydroxyzine
Vitamins, 289
Vitus chorea, 13, 14
Vivactil. *See* protriptyline HCL
Voltmeter, 292

Water metabolism, 88
Waynsinn, 13–14
Weight loss, 98, 141, 146
Whitely Index of Hypochondriasis, 238
Will, 4

Witchcraft, 13, 112
Work, 98, 276

Xenophobia, 135
XYY abnormality, 69

Yielding compulsion, 150
Yoga, 292

Zactane. *See* Ethoheptazine
Zen, 294
Zoophobia, 135